T0180484

Practice-Based Clinical Inquiry in Nursing for DNP and PhD Research

Joan R. Bloch, PhD, CRNP, is associate professor of nursing, and has held secondary appointments as associate professor of Nutritional Science and Public Health at Drexel University. In her more than 30 years of experience as an educator, she has extensive experience in supervising master's- and doctoral-level students in the field of women's health. Since 1981, Dr. Bloch has been practicing as a women's health nurse practitioner and, most currently, practices in a public-funded prenatal clinic. After completing a National Institute of Nursing Research (NINR) postdoctoral research fellowship, Dr. Bloch has maintained an active program of perinatal health disparities research. She has served as a principal investigator on multiple funded and unfunded research projects. Dr. Bloch has authored many refereed/nonrefereed journal articles, book chapters, and refereed paper and poster presentations. She has served on multiple research-related committees at the university and in professional nursing and public health organizations. This includes the National Organization of Nurse Practitioner Faculties (NONPF), the Association of Women's Health, Obstetric and Neonatal Nurses (AWHONN), and the Public Health Management Corporation (PHMC).

Maureen R. Courtney, PhD, APRN, FNP-BC, is associate professor, University of Texas at Arlington College of Nursing and Health Innovation, where she teaches clinical research to doctoral students and supervises Doctor of Nursing Practice (DNP) projects and PhD dissertations, as well as advanced role and clinical courses in the family nurse practitioner (FNP) curriculum. Dr. Courtney has served as a principal investigator for numerous nationally funded community-based primary care projects. Since 1983, Dr. Courtney has been practicing as an FNP, and most currently, practices in a family practice clinic. The most notable of the many awards she has received are as follows: Outstanding NP in the State of Texas (American Academy of Nurse Practitioners), Primary Care Policy Fellowship (U.S. Department of Health and Human Services), and Distinguished Practitioner, National Academy of Nursing, in addition to research awards. Dr. Courtney is an active researcher, having served as the PI on multiple funded and unfunded research projects, and has published many papers and technical research reports. She has made more than 100 national presentations and published several abstracts/proceedings. She is certified by the International Joanna Briggs Institute in the following three areas: conducting quantitative systematic reviews, qualitative systematic reviews, and cost-effectiveness systematic reviews. Dr. Courtney is active in many professional organizations and has served on the Research Advisory Committee to the American Association of Nurse Practitioners, and co-chair of the Research Special Interest Group at NONPF.

Myra L. Clark, PhD, RN, FNP-C, is associate professor, the FNP program, The University of North Georgia, to which she has returned after teaching at the University of Virginia (UVA) School of Nursing for the past 5 years. She is the director of research for the College of Health Sciences and Professions at The University of North Georgia. Prior to returning to The University of North Georgia, she practiced as an FNP at the Charlottesville Free Clinic. Dr. Clark is the recipient of several professional awards, including being inducted as a distinguished educator into the Hall of Honor, Mercer University School of Nursing, the Verhonick Dissertation Award, and the Outstanding Graduate Student Award. She has published multiple peer-reviewed articles. Dr. Clark's funded research (National Institutes of Health and UVA) focuses primarily on diabetes. She has presented both nationally and internationally on various aspects of diabetes and diabetes self-care. She is professionally active in many nursing organizations, including the American Nurses Association, Southern Nursing Research Society, American Association of Nurse Practitioners, the National Organization of Nurse Practitioner Faculty, the Virginia Diabetes Council, and the National Rural Health Association, among others, and is co-chair of the NONPF Research Special Interest Group.

Practice-Based Clinical Inquiry in Nursing for DNP and PhD Research

LOOKING BEYOND TRADITIONAL METHODS

Joan R. Bloch, PhD, CRNP

Maureen R. Courtney, PhD, APRN, FNP-BC

Myra L. Clark, PhD, RN, FNP-C

Editors

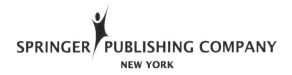

SPRINGER PUBLISHING COMPANY

NEW YORK

Springer Publishing Company, LLC
11 West 42nd Street
New York, NY 10036
www.springerpub.com

Acquisitions Editor: Margaret Zuccarini
Composition: Westchester Publishing Services

ISBN: 978-0-8261-2694-8
e-book ISBN: 978-0-8261-2699-3

16 17 18 19 / 5 4 3 2 1

The author and the publisher of this Work have made every effort to use sources believed to be reliable to provide information that is accurate and compatible with the standards generally accepted at the time of publication. Because medical science is continually advancing, our knowledge base continues to expand. Therefore, as new information becomes available, changes in procedures become necessary. We recommend that the reader always consult current research and specific institutional policies before performing any clinical procedure. The author and publisher shall not be liable for any special, consequential, or exemplary damages resulting, in whole or in part, from the readers' use of, or reliance on, the information contained in this book. The publisher has no responsibility for the persistence or accuracy of URLs for external or third-party Internet websites referred to in this publication and does not guarantee that any content on such websites is, or will remain, accurate or appropriate.

Library of Congress Cataloging-in-Publication Data

Practice-based clinical inquiry in nursing for DNP and PhD research : looking beyond traditional methods / Joan R. Bloch, Maureen R. Courtney, Myra L. Clark, editors.
    p. ; cm.
  Includes bibliographical references.
  ISBN 978-0-8261-2694-8 (hardcopy : alk. paper) — ISBN 978-0-8261-2699-3 (ebook) — ISBN 978-0-8261-3345-2 (powerpoint)
  I. Bloch, Joan R., editor. II. Courtney, Maureen R., editor. III. Clark, Myra L., editor.
  [DNLM: 1. Clinical Nursing Research—methods.   2. Education, Nursing, Graduate.   3. Advanced Practice Nursing—education.   4. Research Design. WY 20.5]
  RT76
  610.73071—dc23
                                                                    2015035666

Special discounts on bulk quantities of our books are available to corporations, professional associations, pharmaceutical companies, health care organizations, and other qualifying groups. If you are interested in a custom book, including chapters from more than one of our titles, we can provide that service as well.
For details, please contact:
Special Sales Department, Springer Publishing Company, LLC
11 West 42nd Street, 15th Floor, New York, NY 10036-8002
Phone: 877-687-7476 or 212-431-4370; Fax: 212-941-7842
E-mail: sales@springerpub.com

Printed in the United States of America by McNaughton & Gunn.

CONTENTS

CONTRIBUTORS

Patricia Abbott, PhD, RN, FAAN, FACMI   Associate Professor, Director of the Hillman Scholars, School of Nursing, University of Michigan, Ann Arbor, Michigan

Joan R. Bloch, PhD, CRNP   Associate Professor, College of Nursing and School of Public Health, Drexel University, Philadelphia, Pennsylvania

Susan Weber Buchholz, PhD, ANP-BC, FAANP   Professor, College of Nursing, Rush University, Chicago, Illinois

Myra L. Clark, PhD, RN, FNP-C   Associate Professor, Family Nurse Practitioner Program, The University of North Georgia, Dahlonega, Georgia

Sarah Cordivano, MUSA   Spatial Data Analyst, Project Manager, Data Analytics, Azavea, Philadelphia, Pennsylvania

Maureen R. Courtney, PhD, APRN, FNP-BC   Associate Professor, College of Nursing and Health Innovation, University of Texas, Arlington, Texas

Maria Elayne DeSimone, PhD, NP-C, FAANP   Clinical Professor, School of Nursing, Widener University, Chester, Pennsylvania

Shirlee M. Drayton-Brooks, PhD, FNP-BC, FAANP   Professor, Director, Doctor of Nursing Practice Program, School of Nursing, Widener University, Chester, Pennsylvania

Judy Faust, RN, MBA   Administrator/Clinical Director Women and Children, Einstein Medical Center Philadelphia, Philadelphia, Pennsylvania

Louis Fogg, PhD   Associate Professor, College of Nursing, Rush University, Chicago, Illinois

Jane T. Garvin, PhD, APRN, FNP-BC   Assistant Professor, College of Nursing, Augusta University, Augusta, Georgia

Mary Ellen Smith Glasgow, PhD, RN, ACNS-BC, FAAN Dean and Professor, School of Nursing, Duquesne University, Pittsburgh, Pennsylvania

Paula Gray, DNP, FNP-C Clinical Assistant Professor, Director Family Nurse Practitioner Programs, School of Nursing, Widener University, Chester, Pennsylvania

Mary Elizabeth "Betsy" Guimond, PhD, RN, WHNP-BC Assistant Professor, Coordinator, Doctor of Nursing Practice, School of Nursing, Duquesne University, Pittsburgh, Pennsylvania

L. Michele Issel, PhD, RN Professor, Director, Public Health Sciences, College of Health and Human Services, University of North Carolina at Charlotte, Charlotte, North Carolina

Kathleen J. Jackson, DNP, MA, APRN Assistant Professor, School of Nursing, Rutgers University, Camden, New Jersey

Bonnie Jerome-D'Emilia, PhD, MPH, RN Associate Professor, School of Nursing, Rutgers University, Camden, New Jersey

Catherine Johnson, PhD, FNP, PNP Chair, Advanced Practice; Executive Director of Community-Based Health and Wellness Centers, School of Nursing, Duquesne University, Pittsburgh, Pennsylvania

Denise M. Linton, DNS, FNP-BC Associate Professor, College of Nursing and Allied Health Professions, University of Louisiana at Lafayette, Lafayette, Louisiana

Amber B. McCall, PhD, APRN, FNP-BC Assistant Professor, College of Nursing, Augusta University, Augusta, Georgia

Marcia Murphy, DNP, ANP, FAHA Associate Professor, College of Nursing, Rush University, Chicago, Illinois

Georgia L. Narsavage, PhD, RN, APRN, FAAN, FNAP Professor, School of Nursing, West Virginia University; Director, Interprofessional Education, West Virginia University Health Sciences Center, Morgantown, West Virginia

Michael E. Schoeny, PhD Assistant Professor, Rush University, College of Nursing, Chicago, Illinois

Beth A. Staffileno, PhD, FAHA Associate Professor, College of Nursing, Rush University, Chicago, Illinois

Devita T. Stallings, PhD, RN Assistant Professor, School of Nursing, Saint Louis University, St. Louis, Missouri

Boqin Xie, PhD, RN Postdoctoral Research Fellow, School of Nursing, University of Michigan, Ann Arbor, Michigan

PREFACE

In this book we build strategically upon traditional nursing research methods textbooks to create a critically needed textbook for PhD and Doctor of Nursing Practice (DNP) nursing students. This book serves those who wish to bring practice-based clinical inquiry into their doctoral studies by building upon the readers' existing knowledge of the research process, methods of scientific inquiry, and analytic techniques. This advanced-methods textbook pulls from an array of frequently used interdisciplinary translational research approaches that have gained popularity over the past decade.

Practice-based research approaches provide the nursing profession with unprecedented opportunities for collaboration among nurses in academe and practice. The exponential growth of DNP programs provides great promise to rapidly accelerate the advancement of nursing science and nursing practice through productive PhD–DNP collaborations. As a result, nurses are now poised to lead the scholarly approaches to generate, advance, and disseminate knowledge that is essential to improve patient well-being and outcomes. It is noteworthy that the same Institute of Medicine (IOM) report that gave rise to the DNP degree, *Crossing the Quality Chasm: A New Health Care System for the 21st Century* (2001), also brought greater respect and support for practice-based research approaches. Additionally, newer practice-based research approaches were brought about in ways that allow the incorporation of technology and knowledge from numerous other disciplines.

Although this is a truly exciting time for nurse scholars, with opportunities for intradisciplinary and interdisciplinary research collaborations, the realities of continued significant disease burden in the presence of an excess of research evidence that could guide evidence-based solutions tempers our overall enthusiasm. As scholars, we must join with our colleagues to foster the science of translating evidence to practice where it will stick. Moreover, we need to apply our nursing science to advance practice-based evidence.

Nurse scholars must participate in robust research teams that aim at improving the overall health of the population. The complexity of health care systems and technology gives rise to both new challenges and new opportunities for clinical inquiry. Will our colleagues in public health, behavioral economics, or computer and information science, for example, think of including nurses in their research team to develop, implement, and evaluate innovation at the bedside and in the community?

Do nurse scholars understand the value of interdisciplinary teams? Do they know how to reach out to other disciplines to create interdisciplinary teams? These collaborations can be enhanced by incorporating the evolving compendium of evidence-based and practice-based methods presented in this textbook into doctoral nursing education.

In this spirit, as faculty teaching in both PhD and DNP programs, we have looked for a textbook that would acquaint our doctoral students with an array of practice-based approaches for clinical inquiry that typically have not yet been integrated into doctoral programs. As each of us is a member of interdisciplinary research teams and a practicing clinician, we recognized that these practice-based approaches—some already well known and practiced in other disciplines—were not yet commonly presented in our doctoral curricula. For this reason, we have developed this textbook.

KEY FEATURES OF THIS BOOK

- Concise resources for research methodologies that are useful in evidence-based and practice-based clinical scholarship and research
- Description of practice-based interdisciplinary health care methodologies needed for evidence-based improvement in health and health care systems
- Source book for determining practice-based research approaches for DNP and PhD nurse scholars
- Chapters written by experienced academic and practice scholars, who have expertise in their topics, from across geographic areas and institutions in the United States

HOW TO USE THIS BOOK

Each chapter is organized strategically to provide a guide on why and how to use the particular scholarly approach. With a consistent organization for each chapter, the reader can toggle back and forth throughout the book to compare and contrast the approaches, enabling deeper and better understanding of scholarly approaches that best meet his or her clinical inquiry needs. Each chapter begins by highlighting the importance of the method and its description. Reasons for using that particular method for doctoral nursing work are identified, followed by practical information about how to use the method. Then, ways to use the method are described, along with examples of the particular method from the published literature.

The chapters in this book are organized into three parts:

- Existing Practice-Based Methods for Clinical Inquiry
- Evolving Practice-Based Research Methods
- A Toolbox for Greater Impact and Success

In Part I, each chapter describes an existing method used extensively among interdisciplinary health scholars to improve clinical and population health. These chapters provide practical information about (a) program planning and evaluation;

(b) patient-engaged and community-based participatory research (CBPR); (c) systematic reviews; and (d) quality improvement.

In Part II, the chapters include innovative emerging science and methods that have evolved in response to the global need to translate science to practice and practice to science more effectively. The chapters cover emerging science and research in regard to (a) big data, (b) dissemination, (c) implementation, and (d) comparative effectiveness research.

Part III concludes the book by providing a toolbox of practical tips for doctorally prepared nurses to consider for impact and success in research and program proposals. The chapters cover (a) a statistical toolkit; (b) the use of geographical information systems (GIS) in health research; and (c) the design of logic models.

It is our hope that this book will enhance practice-based clinical inquiry for practice and research scholars to advance nursing science and achieve desired patient and population health outcomes. Working collaboratively within nursing and with other disciplines can help in improving the quality and effectiveness of health care for all.

Joan R. Bloch
Maureen R. Courtney
Myra L. Clark

ACKNOWLEDGMENTS

We express our profound gratitude to all authors for their expert contributions to this textbook. We believe this unique textbook will educate DNPs and PhDs to be more effective scholars in their respective areas, and that, ultimately, the patients we all serve will benefit.

We are also grateful to our many colleagues and students who have enriched our research knowledge and endeavors along the way. Lastly, this book would have never been possible if it was not for the immediate interest, encouragement, and support from Margaret Zuccarini of Springer Publishing Company—so, thank you!

PART I

EXISTING PRACTICE-BASED METHODS FOR CLINICAL INQUIRY

CHAPTER ONE

HEALTH PROGRAM PLANNING AND EVALUATION: WHAT NURSE SCHOLARS NEED TO KNOW

L. MICHELE ISSEL

OBJECTIVES

After reading this chapter, readers will be able to:

1. Outline the basic steps involved in program planning and evaluation of the program
2. Describe different types of needs and their relevance to planning a programmatic intervention
3. Explain the implications of distinguishing between a program and an intervention
4. Identify appropriate methodologies for each level of program effect evaluation
5. Advocate for nurse scholars as key members of a health program planning or evaluation team

Current trends in health care emphasize population health, health promotion, quality of care improvement, and performance standards. These trends reflect a focus not on the provision of direct, clinical services per se but rather on the health care delivery system. Typically, each of these trends is addressed separately, which need not be the case. Nurses, particularly those with advanced graduate education, will be involved in or managing activities related to each of these trends. To be savvy and make valued contributions to those activities, nurse scholars can bring a unique set of skills to the table, one of which is health program planning and evaluation.

In this chapter, health program planning centers on interventions. An *intervention* is something done intentionally to have a beneficial effect on the recipient (Issel, 2014). This broad definition of an intervention encompasses a continuum of actions, ranging from individually focused actions, such as clinical medical treatments, to population-focused ones, such as a mass media health awareness campaign. A *program* then can be understood as the mechanism and structure used to deliver an intervention or a set of synergistically related interventions. A program can exist as a funded entity; however, it is the actions of a health professional who delivers the actual intervention that makes the program effective. For example, Women, Infants, and Children (WIC) exists as a major federally funded program to improve nutrition for pregnant and lactating women. But the nutritional counseling done by

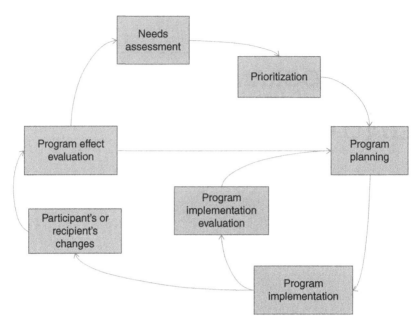

Figure 1.1 The program planning and evaluation cycle: a simplified representation. Adapted from Issel (2014).

the WIC staff and the provision of nutritional supplements constitute the interventions that make WIC a success, meaning an effective program. *Program planning* includes the actions that determine and develop the mechanism for delivery of the intervention as well as the specification of the intervention. Those actions occur after assessing the needs of the target audience and include (a) selecting interventions that have the highest likelihood of addressing the identified and prioritized health problems or needs and (b) developing the organizational structure and mechanisms by which the intervention will be delivered or provided. *Program evaluation* is the application of scientific methods to determine the extent to which the program was implemented as planned and the extent to which the planned effect was achieved. As implied by the definitions of program planning and evaluation, program planning and evaluation constitute a cycle (Figure 1.1) in which the evaluation findings are subsequently used for continued assessment and refinement of the program and its interventions.

THE PUBLIC HEALTH PYRAMID AND HEALTH PROGRAMS

The perspective taken in this chapter is that program planning and evaluation occur at each level of the *public health pyramid* (Frieden, 2010; Issel, 2014). The public health pyramid (Figure 1.2) represents the inverse relationship between the effort and resources needed to make a change and the size of the group reached with the intervention. Starting at the pyramid base, the health care system and community socioeconomic structure form the base with laws, health care workforce, regulations, quality assurance programs, and technological resources that support the delivery of all health care services and programs. Investments in the pyramid base can yield high returns in quality and effective delivery of health care services and programs. Moving

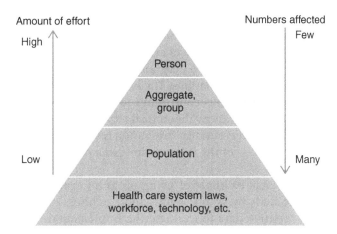

Figure 1.2 The public health pyramid.

up the pyramid, the next level represents a true population that receives interventions designed for populations, with those interventions being the most cost effective; that is, a relatively low cost per each of those persons reached by the program.

Fluoridation of water is a good example of a low cost that reaches entire populations. The middle of the pyramid represents aggregates that are groups with at least one common characteristic. The delivery of interventions to groups and aggregates often entails enabling services, such as transportation services, day care centers, and financial assistance programs. At the apex of the pyramid are individuals and clinical care. Clinical care has the smallest reach and is the costliest. Although clinical care has many benefits to individuals, the limited reach and cost make it less preferable for prevention and health promotion. The current trend of population focus and health promotion puts increasing emphasis on programs that are a broader level in the public health pyramid.

This chapter provides an introductory overview of program planning and evaluation as scholarly activities for doctoral-prepared nurses, and it provides resources for gaining depth of knowledge and skill. This chapter is organized into three main sections. The rationale section outlines the value of program planning and evaluation to nursing scholars. In the methods section, basic content covers types of assessments, implementation considerations, and key evaluation approaches. In the last section, ethical responsibilities and dissemination are reviewed.

RATIONALE FOR UTILIZING PROGRAM PLANNING AND EVALUATION APPROACHES

Nurse scholars need to know about and be able to utilize a program planning and evaluation approach for at least three reasons. Ultimately, each reason relates to advancing nursing knowledge and practice.

Reason 1: Evaluation Research Advances Nursing Research

Evaluation research is the systematic, scholarly application of research methods to assess the extent to which a program was implemented and the magnitude of the intervention effect. The use of randomized controlled trials (RCTs) of new procedures, new treatments, and new care modalities to assess their efficacy and effectiveness can be viewed as a type of evaluation research. Evaluation research, however, more typically is applied to programs with bundles of interventions that are delivered in more real-life situations. The knowledge generated and accumulated through evaluation research thus contributes to the overall evidence for specific interventions, as well as advances theoretical explanations about the causal mechanisms underlying the interventions. Evaluation research has immediate relevance regarding the worthiness of the interventions in a program as the basis for implementation decisions.

One notable example of using program evaluation to advance nursing science is the study by Wand, White, and Patching (2011). They collected qualitative and quantitative data to evaluate the implementation of a mental health nurse practitioner outpatient service. Based on their evaluation data, they generated a set of mid-range theory statements about elements of implementing the program. These statements can then be used to inform and guide development of future programs.

Reason 2: Evaluation Research Contributes to Translational and Implementation Sciences

Systematic implementation of the scientific evidence for a program is consistent with advanced nursing practice. *Translational science* is a field of study focused on understanding how to apply knowledge from basic, laboratory research to the creation of interventions provided to both individual patients and populations. As nurse scholars generate new treatments in nursing laboratories, those interventions need to be translated into nursing care as interventions. Evaluation is one approach to assessing that the translation has occurred. *Implementation science*, sometimes considered an element of translational science, is the systematic study of the factors that influence the extent to which an evidence-based intervention can be put into routine practice. The success of an evidence-based intervention can vary depending upon a wide variety of conditions under which the intervention is provided. Through the process of evaluation and dissemination of the evaluation findings regarding barriers and facilitators to implementation, nursing scholars contribute to advancing translational and implementation science.

Reason 3: Evaluation Research Advances Administration Science

Smart management of the nursing and health care system includes efficient and effective use of resources. Program planning and evaluation can be useful tools for making managerial and administrative decisions about what to support, fund, or endorse. The evaluation, particularly of the implementation of the program, can yield relevant insights to managing health professionals, interdisciplinary teams, and other health systems resources. Such insights contribute to *administration science*, the field of knowledge about creating and managing organizational structures. Nursing scholars who engage in evaluation research and disseminate that known information are essentially advancing administration science.

METHODS FOR PROGRAM PLANNING AND EVALUATION

The methods for program planning and evaluation are presented as three main phases in the planning and evaluation cycle: assessment and planning, program implementation, and effect evaluation. The key concepts and processes involved in each phase are briefly described, with summaries of what the processes are, when the processes of that phase are done, who typically does those processes, how the processes are done, what time and costs are involved, and, lastly, the caveats for nurse scholars to consider.

Assessment and Planning Phase

Needs Assessment

As with the nursing process, program planning begins with assessment of need, characteristics of the health problem, and quantification of the magnitude and seriousness of the problems identified. Unlike assessment of an individual patient, programs often are intended for aggregates, populations, or communities. Thus, the assessment focuses on understanding the needs of individuals, aggregates, populations, or communities. The process begins with defining need. Bradshaw (1972) identified four types of needs, which are particularly relevant for thinking across the public health pyramid. Each ought to be assessed and considered during the program planning stage.

Relative needs are essentially the identification of disparities through comparison of groups. Most of the health disparities literature highlights the relative need of disadvantaged groups. Needs also can be identified as *perceived* by a group. For example, preadolescent boys may perceive a need for a skateboard park, whereas members of the African American community might perceive a need for affordable diabetes supplies. The needs as perceived by various groups may or may not correspond to the *normative needs*, which are needs from the perspective of a health professional. So, the pediatric nurse practitioner might say that the preadolescent boys need to be up to date on vaccinations, and the nurse diabetes counselor might say that preadolescent boys need to access fresh fruits and vegetables. The *expressed needs* are identified though health care seeking and purchasing behavior, and they reveal a different aspect of needs. The expressed needs of the preadolescent boys might be seen in the rate of seeking care at urgent care centers for injuries related to bicycle accidents. The expressed needs of the African American community could be understood through the low rates of mammography screening for women.

Needs assessment is typically done early in the program planning cycle for new programs. Assessing each type of need may reveal the degree of consistency in the pattern of needs. For example, Frank, Kershaw, Chapman, Campbell, and Swinkels (2015) found that residents of two large cities voiced preference for living in walkable settings (perceived need) and those who lived in more walkable neighborhoods walked more (expressed need). In this example, the consistent pattern of both perceived and expressed needs would strengthen the case for a population-level intervention, such as a policy regarding walkable neighborhoods. For ongoing programs, updated needs assessment might occur as a routine activity or as part of a grant renewal process. The techniques and primary focus of needs assessments will vary depending upon the approach taken. Issel (2014) presents four different approaches: an epidemiological approach, a public health approach, a social approach, and an asset approach. Each asks different questions and has a different emphasis. No single approach is inherently better than another. What makes a needs assessment "good" is that it provides insights into the root causes of the health problems, and those insights can form the basis for designing interventions to address those problems.

Needs assessments can be done by nurse scholars by applying diverse methods, such as survey methodology or community focus groups, or analyzing epidemiological data. Ideally, needs assessments involve both individuals who might receive the program and interdisciplinary health and human services professionals. Depending on the approach, needs assessments can be done rapidly, as would be done after a disaster, or over several months, as would be done in a location for the first time and for developing a more complex community health promotion program.

Caveats for nurse scholars are relatively few at this stage in the program planning and evaluation cycle. However, one key caveat is being flexible in the methods used to assess needs while simultaneously guiding stakeholders toward the most scientifically rigorous method. Nurse scholars have a history of involvement in assessing population needs. Table 1.1 summarizes a few examples of the relationship between nursing and needs assessment across the public health pyramid.

Prioritization

Prioritization is the overall process of choosing which need to address. Prioritizing the needs uses the needs assessment data to determine the severity and prevalence of problems as the basis for selecting which need to address. Information about possible effective interventions and preferences of the target audience are taken into consideration. Stakeholders will have different views on which needs are the most important and deserving of attention, which data are the most relevant, and which criteria are to be used for prioritization. These different views can lead to potential conflicts. Thus, part of the prioritizing process involves agreeing upon a philosophical and ethical framework to guide the prioritization. The agreed-upon framework then guides a systematic, quantitative approach to prioritizing needs and selecting the need that will be addressed through a health program.

Prioritization can be done by the group charged with addressing the problem. Ideally, stakeholders for whom the needs are salient are included, whether these are the grant proposal writers or the clinical quality improvement team. Several different systematic, rational approaches exist to arrive at a prioritized list of needs (Issel, 2014). The choice of the prioritization approach depends on the urgency to make a decision, the expertise among the decision makers, and the need for transparency in the process. Generally, the costliest and most time-consuming aspect of prioritization is the effort to gain consensus across the stakeholders.

Caveats for nurse scholars relate mostly to balancing professional biases with the data and the preferences of stakeholders. As health professionals, nurse scholars may prioritize needs differently from other health professionals involved in the planning process, perhaps aligning more closely with objective normative and relative needs. Being politically savvy and culturally sensitive may require patience in helping stakeholders balance perceived needs with relative and expressed needs.

TABLE 1.1 Examples in the Published Literature of Needs Assessments Related to Nursing

Example	Pyramid Level	Purpose	Data Collection	Findings
Filbert, Chesser, Hawley, and St. Romain (2011)	Individual	Determine extent of obesity in a county	Height and weight measurements	Percentage of boys and girls with BMI higher than 85th percentile
Hayff and Secor-Turner (2014)	Individual	Staff perceptions of health care needs of homeless	Interviews	List of needs and barriers to care
Buran, Sawai, Grayson, and Criss (2009)	Family, aggregate	Understand needs of parents of child with cerebral palsy	Questionnaire used in survey	List of parents' service needs, information needs, and obstacles to treatment
McDermott-Levy and Weatherbie (2012)	Population	Understand the health needs as perceived by members of a Nicaraguan community and resource needs of the promotores	Interviews of promotores and qualitative analyses	List of common health problems; supplies needed by the promotores
Aronson, Wallis, O'Campo, and Schafer (2007)	Population	Examine local context of community health program and describe features that affect the target population and health outcomes	Geocoding of physical features in census tracts	Identify high-risk geographical areas and create composite risk scale

BMI, body mass index.

Program Objectives

Having decided upon the need to be addressed, the next step is to establish what will be accomplished by a health program. Although the terms *goals* and *objects* are used inconsistently, *goals* are best thought of as the overarching statement about what will be achieved in the long term. *Objectives*, in contrast, specifically state the short-term achievements in measurable terms, and they thus provide more guidance for what will be measured. Both goals and objectives guide the development of the intervention and the subsequent program monitoring and evaluation. *Process objectives* focus on what will be done, whereas *outcome,* or *effect, objectives* focus on the benefits that program participants will achieve. Issel (2014) suggests writing process objectives using the TAAPS format: Time frame, Amount of what Activities done by which Program Staff/Participants. Using a parallel format, when writing effect objectives, use the TREW format: In what Time frame, what portion of Recipients experience what Extent of Which type of change (Table 1.2). Both the TAAPS and

TABLE 1.2 Examples of Process (TAAPS) and Effect (TREW) Objectives

	Process Objective	Effect Objective
Acronym	TAAPS: Time frame, amount, activities, program staff/participants	TREW: Time frame, recipients, extent, which change
Objective format	By when (time), how many (amount) of what types of outputs, products, actions, or interactions will be created or finalized (activities) by whom (program staff)?	In what time frame, what portion of recipients experience what extent of which type of change?
Example A	By September 1, the participant eligibility screening form will be made completely accessible online by the information technology department.	After completing 50% of the educational sessions, 80% of the participants will be able to correctly name four high-fiber foods.
Example B	After three training sessions, 95% of the program volunteers will have a grade of at least 80% on the quiz that assesses readiness to lead the group.	By the fifth week of the stress reduction program, 75% of participants who attended all sessions will have a 20% decrease in systolic blood pressure from the baseline.
Example C	At the end of the last session, 90% of program participants will answer 100% of the satisfaction questionnaire items.	At 3 months after implementation of the immunization reminder text messaging, 95% of all adult and high-risk clinic patients will be 100% up to date on influenza and tetanus immunizations.

the TREW objectives follow the generic format "by when, who will do what to what extent," although the TAAPS and TREW both provide greater specificity and measurement parameters. In particular, the effect objective ought to indicate the degree or amount of beneficial change, given a specific intervention dosage. The measurement indicator then naturally flows from the extent and type of activity or benefit. The final achievement level ought to be stated as a specific value, rather than stated as "improve" or "reduce," which is less precise.

Development of both process and effect objectives occurs during the planning stage and can be done with the input of future program staff, potential participants, and organizational stakeholders. Objective measures can be used as points of reference for keeping programs aligned with the original intent and for determining the need for program improvements. The approach to measuring objectives is actually stated within the objectives, as the AA in the TAAPS objectives and as the EW in the TREW objectives. The number of both process and effect objectives ought to reflect the complexity of the program, the length of its planned implementation, and the logistic and cost realities of collecting the data specified in the objective measures. The inclination to write many objectives needs to be balanced against those realities.

Caveats for nurse scholars with regard to developing objectives fall into two categories: sufficiency and specificity. Sufficiency encompasses having enough objectives to inform the implementation and evaluation of the program, without becoming burdensome in number. This leads to specificity as a means to determine sufficiency.

The greater the specificity of the objectives, the greater the likelihood that they will be informative once measured. Specificity includes having realistic, data-informed target numbers for the extent of change, the amount of effort required, and the time frame for changes to occur.

Intervention Considerations

In the context of health programs, the choice of interventions needs to consider the strength of the evidence that the actions will have the desired effect. In addition to choosing evidence-based interventions, program planners ought to consider the extent to which the intervention can be done with fidelity to the empirically supported action. Ideally, the intervention shown to be effective in research ought to be replicable by the program staff. Variations from the empirically tested intervention can diminish the potential effect of the intervention as implemented. Also, the dosage of the intervention needs to be specified, again replicating the dosage shown by research to be effective. For example, to address physical activity among the elderly, the physical activity class (as the intervention) ought to match the dosage used in the research, which would include the number of weeks of sessions, number of minutes per session, the type of movements in each session, and the extent of instruction and explanation. Both intervention dosage and fidelity ought to be reflected in some of the TAAPS objectives.

Program Implementation Phase

Program Implementation

Program implementation is the set of activities done to provide the interventions via the structure developed to do so. One should note that this definition puts the interventions at the center with the program structure as the support required to deliver those interventions. Implementation begins after finalizing the TAAPS and TREW program goals and objectives, as well as the details and logistics about how the intervention will be provided. Implementation begins with the recruitment and enrollment of program participants or recipients. The actual *recipients* of the program are those who receive the intervention; *participants* actively partake in the intervention; and the program *targets* are those for whom the program is intended. *Recipients* is a more appropriate terminology when the intervention occurs at the population level and individuals receive the intervention without having to take any action, as would be the case in health policy or environmental change. Participants actively make a choice to be involved in the intervention and need to take some action to receive the intervention, whether that is scheduling a home visit or going to a grief management support group. These distinctions become helpful in determining numbers used as numerators and denominators to calculate program reach, as well as over-inclusion and under-inclusion of individuals in the program (Issel, 2014).

Implementation of a program often involves a number of individuals with different supportive skills and knowledge. The one who delivers the intervention must be trained and qualified to do so, whether that is a lay person (i.e., a doula) or a licensed health professional (i.e., RN or licensed clinical social worker [LCSW]). That person or team of professionals is expected to provide the intervention as developed and refined during the planning phase. Ostensibly, the intervention has been developed to have the maximum potential benefit at a reasonable cost. The maximum benefit would be achieved by following the procedure that details how the intervention is to be delivered. Inputs that might be needed to provide the intervention include human resources (i.e., staff, volunteers, administrative personnel), physical resources (i.e., room, chairs, sphygmometer, handouts), money resources, marketing resources, managerial resources, operational or procedure manual, information systems resources, and time. The amount of each of these resources that is needed will be determined by the scope, duration, and intensity of the intervention and overall size of the program structure.

Implementation Monitoring and Evaluation

The old adage that nothing goes as planned applies to health programs. Thus, some attention must be given to how the program and the intervention are being implemented. The simplest approach is *implementation documentation*, which refers to tallying a count of the different activities and processes done to implement the program. Implementation documentation provides information regarding how much of what was done, but not on the quality of those activities. It includes a count of participants or recipients. The TAAPS objectives guide which activities are tallied for implementation documentation. It is the least expensive and the least intrusive approach. The next, more informative approach is *implementation assessment*, which occurs nearly in real time and is an ongoing act of gathering data about the implementation. The purpose of an implementation assessment is to determine whether timely corrections or modifications are required regarding the way in which the program is delivered or which resources are needed for the program. Implementation assessment is referred to as *process monitoring* in some program planning literature. Last of all, to determine both the extent to which the program and its interventions were delivered as designed and whether variations in the intervention delivery might alter the program effect, an *implementation evaluation* is conducted. Implementation evaluation, often referred to as *process evaluation*, involves systematic research and answers the questions regarding to what extent the program was delivered as intended and to which segments of the target audience.

Implementation documentation, assessment, and evaluation can be done by trained staff, with much of the data collection integrated into routine information gathering about who participated and what was done. Once the data have been converted into a format for ease of inspection, such as graphs, charts, and tables, various stakeholders can assist in interpreting the data, particularly with reference to the TAAPS objectives. They can also make recommendations for improving the implementation of the intervention. For most programs, implementation monitoring activities will continue for the duration of the program, whether that is weeks or decades.

Caveats for nurse scholars regarding implementation monitoring are relatively few. Nurse scholars likely have insights into which intervention elements deserve the most attention, as well as relevant suggestions for keeping the intervention delivery true to the plan (i.e., implementation fidelity). Importantly, nurse scholars contribute to the scientific literature about program implementation. As demonstrated in Table 1.3, nurse scholars have contributed to the science of health program development, implementation, and monitoring. One example of implementation assessment is the study conducted by Goulet et al. (2009) regarding a program to prevent shaken baby syndrome. They assessed patients' perceptions of nurses' skill and comfort with

TABLE 1.3 Examples in the Published Literature of Health Program Development, Implementation, and Monitoring Related to Nursing

Example	Pyramid Level	Purpose	Intervention	Process	Findings
Whittemore et al. (2013)	Individual	Assess implementation of a modified EB diabetes prevention program	Education in classes and behavioral support	Interviewed community health workers who delivered the intervention	Intervention protocol followed but program attendance declined over time
Mueller et al. (2009)	Individual	Implement an HIV risk reduction program and propose modifications	Culturally appropriate promotion of abstinence and condom use among Latino adolescents	Student feedback	Identified issues with parental involvement and student baseline knowledge
DeRosa et al. (2012)	Aggregate	Tailor action to improve school implementation of teen pregnancy and STD prevention intervention	School policy of making condoms available	Worked with schools to address program deficiencies at intervention	Across-time awareness and condoms acquired increased
Olds et al. (2013)	Aggregate	Improve existing nurse–family partnership program	Standardized nurse home visiting of first-time pregnant women	Mixed methods using existing program data and data from previous evaluations; staff interviews	List of possible improvements and challenges to making those improvements
Baisch (2012)	Populations	Document population-level interventions	Varied	Used an electronic health system	Demonstrated possible taxonomy of population-level nursing interventions

EB, evidence-based; STD, sexually transmitted disease.

the program interventions and of the intervention format. They then used those data to determine how best to improve the program and the intervention delivery.

Measuring Health Program Effects: Evaluation Phase

Ultimately, we want to know whether the intervention made a difference and, if so, by how much; in other words, we want an *effect* evaluation. The effect of a program can occur over the short and long term. *Outcomes* refer to the more immediate effects that can be linked to the intervention through a direct cause. In contrast, *impact* refers to the more temporally and causally distant effects arising from the intervention. To understand the effect of an intervention, focus must first be on the program outcomes, with the program impact being assumed through logic and, perhaps, evidence gathered over the long term.

As with implementation evaluation, understanding the link between the intervention and outcomes can entail varying degrees of complexity and scientific rigor. Each level of complexity addresses a slightly more sophisticated question about the program outcomes and, thus, requires slightly more sophisticated scientific approaches. The trade-off for having a greater ability to attribute an effect to the intervention is that the design becomes more complex and, thus, more costly. The most rigorous effect evaluation, an outcome evaluation, will likely be out of reach for the majority of health programs and typically falls within the domain of evaluation research.

Level 1 Effect Evaluation

A Level 1 effect evaluation answers the most basic question as to what the extent to which of the outcomes, TREW, objectives were met. Data collection methods used to conduct a Level 1 effect evaluation are chosen based on the health status indicator within the TREW objectives. The Level 1 effect evaluation requires the least effort, the simplest design, and does not go beyond determining that the TREW objectives were met. Several designs would be considered Level 1 effect evaluation designs: one group with post-test only, two or more groups with post-tests only, and one group with pretest and post-test (Issel, 2014). As can be inferred from this list of designs, the ability to make claims about changes being attributable to the intervention does not exist. The methods typically used for Level 1 effect evaluations would be survey or physical measures of participants or recipients, as indicated by the TREW objectives.

The deficits of conducting a Level 1 effect evaluation are evident in the report by Rantz et al. (2014). They evaluated the health outcomes of an aging in place intervention that involved providing seniors with a set of interventions: ongoing care coordination, health assessments, and exercise and strength training classes. Four waves of data were collected annually about the health and cognitive status of participants. The findings showed a decline in the outcome measures. Without a control group, the researchers were unable to determine whether the decline was less than a normal aging trajectory for individuals in their mid-80s (Rantz et al., 2014).

Level 2 Effect Evaluation

A Level 2 effect evaluation seeks to answer whether an association exists between participating in or receiving the intervention and an observable health status change.

The data collected will be the indicators as specified in the TREW objectives, but the time frame will likely refer to a period after the completion of the health program. The Level 2 effect evaluation goes a step further than Level 1 by adding methods and analyses that can identify a connection between the implementation data (intervention dosage) and the health status measure. A TREW objective that specifies a higher dose of intervention as being related to a greater change would require an effect assessment evaluation.

The design used to conduct Level 2 effect assessment evaluation would essentially be a pretest and a post-test to determine the amount of change within a given period. The majority of research designs are effect assessment designs. Specifically, the designs include two group retrospective (case control design), two group prospective (cohort design), one group time series, multiple group time series, two groups with pretest and post-test without random assignment to the intervention, and two groups with post-test only with random assignment (Issel, 2014). The design choice depends on whether the intervention is population or individual based and on whether a comparison group can be identified before the intervention. The measure(s) used for the evaluation must be sensitive to subtle changes and should have demonstrated validity and reliability with the participant or recipient population.

Level 3 Effect Evaluation

Finding an association between receiving the intervention and a health status change is not the same as being able to say that the program caused the health status change. A Level 3 effect evaluation seeks to attribute changes in health status to having received the intervention, and, thus, being able to say that the program, and nothing else, caused the changes. Accordingly, data collection and sample selection must be able to detect changes due to the program and other potentially influential factors that are not part of the program. This highly rigorous requirement makes a Level 3 effect evaluation similar to basic research (especially clinical trials) into the causes of health problems and the efficacy of interventions.

Only one design can answer the Level 3 effect evaluation question: two groups with random assignment to the intervention with both pretest and post-test intervention data collection from both groups. In other words, an RCT is necessary. The methods and data collection tools would likely be the same as for closely related Level 2 effect evaluation designs.

Caveats exist for nurse scholars regarding participation in effect evaluations of health programs. Nursing scholars have a role in conducting and disseminating health program effect evaluations (Table 1.4), and in doing so for programs that span the public health pyramid. Nonetheless, nurse scholars need to consider their role as both program implementers and evaluators. Being both is a potential conflict of interest. Nurse scholars bring a wealth of knowledge to evaluation regarding appropriate, reliable, and valid measures across a broad spectrum of health conditions and states. This information becomes an invaluable asset to a health program planning team. Furthermore, nurse scholars bring to a team a sensitivity about the target population, which might further inform both the evaluation design and the optimal data collection methods. Nurse scholars, however, need to act upon their confidence in developing programs and effect evaluations, and take a leadership role in furthering the science and evidence about how best to address the health problems.

TABLE 1.4 Examples in the Published Literature of Health Program Effect Evaluation Related to Nursing

Example	Pyramid Level	Intervention	Evaluation Design	Findings
Koh, Nelson, and Cook (2011)	Individual	Cancer patient navigation to coordinate care	Matched historical controls (Level 2)	No significant differences between groups
Vasquez et al. (2010)	Aggregate, family	7-week parent–adolescent, curriculum-based family strengthening	Random assignment to control or experiment with pretest and post-test of both groups (Level 3)	Significant difference in some of the parenting outcome measures
Pence, Nyarko, Phillips, and Debpuur (2007)	Population	Four-arm, community-level, alternative organizational strategies for community health services	Trends based on 2 years pre-intervention and 4 years post-intervention (Level 2)	One intervention arm (locating nurses in villages for easy access) had the most effect on child mortality.

INTERPRETATION AND PRESENTATION OF SCHOLARSHIP PERTAINING TO PROGRAM PLANNING AND EVALUATION

Ethical Responsibilities

Nurse scholars engaged in health program planning, implementation evaluation, and especially effect evaluation must comply with the federal requirements for the protection of human subjects and the Health Information Portability and Accountability Act (HIPAA). The protection of human subjects, which often falls under the purview of institutional review boards (IRBs), becomes most salient if any possibility exists that a member of the health program team might desire to publish findings from any aspect of the health program. Gaining IRB approval for the project would involve having informed consents from the health program participants, and, perhaps, from program staff for process evaluations. All elements of informed consent would be required and, preferably, written at an eighth-grade level. The ethics of who is eligible to participate, how enrollment occurs, how the intervention is delivered, and whether benefits outweigh risks influence the program and intervention design. Thus, examining the ethics and possible scientific value of the program and its evaluation would most appropriately be considered during the planning stage. The program planners, program staff, and possible consultants need to plan for and incorporate the protection of human subjects into all aspects of providing the health program.

More specific to program evaluations, in 2011, the American Evaluation Association (AEA) established a set of five evaluation standards. The first standard is utility: The evaluation ought to be useful and valuable to stakeholders and future program planners. The second standard is feasibility: The evaluation must be doable and, thus, be both efficient and effective. The third standard is propriety:

The evaluation must meet legal, moral, ethical, and just considerations. The fourth standard is accuracy: The evaluation must use valid and reliable measures and designs that increase the truthfulness and dependability of the findings. The last standard is evaluation accountability: The evaluation ought to be disseminated in a manner consistent with advancing the discipline of evaluation and the science about the health problem addressed by the health program. Each AEA evaluation standard applies to all evaluations, regardless of the discipline of the evaluator.

Reporting and Dissemination

Reporting responsibility includes considering what is needed and appropriate for each of the various health program audiences: community stakeholders, program and evaluation funders, lay and scientific journal editors, organizational members, and program personnel. Each will be expecting different information, and the information should be presented in language at a level of sophistication that they will understand. Often, an executive summary is part of the reporting. An *executive summary* presents the background, the accomplishments, and the next steps in a concise manner. Executive summaries ought to be less than four pages.

Reports stemming from either the program implementation or the effect evaluation will often include recommendations. Regardless of whether the recommendations focus on the program implementation or the program effect, developing recommendations should consider the following elements. First, be specific about which program objectives the recommendation addresses. Second, draw upon a variety of sources and resources to explain and justify the recommendation. Third, present a balance of recommendations asking for major changes along with recommendations for keeping what is working well. Fourth, contextualize the recommendations with information about external factors that are relevant or that need to be considered for implementing the recommendations. Lastly, make realistic and feasible recommendations from the perspective of the program personnel and the funder.

Nurse scholars have a responsibility to disseminate program evaluations, particularly Level 3 effect evaluations, to interdisciplinary health care audiences who have an interest in the health problem or interventions used to address that health problem. Implementation science, as an interdisciplinary effort, could benefit from the contributions of nurse scholars who have studied the effects of particular health programs. Accordingly, reports of both scholarly implementation evaluation and effect evaluation can be submitted to a wide range of health journals.

SUMMARY

The planning and evaluation of health programs benefits from the participation of nurse scholars, and nursing scholarship also benefits from that involvement. Table 1.5 provides a summary of key health program planning and evaluation terms. The population focus pervading the current health care environment creates new opportunities for nurse scholars to contribute significantly to health improvement of populations, not only individuals. Planning programs as mechanisms for the delivery of interventions to individuals, families, aggregates, or populations uses the assessment and organizational skills that accompany advanced graduate education. Through the formal evaluation of both the implementation of the health program

TABLE 1.5 Summary of Key Health Program Planning and Evaluation Terms and Corresponding Definitions

Key Terms and Concepts	Definitions
Effect	The consequence, whether beneficial or harmful, of receiving the intervention
Level 1 effect evaluation	Quantifies the extent to which the outcome, TREW, objectives were met, without making any association or attribution to the program intervention: basic evaluation designs at the lowest cost and simplest information about the effect of a health program
Level 2 effect evaluation	Identifies associations between participating in or receiving the intervention and an observable health status change; the most common evaluation designs and available at the most reasonable cost
Level 3 effect evaluation	Establishes that receiving the intervention led to the health status change or that the program caused the health status change; most rigorous and costly evaluation of the effect of a health program
Effect objectives	Statements that focus on the benefits that program participants will achieve or experience; written in the TREW format
Evaluation research	The systematic, scholarly application of research methods to assess the extent to which a program was implemented and the magnitude of the intervention effect
Goals	Overarching statements about what will be achieved in the long term and in nonmeasurable terms
Impact	Temporally and causally distant consequences arising from having received the intervention
Implementation assessment; process monitoring	Nearly real-time and ongoing act of gathering data about the implementation
Implementation documentation	Tallying a count of the different activities and processes done to implement the program
Implementation evaluation; process evaluation	Systematic research and answers the question of to what extent the program was delivered as intended
Implementation science	Systematic study of the factors that influence the extent to which an evidence-based intervention can be put into routine practice
Intervention	Something done intentionally to have a beneficial effect on the participant or recipient
Objectives	Statements describing either the short- or long-term program achievements; these include measurement parameters for the accomplishments
Outcome	The immediate effects from the intervention
Participants	Individuals who make a choice to be involved in the intervention and need to take some action to receive the intervention

(continued)

TABLE 1.5 Summary of Key Health Program Planning and Evaluation Terms and Corresponding Definitions (*continued*)

Key Terms and Concepts	Definitions
Process objectives	The statements describing what will be done by which program staff to what extent and within what time frame; written in the TAAPS format
Program	The mechanism and structure used to deliver an intervention or a set of synergistically related interventions
Program components	The separate structural and intervention elements that collectively comprise the program
Program evaluation	Application of scientific methods to determine the extent to which the program was implemented as planned and the extent to which the planned effect was achieved
Program fidelity	The extent to which the delivery and dosage of the intervention is consistent with the design of the intervention or with the evidence-based description of how to deliver the intervention
Program implementation	Set of activities done to provide the interventions via the structure developed to do so
Program planning	A set of actions that set priorities and decide on the logistics of the delivery of the intervention
Program stakeholders	Individuals, organizational members, or organizations involved in any aspect of the health program or who might be program participants or recipients
Public health pyramid	The inverse relationship between the effort and resources needed to make a change and the size of the group reached with the intervention
Recipients	Those who receive the intervention
Targets	Those for whom the program intervention is intended
Translational science	Field of study focused on understanding how to apply knowledge from basic, laboratory research to the creation of interventions provided to both individual patients and populations

TAAPS, time frame, amount, activities, program staff/participants; TREW, time frame, recipients, extent, which change.

and its effects, nurse scholars have an opportunity to contribute to the science of the health problem and to implementation science. These activities require that nurse scholars collaborate with interdisciplinary team members, various stakeholders in the health program, and the program participants or recipients. Cumulatively, nurse scholars have a responsibility to contribute by way of nursing theory, knowledge, and expertise to the health program planning and implementation.

REFERENCES

American Evaluation Association. (2011). *The program evaluation standards: Summary form*. Retrieved from http://www.eval.org/p/cm/ld/fid=103 accessed Nov. 5, 2015

Aronson, R. E., Wallis, A. B., O'Campo, P. J., & Schafer, P. (2007). Neighborhood mapping and evaluation: A methodology for participatory community health initiatives. *Maternal and Child Health Journal, 11*, 373–383.

Baisch, M. J. (2012). A systematic method to document population-level nursing interventions in an electronic health system. *Public Health Nursing, 29*, 352–360.

Bradshaw, J. (1972). The concept of social need. *New Society, 30*, 640–643.

Buran, C. F., Sawai, K., Grayson, P., & Criss, S. (2009). Family needs assessment in cerebral palsy clinic. *Journal for Specialists in Pediatric Nursing, 14*(2), 86–93.

DeRosa, C. J., Jeffries, R. A., Afifi, A. A., Cumberland, W. G., Chung, E. Q., Kerndt, P. R., . . . Dittus, P. J. (2012). Improving the implementation of a condom availability program in urban high schools. *Journal of Adolescent Health, 5*, 572–579.

Filbert, E., Chesser, A., Hawley, S. R., & St. Romain, T. (2011). Community-based participatory research in developing an obesity intervention in a rural county. *Journal of Community Health Nursing, 2*, 35–43.

Frank, L. D., Kershaw, S. E., Chapman, J. E., Campbell, M., & Swinkels, H. M. (2015). The unmet demand for walkability: Disparities between preferences and actual choices for resident environments in Toronto and Vancouver. *Canadian Journal of Public Health, 106*(1)(Suppl. 1), eS12–eS20.

Frieden, T. R. (2010). A framework for public health action: The health impact pyramid. *American Journal of Public Health, 100*, 590–595.

Goulet, C., Frappier, J. Y., Frotin, S., Deziel, L., Lampron, A., & Boulanger, M. (2009), Development and evaluation of a shaken baby syndrome prevention program. *Journal of Obstetric, Gynecological and Neonatal Nursing, 38*(1), 7–21.

Hayff, A. J., & Secor-Turner, M. (2014). Homeless health needs: Shelter and health service provider perspective. *Journal of Community Health Nursing, 31*, 103–117. doi:10.1080/07370016.2014.901072

Issel, L. M. (2014). *Health program planning and evaluation: A practical, systematic approach for community health* (3rd ed.). Sudbury, MA: Jones & Bartlett Publishers.

Koh, C., Nelson, J. N., & Cook, P. F. (2011). Evaluation of a patient navigation program. *Clinical Journal of Oncology Nursing, 15*, 41–48.

McDermott-Levy, R., & Weatherbie, K. (2012). Health promotores' perceptions of their communities' health needs, knowledge and resource needs in rural Nicaragua. *Public Health Nursing, 30*, 94–105.

Mueller, T. E., Catanenda, C. A., Sainer, S., Martinez, M., Herbst, J. H., Wilkes, A. L., & Villarrueal, A. (2009). The implementation of a culturally based sexual risk reduction program for Latino youth in a Denver area high school. *AIDS Education and Prevention, 21*(Suppl. B), 164–170.

Olds, D., Donelan-McCall, N., O'Brien, R., MacMillan, H., Jack, S., Jenkins, T., . . . Beeber, L. (2013). Improving the nurse–family partnership in community practice. *Pediatrics, 132*, S110–S117.

Pence, B. W., Nyarko, P., Phillips, J. F., & Debpuur, C. (2007). The effect of community nurses and health volunteers on child mortalilty: The Navrongo community health and family planning project. *Scandinavian Journal of Public Health, 35*, 599–608.

Rantz, M., Popejoy, L. L., Galambos, C., Phillips, L. J., Lane, K. R., Marek, K. D., . . . Ge, B. (2014). The continued success of registered nurse care coordination in a state evaluation of aging in place in senior housing. *Nursing Outlook, 62*, 237–246.

Vasquez, M., Meza, L., Almandarez, O., Santos, A., Matute, R. C., Canaca, L. D., . . . Saenz, K. (2010). Evaluation of a strengthening families (familias fuertes) intervention for parents and adolescents in Honduras. *Southern Online Journal of Nursing Research, 10*(3).

Wand, T., White, K., & Patching, J. (2011). Realistic evaluation of an emergency department-based mental health practitioner outpatient service in Australia. *Nursing and Health Services, 13*, 199–206.

Whittemore, R., Rosenberg, A., Gilmore, L., Witley, M., & Brault, A. (2013). Implementation of a diabetes prevention program in public housing communities. *Public Health Nursing, 31*, 317–326.

CHAPTER TWO

PATIENT-ENGAGED AND COMMUNITY-BASED PARTICIPATORY RESEARCH

BONNIE JEROME-D'EMILIA AND KATHLEEN J. JACKSON

OBJECTIVES

After reading this chapter, readers will be able to:

1. Define patient-engaged participatory research (PEPR) and community-based participatory research (CBPR)
2. Define the concept of *community* in CBPR
3. Describe the key principles that define CBPR
4. Explain the steps of the CBPR process

Kurt Lewin (1890–1947), the psychological researcher who is well known for the development of field theory, was also a firm believer in action research, in which social science can be used to help solve social problems (Adelman, 1993). Lewin justified action research in this way: "no action without research, no research without action" (Adelman, 1993, p. 7), and he suggested that this kind of research could help vulnerable populations achieve "independence, equality and cooperation" by "overcoming forces of exploitation" (Adelman, 1993, p. 8). For Lewin, action research began with the affected group discussing their problems and solutions. Active participation by this group of people in identifying problems, recommending solutions, carrying out interventions, and evaluating the process was required. Lewin went further to define participant action research as a method of study in which the residents of an affected community, who would be expected to take part in an intervention, would be involved in the research process from the beginning (Adelman, 1993).

Lewin's process of action, reflection, and experiential learning can be considered the foundation of participatory action research (PAR) as it is conducted today (Faridi, Grunbaum, Gray, Franks, & Simoes, 2007). PAR, whether patient or community based, involves the co-creation of research between researchers and those affected by the issue or intervention under study (patients, communities; Jagosh et al., 2012). PAR is an approach to translational research, developing, implementing, and disseminating effective interventions across diverse communities through strategies to reduce power inequities and to promote reciprocal knowledge and mutual benefit between community and academic partners (Wallerstein & Duran, 2010). PAR can be considered an umbrella term that describes research methodologies that pursue action (or change) and research (or understanding) through the same process and at the same time (Tapp, White, Steuerwald, & Dulin, 2013). PAR is effective in fostering sustainable change, as those who will be affected by the change are actively involved in the process (Tapp et al., 2013).

A range of terms has been used in the past few decades to describe this body of research: *action research, participatory research, participatory action research, community-based research, action science, action inquiry*, and *cooperative inquiry*. All of these descriptors emanate from the same ontological paradigm defined by a participative reality (Holkup, Tripp-Reimer, Salois, & Weinert, 2004). According to Holkup et al. (2004, p. 162), all participatory research relies on "an epistemology of experiential and participative knowing informed by critical subjectivity and participatory transaction." The linkage between action and research, and the collaboration between researcher and research participant, must be present to consider a PAR study.

Lapses of quality in health care delivery, such as poor patient outcomes and health inequities, as well as the extended time it takes for research findings to translate into practice, provide a compelling ethical rationale to include patients, their families and caregivers, and communities in health care research. Traditional research views any phenomenon under study in isolation from "real life." This traditional approach may neglect or inadequately address the health and social complexities of participants, thus potentially missing important social, cultural, and even physical implications of an intervention or a research study. Participatory research gives voice to the individual or group and provides a formal pathway to incorporate local knowledge and priorities into research (Wallerstein & Duran, 2010).

PURPOSE OF PAR

PAR changes the role of the patient or community from passive (that of a data point) to active (patient or community members as research partners). PAR changes the relationship between researcher and research subject. The traditional research process relies on a researcher identifying a research problem, determining the research design, conducting the research, and disseminating the results, whereas in PAR the researcher and the research subject share ownership of the research process and responsibility for the implementation of research findings (Minkler & Wallerstein, 2003). Table 2.1 compares the steps of the research process for traditional and PAR. At every step in the process, as well as before and after the formal study is complete, collaboration is emphasized. Active participation in research by those who are being studied can lead to better, more effective research through the generation of research topics that are particularly relevant to the patients' or communities' concerns. This can result in higher rates of subject enrollment and retention, as well as in greater applicability of the findings to the patients or communities. Participant engagement in the planning and implementation of research may also improve its translation into clinical practice or community life. There is growing agreement about the important role of patient and community involvement in research, with the expectation that participatory research could improve the value of health care research (Domecq et al., 2014). With this growing interest in PAR, there is a need for researchers to learn how to successfully engage and conduct research with patient and community partners in various settings.

TABLE 2.1 Comparison of Traditional Research Methods to CBPR

Stages	Traditional Research	CBPR
Planning	Researchers plan projects, determine objectives, and formulate the team.	Local champions and potential partners are identified. CAB is established. Community members and researchers meet to set priorities, determine objectives, and build a team.
Design development	Researchers plan design based on scientific knowledge as well as previous research, evidence, and methodological feasibility.	Community members and researchers determine design based on community priorities, emphasizing community feasibility, acceptability, context, cultural factors, and local knowledge.
Funding	Researchers determine potential funding sources, write grants, and develop and control budget.	Community members and researchers determine potential sources of funding, collaborate in grant writing and control of budget with equitable division of funds based on contributions to project.
Implement study, collect and analyze data	Researchers conduct study, collect and analyze data.	Community members and researchers collaborate on all facets of study: subject identification, instrument choice, implementation, and data collection. Community-driven questions based on social and cultural factors and local knowledge and local relevance of findings
Disseminate findings	Disseminate to academic audiences via presentations and publications.	Disseminate to academic and lay audiences. Findings are presented to research participants and the CAB, community stakeholders, and policy makers.
Translate research into practice/policy	Not under purview of researchers.	Community members and researchers collaborate to mobilize the community to use findings to improve community life and advocate for policy change.
Sustain team	Researchers move on to new project that may be related to previous study or follow up on findings.	Sustainability plan built into initial team building. CAB collaborates with researchers on next steps.

CAB, community advisory board; CBPR, community-based participatory research.
Source: Horowitz et al. (2009).

DESCRIPTION OF PAR

PAR is an orientation to research rather than a set of specific research methods or techniques. The crucial aspect of PAR is the focus on the relationship between research partners, research participants, and the goals of societal transformation

(Cornwall & Jewkes, 1995). PAR has two main foci: engagement of patients, their caregivers, and significant others in clinically based research and engagement of community members in a study of issues of local (community-based) concern. PEPR involves the active participation of patients, their families, caregivers, and stakeholders in research: designing, implementing, and evaluating health issues and/or health care services (inpatient and outpatient), with the goal of improving the quality of health care and health outcomes. Patients, their families, caregivers, and researchers actively collaborate in all aspects of the research process, including the (a) prioritization of research topics; (b) application for funding; (c) development of study design and procedures; (d) subject recruitment; (e) data collection; and (f) data analysis, as well as in summarizing, disseminating, and applying the findings. PEPR, conducted in multi-professional teams (that include the patient/family/caregiver and relevant stakeholders), aims to apply the knowledge produced to improve health care practice and administration. PAR empowers patients by encouraging active involvement in their own health care. This can lead to higher quality care, with less chance of error, better patient outcomes, and a more positive patient-level view of the health care system (Domecq et al., 2014).

CBPR, by considering a wide range of issues that may impact the public health and welfare of a community of individuals, takes a broad view of health and health care. CBPR is different from simply collecting data in a community setting, with little or no input from the community members. CBPR research is conducted with the community, which is recognized as a social and cultural entity with an active interest and involvement in the research process (Israel, Schulz, Parker, & Becker, 2001). The CBPR process requires the sharing of power, knowledge, and resources with the community (Schmittdiel, Grumbach, & Selby, 2010). In that the community is invested in the research process, the likelihood of translating research into practice is increased in CBPR (Faridi et al., 2007). A byproduct of this research process is the development of a community's problem-solving capacity. The W.K. Kellogg Foundation's Community Health Scholars Program definition for CBPR has been widely used:

> a collaborative approach to research that equitably involves all partners in the research process and recognizes the unique strengths that each brings. CBPR begins with a research topic of importance to the community and has the aim of combining knowledge with action and achieving social change to improve health outcomes and eliminate health disparities. (Faridi et al., 2007, p. 2)

Community—Broadly Defined

Community, for the purposes of CBPR, is defined as a group of people united by at least one common characteristic. A community could be defined geographically (your town); it could be a group with a common identity or characteristic (i.e., men who smoke cigarettes; immigrant Hispanic women) or a group with specific concerns or interests (i.e., a coalition of churches concerned with crime in the local community; Horowitz, Robinson, & Seifer, 2009). Critical to the definition of *community* is who is included and who is excluded. An individual can belong to more than one community at a time or community membership may change over time. It is important to understand an individual's feelings and perceptions about community

TABLE 2.2 Five Core Elements of Community

Element	Description
Locus	A geographic entity ranging from a local neighborhood to a city, or a particular place (church or recreation center) around which people gather
Sharing	A collection of individuals with common interests and values that may cross geographic boundaries
Joint action	Activities that are not focused on a goal of building a sense of cohesion; rather, that sense of cohesion may occur randomly through participation
Social ties	Relationships that create an ongoing sense of cohesion, such as membership, in a religious institution-based social action club
Diversity	The social complexity within communities in which multiple diverse populations of individuals reside

Adapted from MacQueen et al. (2001).

membership, as these may influence his or her willingness or ability to participate in a research effort.

MacQueen et al. (2001) asked individuals involved with HIV vaccine trials to describe what a community meant to them. These researchers identified five core elements of a community (Table 2.2). From these descriptions, it should be apparent that the idea of a community is fluid and can change depending on who is drawing the boundary lines. What is crucial in CBPR development is that the researcher has a clear definition and understanding of the community with which he or she is planning to partner. The experience of community members should weigh heavily in the determination of the issue to be studied and the methods of studying that particular issue.

Partnership Between Academic Researchers and Community Stakeholders

True CBPR includes a partnership or coalition between academic and community stakeholders that involves researchers and community members in all phases of the research process. This coalition development has been described by Lasker, Weiss, and Miller (2001) as *partnership synergy*, which is defined as the combination of perspectives, resources, and skills to create a new whole that is greater than the sum of its parts (Lasker et al., 2001). Partnership synergy, these authors suggest, allows the research partnership to study and solve difficult issues more effectively than the individual partners could on their own. Israel, Schulz, Parker, and Becker (1998, p. 177) suggest that the partners conducting a CBPR study "contribute unique strengths and shared responsibilities to enhance understanding of a given phenomenon and the social and cultural dynamics of the community, and integrate the knowledge gained with action to improve the health and well-being of community members."

Israel et al. (1998) conceptualized nine key principles that define a true CBPR study.

The CBPR process:

1. Recognizes the community as a unit of identity
2. Builds on strengths and resources within the community
3. Facilitates collaborative, equitable involvement of all partners in all phases of the research
4. Integrates knowledge and action for mutual benefit of all partners
5. Promotes a co-learning and empowering process that attends to social inequalities
6. Involves a cyclical and iterative process
7. Addresses health from both positive and ecological perspectives
8. Disseminates findings and knowledge gained by all partners
9. Involves a long-term commitment by all partners

Although CBPR studies have been found to vary widely in purpose and design, common themes can be expected. CBPR (Agency for Healthcare Research and Quality [AHRQ], 2004):

1. Recognizes the importance of social, political, cultural, and economic systems to health behaviors and outcomes
2. Engages community members in choosing research topics, developing projects, collecting data, and interpreting results
3. Emphasizes both qualitative and quantitative research methods
4. Places high priority on translation of the findings of basic, intervention, and applied research into changes in practice and policy

Development of CBPR includes building trust and enabling co-learning, sharing decision making and ownership, recognizing the expertise of all partners, and finding a balance between research and action (Minkler & Wallerstein, 2003). This synergistic partnership between researcher and community empowers the community, by incorporating local knowledge and culture in the understanding of health problems and the design of research interventions. The partnership is invested in the dissemination and application of research findings to improve community health and to reduce health disparities.

Community-Campus Partnerships for Health (CCPH) is a national network of academic–community partnerships working together to encourage community-based research and opportunities for student service learning. CCPH has formulated nine principles, listed next, which they suggest would facilitate and strengthen academic–community partnerships:

1. Partners have an agreed-upon mission, values, goals, and measurable outcomes for the partnership.
2. The relationship between partners is characterized by mutual trust, respect, genuineness, and commitment.
3. The partnership not only builds on identified strengths and assets but also addresses areas that need improvement.
4. The partnership balances the power among partners and enables resources among partners to be shared.

5. There is clear, open, and accessible communication between partners, making it an ongoing priority to listen to each need, develop a common language, and validate/clarify the meaning of terms.
6. Roles, norms, and processes for the partnership are established with the input and agreement of all partners.
7. There is feedback to, among, and from all stakeholders in the partnership, with the goal of continuously improving the partnership and its outcomes.
8. Partners share the credit for the partnership's accomplishments.
9. Partnerships take time to develop and evolve over time. (Community-Campus Partnerships for Health, 2015)

Wallerstein and Duran (2006, p. 313) stress the importance of full community collaboration in the research process. CBPR should not be limited to a community outreach focus, but should be seen as a "systematic effort to incorporate community participation and decision making, local theories of etiology and change, and community practices into the research effort."

IMPORTANCE OF PEPR AND CBPR

It has become clear in recent decades that the social environment in which we live has implications for our health. In addition to an individual's lifestyle and behavior, the environment in which he or she lives may increase or decrease the risk of illness or maladaptive health-related behaviors (IOM, 1988). Furthermore, evidence shows that when individuals become involved in their community and collaborate with their neighbors to effect change, their health and the health of the community may improve (Hanson, 1988). These findings about public health demonstrate the importance of engaging the community in decisions about health and health care and encouraging community participation in health promotion and disease prevention (Fawcett, Paine-Andrews, Francisco, & Vliet, 1993).

CBPR was highlighted as a core strategy in the first (2008) National Institutes of Health (NIH) Summit to Eliminate Disparities (Dankwa-Mullan et al., 2010). Health inequities faced by low-income and minority populations, defined by premature death, increased burden of disease, and inadequate access to quality health care (Nolte & McKee, 2008), are pervasive in the health care system. According to Dankwa-Mullan et al. (2010), improving and sustaining improved health outcomes for vulnerable populations requires community engagement and cross-disciplinary research. The conclusions drawn by Summit participants included the mandate that social determinants of health be an integral component of health care research, and that research should be collaborative with communities and promote community engagement, sustainable partnership models, and infrastructure and capacity building. Health disparities are a significant financial and social burden on our health care system and life in the United States and so must be addressed. CBPR offers a means of developing and implementing more effective interventions that focus on reducing disparities and health inequities; therefore, this methodology is likely to become more commonly used and funded in the near future (Horowitz, Robinson, & Seifer, 2009).

As Green and Mercer (2001) have noted, CBPR participants do more than give informed consent; rather, they share their knowledge and experience in helping to identify key problems to be studied, formulate research questions in culturally sensitive ways, and use study results to help support relevant program and policy development or social change. This is particularly important in the communities of low-income minority individuals in which much of CBPR takes place, as these individuals are often misrepresented or underrepresented in health services research (George, Duran, & Norris, 2014; Minkler, Blackwell, Thompson, & Tamir, 2003).

Reasons for Using PEPR and CBPR

PAR not only offers many benefits to participants, both academic and patient or community, but can also be extremely time consuming and does require the development of a potentially new set of skills not routinely taught in graduate nursing programs. Despite these potential challenges, it can be valuable and rewarding for the nurse researcher to spend his or her time searching out and developing relationships with members of vulnerable communities.

PAR can benefit the nurse researcher by providing entry into an underrepresented population that may be struggling with a significant health deficit. Shoultz et al. (2006) describe the methods they used to learn about a sensitive issue in a diverse and hard-to-reach population. Clinicians and researchers from the University of Hawaii wanted to learn about and respond to the incidence of intimate partner violence (IPV) in a population that included Native Hawaiians, Micronesians, Filipinas, and women who worked in the sex industry. Previous research in these communities had left residents feeling exploited and had failed to have an impact on issues of concern to community members. IPV is a complex issue with social and cultural implications and the potential for stigma not just for the involved couple but also for their extended families and children. Culturally relevant care requires an understanding of the social and cultural aspects of IPV (Schoultz et al., 2006). Viswanathan et al. (2004) suggest that using CBPR methodology in such a situation and with such a population can result in a deeper understanding of a community's unique circumstances and a more feasible foundation for trying out and adapting the best practices to fit the community's needs.

The goal of the project by Schoultz et al. (2006) was to help local community health centers to develop the needed expertise to encourage patient disclosure of IPV and to plan for effective services to be provided once IPV was reported. Through the development of a CBPR framework, researchers were able to develop long-term relationships with the community health centers. The centers' staff members subsequently would have increased access to expert resources, and researchers would be able to obtain a deeper understanding of how services were being provided to these populations. An agreement was reached to continue the collaboration between academia and practice, allowing students to participate in future research and providing researchers with access to study sites and enthusiastic research partners. The health centers are now more likely to participate in research and to improve practice based on research findings, due to the trusting relationship formed with the University. As Goldstein, Robson, and Botnick (1998) suggest, scholarly excellence can develop when there is synergy between research, education, practice, and community involvement.

By its very nature, PAR must also offer benefits to the community or patient research participants. By including those who are affected by a clinical issue or disparity in the research process, PAR empowers these vulnerable individuals by providing them with the agency to investigate and solve their own problems (Holkup et al., 2004). *Capacity* is defined by the United Nations Development Program (Department for International Development [DFID], 2008) as "the ability of people, institutions and societies to perform functions, solve problems, and set and achieve objectives." Capacity development is the process by which communities enhance their ability to mobilize and use resources to achieve objectives and sustain achievements (DFID, 2008). Communities of vulnerable populations, such as those most likely to participate in CBPR, are, by definition, communities with the need for capacity building and infrastructure and resource development. Building capacity would include developing the resources needed to meet specific challenges such as collecting needed data to identify problems or actually intervening and trying out alternatives to solve community problems. Capacity building in this regard can also translate into improvements in the community's capacity to help itself by identifying community members with various skills and talents, bringing interested residents together to achieve a specific objective, and teaching community members how to apply for funding or locate external resources to meet local needs. By developing a sustainable relationship between researcher and community, interested community members have access to information and expertise with which to tackle future problems.

Challenges to CBPR

Many valuable research findings either take years to disseminate or are never tested and evaluated as means to solve problems in vulnerable communities. Six core challenges have been identified that prevent the rapid translation of research findings into practice. The CBPR process facilitates a more rapid translation of research into practice by countering each of these challenges through the collaboration and co-learning of community–academic partnerships (Wallerstein & Duran, 2010). The challenges are as follows:

1. The need for external validity
2. The determination of adequate evidence
3. The incompatible language used in academia and practice
4. The "business as usual" attitude within universities
5. The lack of sustainability after research funding is exhausted
6. The lack of trust between researchers and clinicians

External validity refers to the ability to generalize findings from small samples to larger populations. If a proposed study or intervention does not seem to be a ready fit with the prevailing social and cultural norms of a community, it will likely not make sense to the community partners and so the work will not go forward. If aspects of local knowledge, customs, and values can be incorporated into a study so as to make the intervention more acceptable, uptake will be improved.

The second challenge, the determination of adequate evidence, implies an imbalance between research findings and what Wallerstein and Duran (2010) refer to as *indigenous knowledge*, which is defined as the knowledge that is local and unique to a specific culture and is focused on methods of problem solving appropriate to that culture. Indigenous knowledge is the basis of community decision making. The evidence of a successful intervention in CBPR would require that both community and academic partners perceive a positive outcome. CBPR endorses the integration of culturally based evidence and indigenous problem solving into research methodology, thus allowing researchers to examine how communities can successfully use their own resources to problem solve. Evidence of success is community based, and this can sometimes limit the generalizability of CBPR studies to other community settings.

The third challenge is language, the different names that academicians and community members may give to phenomena. Resistance can be triggered by a researcher's inability or refusal to use the language that the community finds the most appropriate. Community members do not want to take a subservient position to researchers in a collaborative relationship, and so academicians may be forced out of their comfort zone to accommodate the partnership. CBPR changes the terminology of research discourse: from "research subject" to "research participant," or from "targeting community members" to "engaging community partners" (Wallerstein & Duran, 2010).

The fourth challenge is business as usual, which is defined as the total control that academics traditionally maintain over the budget, resources, and research process (Wallerstein & Duran, 2010). CBPR, by definition, requires engagement of the community in each facet of the research process, including control of the budget, and so requires researchers to rethink the status quo of traditional research. This can be facilitated by the inclusion of ethnically or racially diverse researchers, specifically of the same race or ethnic group as the community members, thus attempting to alleviate a sense of a racial or ethnic power imbalance. Universities can upend the research status quo by amending institutional review board processes to require community benefits or by changing tenure and promotion requirements to take into account the length of time required to develop a true community–academic partnership (Wallerstein & Duran, 2010).

When a CBPR proposal is being considered for funding, questions such as "Is there evidence of participation of community members throughout the research?" "Has an adequate structure been developed to facilitate participation?" and "Is there evidence of collaborative decision making?" will challenge the traditional research model to demonstrate a true research partnership.

The fifth challenge to the translation of research is sustainability—are there any financial considerations that can allow for the research team to go forward and put the findings into practice? One of the major principles of CBPR is capacity building—helping the community to obtain the needed skills and resources to continue to improve its standard of living. CBPR always includes action in the research trajectory, and so after data collection and analysis it is expected that effort will be put forth to test the recommended change and institutionalize successful change efforts.

The final challenge is that of lack of trust. Trust is often an issue in research studies, particularly when diverse populations are being studied (Cook, Kosoko-Lasaki, & O'Brien, 2005). Wallerstein and Duran (2010) suggest that policies that equalize power can create an atmosphere of trust, such as the NIH–Indian Health Service partnership Native American Research Centers for Health, which situate the primary investigator within the tribal organization with tribal oversight. Shoultz et al. (2006) describe the establishment of defined roles for each team member and policies of operation for the team as methods of encouraging trust. Matsunaga et al. (1996) talk about conflict as an inevitable part of the collaborative research process in CBPR. These authors suggest that the effort to develop a trusting environment will allow the team to successfully negotiate the inevitable conflict.

METHODS OF CREATING PEPR AND CBPR

The steps of CBPR include team building, study design, implementation, data analysis and interpretation, dissemination of findings, translation of research into practice and/or policy, and institutionalization of successful change in the community (Horowitz et al., 2009). Team building is the important first step that differentiates CBPR from more traditional research methods. Team building may begin with a researcher looking for community members who are willing to participate in the research process or with concerned community members seeking out a researcher with expertise in an issue the community is facing. Researchers share their scientific knowledge and expertise with community members while relying on their community partners to teach them about the local cultural and social norms and help them avoid offending community members (Horowitz et al., 2009).

Researchers may find willing partners by first reaching out to local public health agencies such as Area Health Education Centers (AHECs); these academic–community partnership-based agencies facilitate access to health care to improve the distribution, diversity, and supply of the primary care health professions workforce who work in underserved health care delivery areas (Health Resources and Services Administration [HRSA], n.d.). Researchers can find local AHEC programs by searching the HRSA Data Warehouse. Other ways to locate community partners are through local clinics, churches, or community coalitions or through connections with academics in other departments who may be working with community members (i.e., social work, business, psychology, etc.).

The formation of a community advisory board (CAB) is often one of the first steps in the development of a community–academic partnership. The CAB, which may include community members, local clinicians, and representatives of local community-based organizations or agencies (Israel, Eng, Schultz, & Parker, 2005), can help solidify a researcher's connection with a community, facilitate the development of a research program, and increase the likelihood of research findings becoming translated into practice or policy. Board members should include local champions, those individuals who have a firsthand understanding of the community and its issues, a level of influence among community members, and an interest in creating change in the community. Local champions bridge the gap between researchers and community members by facilitating communication, encouraging trust and participation, and developing the level of enthusiasm needed to accomplish goals. Howell, Shea, and Higgins (2005) describe three roles of the local champion: expressing enthusiasm and confidence about the success of an innovation or change, getting the right people involved, and persisting under adversity. Another definition of *local champion* is a person who is able to inspire and motivate community members, and who is able to advocate for change and influence local organizations (National Institute for Healthy and Clinical Effectiveness, 2008).

Horowitz et al. (2009) suggest including the following categories of individuals in a community partnership: (a) Bridge builders, identified as those who have experience with research and community cultures and who can moderate the process, mediate conflicts, interpret results, and mentor others; (b) "Bringers," identified as those who could help identify new members or resources that could be included in the project; and (c) Historians, identified as those who have a profound understanding of the community, as well as its culture, norms, and values, and therefore help the team understand the challenges of health and health promotion in that setting.

Once a team of interested and motivated community members has been identified, researchers will have to clarify research aims and objectives. Community interests may clash with scientific goals at this stage and throughout the process. If the effort to develop rules for engagement and trust does not start at the beginning with the choice of a mutually agreed-upon research topic, the entire project may be threatened. CBPR, by definition, is expected to address questions that are relevant to the needs and priorities of the community (Resnik & Kennedy, 2010). Community partners who are concerned with meeting community health needs may attempt to collaborate with researchers who have a set plan of study or who are determining a course of study based on a review of current literature. On the one hand, an imbalance in the interests at this time could scuttle the project, and so researchers wishing to develop community networks may have to forgo personal aims at this point. On the other hand, community members may not be aware of significant health risks and may be willing to respond to education. For example, Mills, Cooper, and Kanfer (2005) discuss a situation in which researchers on an HIV treatment study in a sub-Saharan country were interested in studying the effectiveness of anti-retroviral drug therapy, whereas community members were more interested in studying the effectiveness of traditional, herbal remedies (Mills et al., 2005). In sub-Saharan Africa, there are many more traditional healers (1/500 residents) than medical doctors (1/40,000 residents) and up to 70% of the population may receive traditional treatment rather than medical treatment. Thus, the goal of using traditional medicine as a means of treating HIV should not be unexpected if local knowledge and custom are being considered (Mills et al., 2005). Although it may be difficult to confront long-held beliefs about the efficacy of traditional healing as compared with modern medical treatment, it would be beneficial for researchers to collaborate with traditional healers (as a type of local champion) to disseminate information about available medical treatment, while attempting to evaluate the effectiveness or potential harm of traditional practices. Although selection of a research focus likely reflects the scientific bias of the academic researcher, this bias should be appropriately managed in CPBR to prevent the views of the researchers from dominating those of the community collaborators. The research focus chosen should have value for both partners (Resnik & Kennedy, 2010).

At this point, researchers are likely to consider the need to identify potential funding sources. Identifying grants and grant writing should be collaborative processes. CBPR grants are likely to include a level of flexibility for developing concepts that emanate from the community partnership. If funding is found, community partners should receive the financial resources and incentives needed to encourage and facilitate their participation. If research assistants are to be hired, they should be hired from within the community. By sharing the control of the budget and financial resources, researchers are demonstrating their willingness to collaborate and are building trust (Horowitz et al., 2009). Funding sources have been improving for CBPR projects in the recent past (see Table 2.3 for funding agency information).

Another point at which disagreements between community partners and researchers are likely to occur is in the design of the study (Resnik & Kennedy, 2010). Using CBPR for a clinical trial or a study, including placebo, can be very difficult for

---

TABLE 2.3 **Funding Sources for CBPR**

- NIH through the following agencies:
  - National Cancer Institute
  - National Heart, Lung, and Blood Institute
  - National Institute of Alcohol Abuse and Alcoholism
  - National Institute of Child Health and Human Development
  - National Institute on Drug Abuse
  - National Institute on Deafness and Other Communication Disorders
  - National Institute on Dental and Craniofacial Research
  - National Institute of Environmental Health Services
  - National Institute of Mental Health
  - National Institute of Minority Health and Health Disparities
  - National Institute of Nursing Research
  - Office of Behavioral and Social Science Research
  - Office of Research on Women's Health
- A CBPR SIG has been established at the NIH to strengthen communication among federal agencies supporting CBPR.
  - See this webpage for updates: http://obssr.od.nih.gov/scientific_areas/methodology/community_based_participatory_research
- American Cancer Society: Request for proposals to stimulate research on effective interventions to reduce cancer health disparities (at any stage of the cancer continuum) and achieve cancer health equity using CBPR
  - See this webpage for more information: https://obssr.od.nih.gov/scientific_areas/methodology/community_based_participatory_research
- NARCH: Partners with The National Institute of General Medical Sciences and several other NIH Institutes and Centers. The NARCH initiative supports partnerships between AI/AN tribes or tribally based organizations and institutions that conduct intensive academic-level biomedical research. As a consequence of these partnerships, tribes and tribal organizations are able to build a research infrastructure, including a core component for capacity building and the possibility of reducing the many health disparities so prevalent in AI/AN communities.
  - See this webpage for more information: www.nigms.nih.gov/training/NARCH/Pages/default.aspx
- PCOR: Supports research that will provide reliable, useful information to help people make informed health care decisions and improve health care delivery and outcomes. This research is a type of comparative effectiveness research. It includes some large pragmatic studies and large-scale observational studies. We also fund research to address gaps in methodology relevant to PCOR.
  - See this webpage for more information: www.pcori.org/content/research-we-support
- CCPH is a national nonprofit organization supporting CBPR partnerships. The CCPH website: www.ccph.info offers CBPR resources such as tools, reports, presentations, journal articles, syllabi, and course materials.

AI/AN, American Indian/Alaska Native; CBPR, community-based participatory research; CCPH, community-campus partnerships for health; NARCH, Native American Research Centers for Health; NIH, National Institutes of Health; PCOR, patient-centered outcomes research; SIG, scientific interest group.

---

community members to understand or accept. If community norms and values interfere with the scientific rigor of a study, a researcher may need to reconsider whether such a study can be successfully managed in a true CBPR framework. If disagreements about research focus and design occur, researchers should work with their community partners to find mutually acceptable solutions that not only will be appropriate to community norms and values but also will provide scientifically acceptable findings (Minkler, 2004). In cases of disagreement, discussion with the CAB may be helpful.

According to Minkler (2004), disagreements concerning data analysis may also occur. The CBPR process does not mandate or recommend any specific methods of research design or data analysis; therefore, researchers are expected to choose a design and method that will address the research focus with scientific rigor. However, community partners are not likely to know or understand what is expected in a research study, and it is up to the research partner to explain and justify the design and interpretation of the data in ways that the entire research team can appreciate. It is possible that data interpretation can lead to results that do not show community residents in a way that is favorable to the community. Resnik and Kennedy (2010) describe a situation in which an HIV study resulted in findings that the prevalence of HIV within the community was more likely to be found in a certain race or ethnic group of individuals in the community. Community research partners may resist such an interpretation of the data and may be concerned with stigma, whereas the researchers are hoping to use these data to move forward with an intervention. Again, the research team must make every effort to work toward a mutually acceptable solution. It is possible that reframing the findings as a means to an effective end—the development of an intervention, an increased potential for community health promotion funding, and the opening of a clean needle exchange center—may make the results more acceptable to concerned community members. If agreement cannot be found, Resnik and Kennedy (2010) suggest that a future publication reporting the contested results can include the researchers' interpretation of the data as well as an addendum reporting the community members' alternative view of the data. Such a compromise may, however, have implications on the sustainability of the research partnership.

THE INTERPRETATION AND PRESENTATION OF PEPR AND CBPR

The interpretation of CBPR study data should be consistent with data analysis and interpretation norms for the specific type of analysis used. The CBPR framework does not preclude or require any specific research design or data analysis. What would be unique to a CBPR study is a discussion of how the community–academic partnership may have influenced the interpretation of the findings, and the resultant implementation of practice or policy change (Bordeaux et al., 2007).

The next step in the research process is publication and dissemination of the study findings. The main reason for publication is to disseminate new knowledge to improve health. In CBPR studies, publication can help to engage community partners in the research process and help convince community decision and policy makers of the validity and importance of the project. Dissemination of CBPR results can also be helpful to other community–academic partnerships that may benefit from lessons learned (Bordeaux et al., 2007).

A researcher's primary interest is to advance human knowledge by describing, explaining, and predicting natural phenomena (Resnik & Kennedy, 2010). This knowledge has value and is potentially important in policy making and practice. Researchers must adhere to epistemological and ethical norms to ensure that their research findings are valid and reliable (Resnik, 2007). Adhering to these norms and rules may be difficult when collaborating with community partners who will likely be prioritizing their own interests and needs in the conduct of CBPR. Community partners may focus primarily on the benefits they expect to obtain for their community rather than on the research process (Resnik & Kennedy, 2010).

Community partners may oppose making the findings public due to concern about stigma or the community's reputation; this desire would be in opposition to the expectations of the researchers. Sometimes, it may be possible to protect the community from harms related to publication by removing information that could be used to identify the community, such as location or demographic characteristics of the population. However, given that the community plays such an important role in the CBPR process, removal of identifying information relatively invalidates the CBPR framework of the study (Resnik & Kennedy, 2010).

Strategies have been suggested to prevent undue influence from being placed on researchers who work closely with industries that may be funding their research, such as pharmaceutical companies. These same strategies may be helpful if the interests and goals of the community partners run counter to those of the researchers. Some of these strategies, such as managing conflicts of interest, obtaining independent reviews of research design and data analyses, and the preparation of formal agreements for publication and dissemination, could be applied to CBPR (Resnik & Kennedy, 2010). The development of a formal agreement at the beginning of the study that would identify who among the partners will be responsible for dissemination of the findings and how dissemination will be managed can be very helpful if conflict occurs (Horowitz et al., 2009).

In preparing a manuscript for publication, it is important for the authors to justify why they used a CBPR approach rather than a community setting. It is suggested that researchers begin by defining the CBPR process and differentiating it from "community-placed" research (research conducted in a community setting, but without community partnership; Bordeaux et al., 2007). CBPR is often chosen as the framework for a study, because the community is "disproportionately affected by a health condition, hard to reach, poorly understood, or unchanged after using a traditional research approach to address a health problem" (Bordeaux et al., 2007, p. 284). CBPR manuscripts should define the community and the specifics of the partnership. When defining the partnership, manuscripts should include a description of how the partnership was created, its membership and focus, and the level of involvement of community participants in the research process (noting specific areas of collaboration such as study design, data collection, etc.; Bordeaux et al., 2007).

One aspect of patient-engaged research that is being given funding priority at the current time is patient-centered outcomes research (PCOR). As defined by the Patient-Centered Outcomes Research Institute ([PCORI], a nonprofit, nongovernmental organization authorized by Congress in the Patient Protection and Affordable Care Act of 2010), "[PCOR] helps people and their caregivers communicate and make informed healthcare decisions, allowing their voices to be heard in assessing the value of healthcare options" (PCORI, 2014a). PCORI's mission states that PCORI "helps people make informed healthcare decisions, and improves healthcare delivery and outcomes, by producing and promoting high-integrity, evidence-based information that comes from research guided by patients, caregivers, and the broader healthcare community" (PCORI, 2014b). Specifically, PCOR is comparative effectiveness research focused on and guided by the needs and concerns of patients. Similar to the general principles of PAR, PCOR requires the active involvement of stakeholders to ensure that the research will meet its stated goals. Unlike PAR, PCOR specifies a particular research design and data analysis methodology. PCOR is based on the concept of comparative effectiveness research, a design that is utilized to compare treatment alternatives to improve decision makers' ability to fully understand and weigh alternatives (Gabriel & Normand, 2012). Without research to compare innovations with currently accepted practices, diffusion may be constrained or ineffective methodology may be adopted without adequate evidence. PCOR is designed to answer the following questions (PCORI, 2014a):

1. "Given my personal characteristics, conditions, and preferences, what should I expect will happen to me?"
2. "What are my options, and what are the potential benefits and harms of those options?"
3. "What can I do to improve the outcomes that are most important to me?"
4. "How can clinicians and the care delivery systems they work in help me make the best decisions about my health and health care?"

PCORI was created to support research that can produce this information. Because it was recognized that to be trusted, research must be generated with the use of rigorous, valid, patient-centered methods, PCORI's founding legislation established a 17-member methodology committee, to be selected by the Government Accountability Office. This committee has been charged with the goal of developing and improving the science and methods of comparative clinical effectiveness research (Gabriel & Normand, 2012).

CONSIDERATIONS: CHALLENGES AND ETHICAL ISSUES IN PEPR AND CBPR

PEPR and CBPR inform and enrich the research process as well as provide benefits to the patient and community participants as noted earlier (improved research quality, empowerment, voice, productive partnerships, program extension, improved health/health outcomes, and sustainability). However, this research also poses potential challenges and ethical considerations for both researcher and patient or community participant partners (Domecq et al., 2012, 2014; Jagosh et al., 2012; Shalowitz et al., 2009).

For patients participating in patient-engaged research, frustration may be due to the length of time required for training and consultation sessions and transportation issues (Domecq et al., 2012, 2014). Language barriers for non-native English speakers and the use of academic or medical jargon can impede communication and cause frustration as well. "Tokenism" may be present, in which patients' participation is included to meet the requirements of a grant or increase sample numbers, but participants' contributions, their ideas, and feedback are not incorporated into the research design. This leads to a devaluing of the patients' input (Domecq et al., 2014).

For researchers, the logistics of working within the patient partnership, the extra time needed to complete studies due to training needs and preparation of patient participants, the variation in patient participation levels, and the need to collaborate with patients throughout the research process can cause frustration as well. Additional costs due to patient training and consultation can greatly increase the cost of the research so that additional funding is needed. Several participatory researchers have noted the need to be concerned about "scope creep," a theoretical concern that engaging patients in the research process may result in the inclusion of extraneous concerns and issues that would make the research impractical (Domecq et al., 2012, 2014). Researchers must be cognizant of the appearance of tokenism in their collaboration with patients, as well as of their own learning needs regarding patients' culture and language preferences.

The CBPR process can result in similar concerns for academic and community collaborators, with the additional complications that result from the expectation of long-term commitment that would be required for the service delivery component (action step) of the research process. Much of CBPR takes place with historically underrepresented diverse populations. These communities, often vulnerable or "at-risk," may have felt exploited by previous short-term studies in which researchers had collected data within the community, but had not provided any benefit to the residents (Attree et al., 2011; Michener et al., 2008; Shalowitz et al., 2009). In addition, residents of vulnerable diverse communities may already feel disenfranchised from academia, and may have perceived a power deferential between researchers and community participants that could lead to conflicts between partners (Israel et al., 1998; Shalowitz et al., 2009). Community participants may feel stress or frustration with the time commitments for training and consultation in the research process, and this can impact the team's ability to engage and maintain truly representative community participation (Israel et al., 1998; Shalowitz et al., 2009).

Attree et al. (2011), in a review of the evidence justifying the CBPR process, found that although most community participants found positive benefits from CBPR, there was some evidence of negative consequences such as fatigue, stress, and disappointment (particularly for disabled individuals). Participants complained about the lack of sustainability of the CBPR projects, the feeling that they were not able to actively participate in the research, and the failure of researchers to act on the community participants' suggestions. They also noted perceived disapproval or criticism from other community members for their participation.

Researchers must spend a considerable amount of time with the community to build trust and overcome potential community resistance; this requires a long-term time commitment to the process, of which academics might not be cognizant, at the start. Researchers must be prepared for the long period between the research and dissemination of the CBPR, which can result from allowing true collaboration in the process, but that can negatively influence the promotion and tenure process for the academics. The time required to build a trusting relationship with community collaborators and to foster engagement throughout the research process can have negative consequences for researchers who are faced with publishing pressures (Shalowitz et al., 2009).

Additional concerns for researchers engaging in CBPR follow from the need for a long-time commitment to the community and the project. Team members may leave their positions during the process or burnout of the research team may occur, especially if there is an extra workload of non-research-related duties and little to no funding available (Holkup et al., 2004). Researchers may need to donate volunteer time to community organizations to enhance enthusiasm for community engagement. Finally, there are likely to be concerns related to the change process in the community. Change, even for the better, is usually met with resistance and fear, as residents are unsure of what to expect from the researchers and the research process. Playing an integral role in the change process may be empowering for some community participants, and encouragement from local champions may help defuse resistance that might prevent real benefits from being appreciated in the community.

Holkup et al. (2004) worked with a Native American population to understand and improve care of the elderly in that community. They began the CBPR partnership with a pilot project. First, they investigated what community leaders, elders, and local service providers thought about the issue of elder mistreatment to discover whether this was actually a problem in that community, and if so, how it was being addressed. They asked these opinion leaders whether a form of family conference model might be helpful in improving the lives of the elders in the community. When they had sufficient knowledge of the issue, the team enrolled a family that was willing to experiment with the family conference model. If the model was successful with one family, it could provide a means to diffuse the model throughout the community. In this way, the community was able to see the value of the intervention and enthusiasm for engagement was widely expressed. Federal funding from the National Institute of Nursing Research was received for this project, and members of the community were hired and trained to facilitate the development of the family conference model throughout the reservation.

Research on best methods to achieve engagement is lacking. Nonetheless, potential-suggested solutions to these ethical and other challenges to patient and community-based PAR exist in the literature. Michener et al. (2008) note that resistance to participatory research approaches can originate from all participants, researchers and patients, or communities, and that to overcome this issue "steadfast patience" is necessary (p. 412). For CBPR to result in tangible, lasting health benefits for communities, researchers must balance scientific rigor and community support. This may not be easy to accomplish (Israel et al., 2005). Patience and flexibility are needed for all participants to build mutual trust over time; engage in co-learning, for example, with researchers about the community and community participants about the research process; develop a commitment to long-term involvement; spend time to build reciprocal power while sharing relationships; plan for equitable compensation and credit (between patients, community participants, and researchers); collaborate in developing clear expectations that are explicitly described and documented; attempt to reach and involve representative membership of the community; and learn and exercise productive conflict resolution and negotiation (Anderson et al., 2012; Domecq et al., 2014; Jagosh et al., 2012; Michener et al., 2008, 2012; Shalowitz et al., 2009).

EXAMPLES OF PUBLISHED PEPR AND CBPR

Service User and Carer Group Advising on Research (SUGAR; Simpson, Jones, Barlow, and Cox, 2014) is an example of patient-engaged research that describes the integration of patients and caregivers with researchers and practitioners throughout the mental health research process. The researchers actively recruited mental health patients and their caregivers to advise and contribute throughout the research process. The team collaborated with the patients and caregivers in doing the following things: learning about the research process, formulating research questions, designing the study and collecting data, as well as implementing the study and

TABLE 2.4 Selected Examples From Participatory-Engaged Research Literature

	Study	Design and Objective	Setting	Sample	Outcome	Findings
CBPR: development of a CBPR network	Wynn, Taylor-Jones, Johnson, Bostick, and Fouad (2011)	Case study methodology to provide a detailed account of how the CBPR principles were instrumental in the initiation and promotion of policy change efforts, particularly with tobacco and breast cancer legislation	African American community in Alabama	A group of community health advisors, community-based organizations, businesses, churches, health care facilities, and academic institutions from Tuscaloosa, Alabama	Smoking Cessation Coalition implemented a systematic plan to address the social, economic, and political factors that would potentially exacerbate cancer disparities among Alabama's most underserved communities.	The partnership formed was significant in educating political leaders and in empowering other community members to be active participants in the policy process.
CBPR: intervention study	Newman et al. (2014)	Development and pilot testing of an intervention using community-based Peer Navigators with SCIs to provide health education, reduce preventable secondary conditions and rehospitalizations, and improve community participation	The five-county service area of a disability resource center in South Carolina	73 individuals with SCI who were on the contact list of the South Carolina SCI Association	Preliminary evaluations indicate a positive effect in improvement of pressure ulcers present on enrollment, and increased participation in productive and preferred community activities.	The CBPR framework provides a guide for inclusion of individuals with SCI as research partners in the development, implementation, and evaluation of interventions intended to improve outcomes after SCI.

(continued)

TABLE 2.4 Selected Examples From Participatory-Engaged Research Literature (*continued*)

	Study	Design and Objective	Setting	Sample	Outcome	Findings
PEPR	Boivin, Lehoux, Lacombe, Burgers, and Grol (2014)	Cluster RCT comparing health care improvement priority setting with and without patient involvement	Six communities in a Canadian region	172 individuals from six communities participated in the study, including 83 chronic disease patients and 89 health professionals.	The primary outcome was the level of agreement between patients' and professionals' priorities.	Patient involvement can change priorities driving health care improvement at the population level.
PCOR	Keren et al. (2014)	Retrospective cohort study comparing PICC and oral therapy for the treatment of acute osteomyelitis	Thirty-six participating children's hospitals in the United States	2,060 children and adolescents with osteomyelitis received oral antibiotics at discharge; 1,055 received PICC-administered antibiotics.	The primary outcome was treatment failure. Secondary outcomes included adverse drug reaction, PICC line complication, and a composite of all three end points.	Due to the magnitude and seriousness of PICC complications, clinicians should reconsider the practice of treating otherwise-healthy children with acute osteomyelitis with prolonged intravenous antibiotics after hospital discharge when an equally effective oral alternative exists.

CBPR, community-based participatory research; PCOR, patient-centered outcomes research; PEPR, patient-engaged participatory research; PICC, peripherally inserted central catheter; RCT, randomized controlled trial; SCI, spinal cord injury.

disseminating the findings, including joint presentations, workshops, and as authors of a peer-reviewed article.

The article presents a review of their patient-engaged research process as well as a qualitative reflective evaluation of the processes and outcomes of their participatory method itself. Themes that were derived through a constant comparative analysis of reflective narratives revealed the perspectives of the service user and caregivers on participation in the research process. Examples of identified themes included "growth," "empowerment," and "challenges." The authors noted that user and caregiver discussions and perspectives have enhanced and refined research proposals and activities intended to improve mental health services.

Articles about the CBPR process tend to discuss the process of developing a community–academic partnership. Mishra, DeForge, Barnet, Nitri, and Grant (2012) used CBPR principles to investigate issues around mammography screening and strategies to increase screening in a population of urban women. The authors conducted five focus groups with 41 primarily African American women in Baltimore, Maryland. Using the social determinants of health perspective to conduct a qualitative content analysis, the authors found that the major obstacles to screening were at the individual (pain from the procedure) and structural (cost, convenience) levels. Strategies that were suggested to overcome these barriers included the ability to receive a number of services during one visit to a health provider. The CBPR framework was used to encourage the participation of health center clinicians and patients in the project's conceptualization, design, implementation, analysis, and dissemination. See Table 2.4 for additional examples of PAR from the published literature.

SUMMARY

In summary, in contrast to traditional health care research methods, new methods that engage participants and stakeholders in the research process have emerged. Active participation in research by those who are being studied can lead to better, more effective research through the generation of research topics that are particularly relevant to the patients' or communities' concerns. Likewise, participant engagement in the planning and implementation of research may also improve its translation into clinical practice or community life. With this growing agreement about the important role of patient and community involvement in research, there is a need for nurse scholars to learn how to successfully engage and conduct research with patient and community partners in various settings.

REFERENCES

Adelman, C. (1993). Kurt Lewin and the origins of action research. *Educational Action Research, 1*(1), 7–24. doi:10.1080/0965079930010102

Agency for Healthcare Research and Quality. (2004). *Community-based participatory research: Assessing the evidence* (AHRQ Publication no. 04–E022-2).

Anderson, E. E., Soloman, S., Heitman, E., DuBois, J. M., Fisher, C. B., Kost, R. G., . . . Ross, L. F. (2012). Research ethics education for community-engaged research: A review and research agenda. *Journal of Empirical Research on Human Research Ethics, 7*(2), 3–19.

Attree, P., French, B., Milton, B., Povall, S., Whitehead, M., & Popay, J. (2011). The experience of community engagement for individuals: A rapid review of evidence. *Health & Social Care in the Community, 19*(3), 250–260.

Boivin, A., Lehoux, P., Lacombe, R., Burgers, J., & Grol, R. (2014). Involving patients in setting priorities for healthcare improvement: A cluster randomized trial. *Implementation Science, 9*(4), 1–10. Retrieved from http://www.implementationscience.com/content/9/1/24

Bordeaux, B. C., Wiley, C., Tandon, S. D., Horowitz, C. R., Brown, P. B., & Bass, E. B. (2007). Guidelines for writing manuscripts about community-based participatory research for peer-reviewed journals. *Progress in Community Health Partnerships: Research, Education, and Action, 1*(3), 281–288.

Community-Campus Partnerships for Health. (2015). *Nine principles of partnership.* Retrieved from https://ccph.memberclicks.net/principles-of-partnership

Cook, C. T., Kosoko-Lasaki, O., & O'Brien, R. (2005). Satisfaction with and perceived cultural competency of healthcare providers: The minority experience. *Journal of the National Medical Association, 97*(8), 1078–1087.

Cornwall, A., & Jewkes, R. (1995). What is participatory research? *Social Science & Medicine, 41*(12), 1667–1676.

Dankwa-Mullan, I., Rhee, K. B., Williams, K., Sanchez, I., Sy, F. S., Stinson, N., Jr., & Ruffin, J. (2010). The science of eliminating health disparities: Summary and analysis of the NIH summit recommendations. *American Journal of Public Health, 100*(Suppl. 1), S12–S18.

Department for International Development (DFID). (2008). *Working paper series: Capacity building.* Retrieved from http://www.google.com/url?sa=t&rct=j&q=&esrc=s&source=web&cd=1&ved=0CC AQFjAA&url=http%3A%2F%2Fr4d.dfid.gov.uk%2FPDF%2FOutputs%2FConsultation%2FResearc hStrategyWorkingPaperfinal_capacity_P1.pdf&ei=5Bu9VKLlN4jYggT82IDIDQ&usg=AFQjCNFVk F6hXWYPJKLiIW4NUxA_c0pPfw&sig2=a0LVGpcf_a5XGs7FMVK9BA&bvm=bv.83829542,d.eXY

Domecq, J. P., Prutsky, G., Elraiyah, T., Wang, Z., Nabhan, M., Shippee, N., . . . Murad, M. H. (2014). Patient engagement in research: A systematic review. *BMC Health Services Research, 14*(1), 89.

Domecq, J. P. G., Lopez, G. J. P., Wang, Z., Elraiyah, T. A., Nabhan, M., Brito, J. P. C., . . . Murad, M. H. (2012). Eliciting patient perspective in patient-centered outcomes research: A meta narrative systematic review. In *A Report Prepared for the Patient-Centered Outcomes Research Institute* (pp. 1–164). Rochester, MN: Mayo Clinic. Retrieved from http://www.pcori.org/sites/default/files/Eliciting-Patient-Perspective-in-Patient-Centered-Outcomes-Research-A-Meta-Narrative-Systematic-Review1.pdf

Faridi, Z., Grunbaum, J. A., Gray, B. S., Franks, A., & Simoes, E. (2007). Community-based participatory research: Necessary next steps. *Preventing Chronic Disease, 4*(3), 70. Retrieved from http://www.ncbi.nlm.nih.gov/pubmed/17572974

Fawcett, S. B., Paine-Andrews, A., Francisco, V. T., & Vliet, M. (1993). Promoting health through community development. In D. S. Glenwick & L. A. Jason (Eds.), *Promoting health and mental health in children, youth and families* (pp. 233–255). New York, NY: Springer-Verlag.

Gabriel, S. E., & Normand, S. L. T. (2012). Getting the methods right—The foundation of patient-centered outcomes research. *New England Journal of Medicine, 367*(9), 787–790.

George, S., Duran, N., & Norris, K. (2014). A systematic review of barriers and facilitators to minority research participation among African Americans, Latinos, Asian Americans, and Pacific Islanders. *American Journal of Public Health, 104*(2), e16–e31.

Goldstein, B. D., Robson, M. G., & Botnick, C. E. (1998). Size characteristics of larger academic human environmental health programs in the United States. *Environmental Health Perspectives, 106*(10), 615–617.

Green, L. W., & Mercer, S. L. (2001). Can public health researchers and agencies reconcile the push from funding bodies and the pull from communities? *American Journal of Public Health, 91*(12), 1926–1929.

Hanson, P. (1988). Citizen involvement in community health promotion: A role application of CDC's patch model. *International Quarterly of Community Health Education, 9*(3), 177–186.

Health Resources and Services Administration. (n.d.). *Area health education centers*. Retrieved from http://bhpr.hrsa.gov/grants/areahealtheducationcenters

Holkup, P. A., Tripp-Reimer, T., Salois, E. M., & Weinert, C. (2004). Community-based participatory research: An approach to intervention research with a Native American community. *ANS Advances in Nursing Science, 27*(3), 162–175.

Horowitz, C. R., Robinson, M., & Seifer, S. (2009). Community-based participatory research from the margin to the mainstream: Are researchers prepared? *Circulation, 119*(19), 2633–2642.

Howell, J. M., Shea, C. M., & Higgins, C. A. (2005). Champions of product innovations: Defining, developing, and validating a measure of champion behavior. *Journal of Business Venturing, 20*(5), 641–661.

Institute of Medicine. (1988). *The future of public health*. Washington, DC: National Academy Press.

Israel, B. A., Eng, E., Schulz, A., & Parker, E. A. (2005). Introduction to methods for CBPR for health. In E. A. Parker, T. G. Robins, B. A. Israel, W. Brakefield-Caldwell, K. K. Edgren, D. J. Wilkins, . . . & A. J. Schultz (Eds.), *Methods in community-based participatory research for health* (pp. 3–26). San Francisco, CA: Jossey-Bass.

Israel, B. A., Schulz, A. J., Parker, E. A., & Becker, A. B. (1998). Review of community-based research: Assessing partnership approaches to improve public health. *Annual Review of Public Health, 19*(1), 173–202.

Israel, B. A., Schulz, A. J., Parker, E. A., & Becker, A. B. (2001). Community-based participatory research: Policy recommendations for promoting a partnership approach in health research. *Education for Health, 14*(2), 182–197.

Jagosh, J., Macaulay, A. C., Pluye, P., Salsberg, J., Bush, P. L., Henderson, J., . . . Greenhalgh, T. (2012). Uncovering the benefits of participatory research: Implications of a realist review for health research and practice. *Milbank Quarterly, 90*(2), 311–346.

Keren, R., Shah, S. S., Srivastava, R., Rangel, S., Bendel-Stenzel, M., Harik, N., . . . Parker, A. (2014). Comparative effectiveness of intravenous vs oral antibiotics for postdischarge treatment of acute osteomyelitis in children. *JAMA Pediatrics, 169*(2), 120–128.

Lasker, R. D., Weiss, E. S., & Miller, R. (2001). Partnership synergy: A practical framework for studying and strengthening the collaborative advantage. *Milbank Quarterly, 79*(2), 179–205.

MacQueen, K. M., McLellan, E., Metzger, D. S., Kegeles, S., Strauss, R. P., Scotti, R., . . . Trotter, R. T. (2001). What is community? An evidence-based definition for participatory public health. *American Journal of Public Health, 91*, 1929–1938.

Matsunaga, D. S., Enos, R., Gotay, C. C., Banner, R. O., DeCambra, H. O., Hammond, O. W., . . . Tsark, J. A. (1996). Participatory research in a native Hawaiian community: The Wai'anae cancer research project. *Cancer, 78*(Suppl. 7), 1582–1586.

Michener, L., Cook, J., Ahmed, S. M., Yonas, M. A., Coyne-Besaley, T., & Aguilar-Gaxiola, S. (2012). Aligning the goals of community-engaged research: Why and how academic health centers can successfully engage with communities to improve health. *Academic Medicine, 87*(3), 285–291. doi:10.1097/ACM.0b013e3182441680

Michener, J., Yaggy, S., Lyn, M., Warburton, S., Champagne, M., Black, M., . . . Dzau, V. (2008). Improving the health of the community: Duke experience with community engagement. *Academic Medicine, 83*(4), 408–413.

Mills, E., Cooper, C., & Kanfer, I. (2005). Traditional African medicine in the treatment of HIV. *Lancet Infectious Diseases, 5*(8), 465–467.

Minkler, M. (2004). Ethical challenges for the "outside" researcher in community-based participatory research. *Health Education Behavior, 31*, 684–697.

Minkler, M., Blackwell, A. G., Thompson, M., & Tamir, H. (2003). Community-based participatory research: Implications for public health funding. *American Journal of Public Health, 93*(8), 1210–1213.

Minkler, M., & Wallerstein, N. (2003). Part one: Introduction to community-based participatory research. In *Community-based participatory research for health*. San Francisco, CA: Jossey-Bass.

Mishra, S. I., DeForge, B., Barnet, B., Ntiri, S., & Grant, L. (2012). Social determinants of breast cancer screening in urban primary care practices: A community-engaged formative study. *Women's Health Issues*, 22(5), e429–e438.

National Institute for Healthy and Clinical Effectiveness. (2008). *Community engagement to improve health. NICE public health guidance 9*. London, UK: Author.

Newman, S. D., Gillenwater, G., Toatley, S., Rodgers, M. D., Todd, N., Epperly, D., & Andrews, J. O. (2014). A community-based participatory research approach to the development of a Peer Navigator health promotion intervention for people with spinal cord injury. *Disability and Health Journal*, 7(4), 478–484.

Nolte, E., & McKee, C. M. (2008). Measuring the health of nations: Updating an earlier analysis. *Health Affairs (Millwood)*, 27(1), 58–71.

Patient-Centered Outcomes Research Institute (PCORI). (2014a). *Patient-centered outcomes research*. Retrieved from http://www.pcori.org/content/patient-centered-outcomes-research

Patient-Centered Outcomes Research Institute (PCORI). (2014b). *About us*. Retrieved from http://www.pcori.org/about-us

Resnik, D. (2007). *The price of truth*. New York, NY: Oxford University Press.

Resnik, D. B., & Kennedy, C. E. (2010). Balancing scientific and community interests in community-based participatory research. *Accountability in Research*, 17(4), 198–210.

Schmittdiel, J. A., Grumbach, K., & Selby, J. V. (2010). System-based participatory research in health care: An approach for sustainable translational research and quality improvement. *Annals of Family Medicine*, 8(3), 256–259.

Shalowitz, M. U., Isacco, A., Barquin, N., Clark-Kauffman, E., Delger, P., Nelson, D., . . . Wagenaar, K. A. (2009). Community-based participatory research: A review of the literature with strategies for community engagement. *Journal of Development and Behavioral Pediatrics*, 30(4), 350–361.

Shoultz, J., Oneha, M. F., Magnussen, L., Hla, M. M., Brees-Saunders, Z., Cruz, M. D., & Douglas, M. (2006). Finding solutions to challenges faced in community-based participatory research between academic and community organizations. *Journal of Interprofessional Care*, 20(2), 133–144.

Simpson, A., Jones, J., Barlow, S., Cox, L.; Service User and Carer Group Advising on Research (SUGAR). (2014). Adding SUGAR: Service user and carer collaboration in mental health nursing research. *Journal of Psychosocial Nursing and Mental Health Services*, 52(1), 22–30.

Tapp, H., White, L., Steuerwald, M., & Dulin, M. (2013). Use of community-based participatory research in primary care to improve healthcare outcomes and disparities in care. *Journal of Comparative Effectiveness Research*, 2(4), 405–419.

Viswanathan, M., Ammerman, A., Eng, E., Garlehner, G., Lohr, K. N., Griffith, D., . . . Whitener, L. (2004). *Community-based participatory research: Assessing the evidence*. Evidence Report/Technology Assessment No. 99 (Prepared by RTI-University of North Carolina Evidence-Based Practice Center under Contract No. 290-02-0016; AHRQ Publication no. 04-E022). Rockville, MD: Agency for Healthcare Research and Quality.

Wallerstein, N. B., & Duran, B. (2006). Using community-based contributions to participatory research to address health disparities. *Health Promotion Practice*, 7(3), 312–323.

Wallerstein, N. B., & Duran, B. (2010). Community-based participatory research contributions to intervention research: The intersection of science and practice to improve health inequity. *American Journal of Public Health*, 100(Suppl. 1), S40–S46.

Wynn, T. A., Taylor-Jones, M. M., Johnson, R. E., Bostick, P. B., & Fouad, M. (2011). Using community-based participatory approaches to mobilize communities for policy change. *Family and Community Health*, 34(Suppl. 1), S102–S114.

CHAPTER THREE

SYSTEMATIC REVIEWS

SUSAN WEBER BUCHHOLZ, DENISE M. LINTON,
MAUREEN R. COURTNEY, AND MICHAEL E. SCHOENY

OBJECTIVES

After reading this chapter, readers will be able to:

1. Describe why it is important to use systematic reviews as a part of what informs evidence-based practice (EBP) health care
2. Illustrate the steps that are needed when conducting a systematic review
3. Differentiate between methods that are used to interpret systematic reviews
4. Propose a plan to critically appraise systematic reviews for use in clinical decision making

THE IMPORTANCE OF SYSTEMATIC REVIEWS

The exponential growth of published peer-reviewed research literature has resulted in the inability of clinicians to realistically review the literature in a timely manner. Using the broad search terms *nurse* and *hospital* in the title and/or abstract from the years 1950 to 1999 resulted in 4,402 publications in PubMed (U.S. National Library of Medicine [NLM], 2015). Using the same terms from the years 2000 to 2014 resulted in almost double that amount of publications. However, by adding the search term *systematic review* to the resulting set of 8,224 publications, the publication list was significantly reduced to 79 publications. Although this is still a substantial number of publications, it can become more manageable by adding additional search terms that are specific to the clinician's topic of interest. Clinicians strive to use evidence-based research to assist their efforts to balance quality and cost-effective care, which results in positive outcomes in their patients (Windle, 2010). EBP includes clinical expertise, incorporating patient values and preferences, and using the best research evidence available (Duke University Medical Center Library and the Health Sciences Library at the University of North Carolina at Chapel Hill, 2014; Sackett, Rosenberg, Gray, Haynes, & Richardson, 1996). Systematic reviews provide a powerful tool for clinicians to more easily access reliable literature for making evidence-based decisions (Eden, Levit, Berg, & Morton, 2011).

Research evidence comes from multiple sources, including publications that present and discuss the results of single quantitative or qualitative studies. The strength of the evidence increases, however, when multiple study publications with similar topic variables are synthesized within the context of a systematic review (Melnyk & Fineout-Overholt, 2011). The generic term *literature review* is occasionally used as an overarching term for different types of reviews, including systematic reviews. Specifically, a systematic review provides information regarding a specific research question being examined, how and which databases are used for publication retrieval, which search terms are used, how data are extracted, and how the data are synthesized (Centre for Reviews and Dissemination [CRD], University of York, 2009; Joanna Briggs Institute, 2014). Several systematic review resource website links can be found in Appendix 3.1.

Systematic Reviews in Context of Other Types of Literature Reviews

There are many different types of reviews in addition to systematic reviews that are used to inform health care decisions. These include scoping, umbrella, historical, narrative, economic, and integrative reviews (Conn & Coon Sells, 2014a; Joanna Briggs Institute, 2014). The differences between these literature reviews are depicted in Table 3.1 with examples given from various aspects of one area of research, in this case physical activity research. With all clinical areas, the focus of the review will determine the type of review that will be conducted. This chapter focuses specifically on the systematic review process.

Systematic review is the term given to a review that examines original research in the literature using rigorously defined methods, and it then synthesizes the findings so they can be used in health care decision making. In addition, transparency of the review process should be very obvious. Enough information should always be provided regarding how the systematic review was conducted so that the systematic review can be replicated with very similar results (CRD, University of York, 2009; Joanna Briggs Institute, 2014). Systematic reviews can be both quantitative and qualitative in nature (Higgins & Green, 2011; Joanna Briggs Institute, 2014).

The Importance of Using Both Quantitative and Qualitative Reviews

Although systematic reviews were originally used to provide a synthesis of quantitative research studies, the systematic review field has grown considerably to include qualitative systematic reviews (Cochrane Collaboration, 2014b). The combinations of quantitative and qualitative systematic reviews that are now available provide the clinician with a wide breadth of knowledge to use when addressing health care issues. Quantitative and qualitative studies can also be examined within the same systematic review.

For example, if clinicians seek to understand, assess, and provide recommendations for interventions regarding how caregiver burden is affecting a stroke survivor's family, they could read several systematic reviews. The following reviews provide insight into understanding, assessing, and providing recommendations for caregivers of stroke survivors and are derived from both the qualitative and quantitative research literature:

1. A meta-ethnographic qualitative systematic review by Greenwood and Mackenzie (2010) examines the experiences of caregivers of stroke survivors.

2. A quantitative systematic review by Whalen and Buchholz (2009) reviews caregiver screening tools, including those that have been used with family caregivers of stroke.
3. A quantitative systematic review and meta-analysis by Cheng, Chair, and Chau (2014) evaluates the effectiveness of interventions that can be used with family caregivers of stroke survivors.

In combination with their expert opinion, clinicians can use clinical guidelines, patient preferences and resources, and examination of systematic reviews to quickly appraise the literature to determine what represents the best practice in their setting.

TABLE 3.1 Types of Reviews With Examples From Physical Activity Research

Type of Review	Brief Definitions of Review	Examples of Different Types of Reviews Related to Physical Activity
Scoping review	Examines the number and type of previous studies available on a topic. This is often done before writing a systematic review in order to assess existing studies in the published literature.	Spencer, Rehman, and Kirk (2015)
Umbrella review	Provides a review of existing reviews, including systematic reviews that are already published.	Buchholz, Wilbur, Halloway, McDevitt, and Schoeny (2013)
Historical review	Examines literature in relationship to time, from a chronological perspective.	Berryman (2010)
Narrative review	Provides a descriptive review that often examines a subset of studies on a topic based on what is available or what the writer selects.	Kreichauf et al. (2012)
Economic review	Examines literature that reviews and analyzes costs related to a certain health care question.	Wolfenstetter and Wenig (2011)
Integrative review	Examines the literature on a topic by reviewing studies often conducted using different methodologies, and integrating the findings in a framework, so that a new perspective is developed.	Halloway, Buchholz, Wilbur, and Schoeny (2015)
Qualitative review	Examines qualitative studies, from one qualitative method or multiple methods, to synthesize findings	Stankov, Olds, and Cargo (2012)
Systematic review	Examines the literature rigorously, using a transparent protocol. This review can be replicated with very similar results. The review can include quantitative and/or qualitative papers. Different statistical techniques, including meta-analyses, are used to analyze quantitative systematic reviews. Typically, narrative and tabular formats are used to depict qualitative systematic results.	Buchholz, Wilbur, Ingram, and Fogg (2013); Conn, Hafdahl, and Mehr (2011); Martin, Saunders, Shenkin, and Sproule (2014)

Sources: Arksey and O'Malley (2005); Conn and Coon Sells (2014a, 2014b); Green, Johnson, and Adams (2006); Walker et al. (2012); Whittemore and Knafl (2005).

THREE IMPORTANT REASONS FOR SYSTEMATIC REVIEWS

Three reasons for the importance of systematic reviews are discussed. Systematic reviews are important because they provide:

1. A rigorous appraisal and synthesis of multiple original research studies
2. Evidence for informing clinical decision making
3. Guidance on the types of research that are needed

The systematic review process is a meticulous one that allows for transparency and replication. Given the large number of original research studies that often exist around health care issues and their related variables, systematic reviews provide a manageable method to foster clinician familiarity with health care literature. Literature volume is reduced due to the fact that systematic reviews appraise and synthesize information from multiple research documents into one (Stevens, 2014).

A health issue where a large volume of literature already exists, and where synthesis of research is useful to the clinician, is in regards to tobacco use. Despite the well-known fact that smoking is harmful to an individual's health, tobacco use continues worldwide. Vulnerable groups are at particular risk for tobacco use. Multiple studies have examined smoking barriers to smoking cessation, and how to impact these barriers. To examine the perceived barriers to smoking cessation in vulnerable groups, Twyman, Bonevski, Paul, and Bryant (2014) conducted a review of both the quantitative and qualitative literature. They initially identified 26,249 records in their database search, in addition to 27 records identified through other sources. After duplicates were excluded, they reviewed 21,767 titles or abstracts, from which they chose to retrieve 442 full text articles to assess for eligibility. With the full text review, 377 texts were excluded, which resulted in 65 studies that were included in their synthesis. Although it would be a near impossibility for busy clinicians to work through this amount of literature, this review team was able to synthesize this literature to provide recommendations for individual, community, and social network-level interventions for smoking cessation interventions in vulnerable groups. The clinician benefits from this synthesis by reading a scholarly article that provides part of the evidence that will inform practice. Appendix 3.2 provides a display of selected systematic reviews and guidelines that could be used to provide recommendations for lung cancer screening and smoking cessation.

Globally, clinicians are seeking to provide care that is no longer dictated by traditional practices, or following the path of least resistance, but is instead evidence based (Alliance for Health Policy and Systems Research, 2015; Cochrane Collaboration, 2015). Since an important component of EBP is strong research, systematic reviews have been and are being used to guide clinical decision making. Carefully conducted systematic reviews provide fundamental scientific information for making decisions on the development of these clinical practice guidelines. Given the findings of these systematic reviews in combination with select single research studies, expert opinion, decisions on whether to recommend certain practices, and the degree of certainty given to this recommendation are typically decided (U.S. Preventive Services Task Force, 2014). These guidelines are used by clinicians to make day-to-day decisions on how they provide care for patients. Examples of how systematic reviews have been used in the process of determining testing for and management of diabetes are seen in the work done by the American Diabetes Association (ADA, 2015) in updating their annual standards for providing medical care to diabetics, and by the World Health Organization (2011), which specifically reviewed the use of glycated hemoglobin (HbA1c) in diagnosing diabetes.

Systematic reviews not only influence clinical guidelines but also stand alone as a synthesis of the scientific literature. Guidelines that are influenced by systematic reviews can be used to influence decisions related to health policy by providing documentation of evidence-based approaches for use in clinical practice. Systematic reviews can provide the evidence for developing new policy, as well as for analyzing and further refining current policy (Petticrew & Roberts, 2006). Systematic reviews can also examine the results of health policy implications, as Galbraith-Emami and Lobstein (2013) did. They examined papers and websites from countries around the globe, to assess whether voluntary codes that were in place to limit advertising of certain high-fat and high-sugar food and beverage products to children were effective. They concluded that voluntary codes may be insufficient to reduce exposure of the children to the advertising of these unhealthy food products. This led the authors to provide recommendations that could be used by government agencies to reduce the exposure of children to unhealthy food and beverages.

In addition to demonstrating what is effective in providing health care, systematic reviews also provide evidence of what is ineffective. Systematic reviews can distinguish interventions that are ineffective, harmful, or wasteful (Stevens, 2014). In addition, systematic reviews reveal existing gaps within the literature. When reviewers ask questions about a very specific area of health care, for example, they may encounter a lack of studies that help to answer their question, therefore showing a gap in the literature. Similarly, although many studies may have been conducted in a particular area of health care, these studies may comprise mainly small sample sizes, which limit the generalizability of the outcomes. Studies may also demonstrate a large amount of heterogeneity, making it difficult to draw useful clinical inferences unless the reviewer has carefully taken that heterogeneity into account and adjusted for it statistically. Systematic reviews are, therefore, important in understanding not only what is effective and important for patient care but also what may not be as effective and useful, as well as in identifying the types of research that need to be done in the future.

CONDUCTING A SYSTEMATIC REVIEW

A systematic review, as already noted, follows carefully outlined steps. Thirteen steps involved in conducting a systematic review are presented in Table 3.2. The goal of all systematic reviews is to ultimately produce a summary of key research findings that will guide clinical practice and/or promote primary research. Depending on the nature of the systematic review, the systematic review team may include content experts, information specialists, and statisticians. Typically, two people are designated as the primary reviewers; however, other professionals may be needed. These include experts who can advise on the content that is being explored. It is also very helpful to invite information specialists who are experts at understanding how to search the literature. These information specialists are often the librarians who are located within an academic and/or medical health care setting.

Once a topic area has been identified, a specific clinical question needs to be developed. One method that can be used to guide the development of a quantitatively

TABLE 3.2 Steps in Conducting a Systematic Review
Step 1. Determination of a research question (clearly stated PICO)
Step 2. Protocol development (done a priori)

Step 3. Study retrieval plan (conduct mini-test)
  • Identify databases that will be searched
  • Identify key words that will be used in the search
  • Identify the criteria that will be used to decide whether a retrieved study will be included

Step 4. Literature retrieval
Step 5. Title review (blinded dual decision)
Step 6. Abstract review (blinded dual decision)
Step 7. Full-text review (blinded dual decision)
Step 8. Text mining from reference lists of retrieved papers and other systematic reviews
Step 9. Data extraction (author-developed or standardized tools used)   (include assessment of study variables as well as quality or rigor of each study)
Step 10. Data organization (using a database grid or another method of organization)

Step 11. Synthesizing the data
  • Quantitative data (analytic techniques, including meta-analysis)
  • Qualitative data (various synthesis techniques)

Step 12. Reporting the data and citing major conclusions of the review   (determine how to address heterogeneity)
Step 13. Interpretation of the findings (including limitations)

oriented clinical question is the PICO tool (Joanna Briggs Institute, 2014; Stillwell, Fineout-Overholt, Melnyk, & Williamson, 2010). This carefully developed question supports the structured approach required to investigate the literature. With quantitative research, the "P" represents the population; the "I" refers to the intervention; the "C" refers to the comparison intervention, which is often standard or routine care; and the "O" is the outcome. An example of a PICO question is: (P) In adult patients with type 2 diabetes mellitus (T2DM), (I) does self-monitoring of blood glucose (C) compared with no monitoring result in (O) lower A1C levels? In qualitative research, a PICo mnemonic can be used. Here also, the "P" represents the population, the "I" represents the phenomena of interest, and the "Co" represents the study context (Joanna Briggs Institute, 2014; Stillwell et al., 2010). An example of a PICo question that could be used in qualitative research is: (P) In adult patients with T2DM, (I) what are their experiences (Co) when initiating insulin therapy?

A systematic review is a form of secondary research that requires a clearly defined a priori protocol that is transparent and reproducible. The review protocol outlines the steps that will occur in the review. The review protocol includes the background, which provides the rationale for the review. The aims or objectives of the review are presented, along with the review question that is being answered. A detailed search strategy is provided on the database that will be used, the search terms that will be used and how they will be combined in the search strategy, and the inclusion and exclusion criteria of studies. A description of how studies will be critically appraised and how data will be extracted is given. Analytic techniques for the synthesis are also provided. Depending on whether the reviewers are working independently or in collaboration with a center that produces systematic reviews, the protocol will also be peer-reviewed and approved prior to starting the actual process of study retrieval in the systematic review.

After the question for the systematic review has been developed, the researcher needs to determine which databases will be used to conduct the search and in which order. The researcher may choose to start with the database that is expected to produce the greatest yield of publications initially. Additional databases need to be chosen that will provide new publication titles for review. However, duplicate titles are usually found across databases, as many journals are indexed in multiple databases. The number of databases chosen to retrieve publication titles is dependent on how extensive the reviewers desire the review to be, and/or whether they have the resources to manage an extensive review. In addition to traditional databases that house peer-reviewed journals, the Cochrane Collaboration database can be searched for systematic reviews. Other systematic review databases such as the Joanna Briggs Institute and CRD can also be searched. It can also be useful to search dissertation and theses databases as well. In addition, literature that contains unpublished studies called the *gray literature* should be examined, if a comprehensive search is to be undertaken. This includes searching Google Scholar, Conference Proceedings, and other sources of unpublished literature. An example of a search strategy can be found in a systematic review in a reference from the work of Whalen and Buchholz (2009).

Determining which key words to use, and in which combination, is typically accomplished by identifying appropriate key words that are used in several highly cited or otherwise important or useful publications on the topic. Once general key words have been identified, the reviewer should first assess whether there are MeSH terms published by the National Center for Biotechnology Information and U.S. NLM (2015a) that match either identically or closely to the identified meaning of the key words. MeSH terms are used to index articles in PubMed, and they come from a controlled vocabulary thesaurus. If there are no MeSH terms that can be used for each of the key words, then carefully chosen non-MeSH terms can be used. The reviewer should take great care in identifying search terms and involve an information specialist in this critical step. The Boolean operators are useful when conducting a database search to help narrow or broaden the search results. Boolean operators are AND, OR, and NOT (U.S. NLM, 2013b). Advanced searches can use Boolean logic, history, phrase searching, and truncation (U.S. NLM, 2013a). The reviewer can conduct a mini-test using these terms to determine whether the appropriate titles were retrieved. By testing one or two databases initially, putting in different word combinations, and finding out how key words are being used, the reviewer will have an opportunity to expand or narrow key word searches before embarking on the systematic review process (Holly, Salmond, & Saimbert, 2012). Again, an information specialist is essential to a quality search. An example of how the MeSH term *intensive care units* is displayed is provided in Figure 3.1.

Inclusion and exclusion criteria must be developed to guide the selection of studies for review and are dependent on the nature of the systematic review question. These criteria are decided prior to starting the search. Inclusion and exclusion criteria typically include patient characteristics, study design, topical area, and other

Intensive Care Units
Hospital units providing continuous surveillance and care to acutely ill patients
Year introduced: 1966 (1963)

PubMed search builder options
Subheadings:

☐ classification   ☐ legislation and jurisprudence   ☐ statistics and numerical data

☐ economics   ☐ manpower   ☐ supply and distribution

☐ ethics   ☐ methods   ☐ trends

☐ history   ☐ organization and administration   ☐ utilization

☐ instrumentation   ☐ standards

☐ Restrict to MeSH Major Topics

☐ Do not include MeSH terms found below this term in the MeSH hierarchy

Tree Number(s): N02.278.388.493
MeSH Unique ID: D007362
Entry Terms:

- Care unit, intensive
- Care units, intensive
- Intensive care unit
- Unit, intensive care
- Units, intensive care

All MeSH Categories
   Health Care Category
      Health Care Facilities, Manpower, and Services
         Health Facilities
           Hospital Units

              Intensive Care Units
                Burn Units
                Coronary Care Units
                Intensive Care Units, Pediatric
                  Intensive Care Units, and Neonatal
                Recovery Room
                Recovery Care Units

Figure 3.1 MeSH term: intensive care units.
Source: National Center for Biotechnology Information & U.S. NLM (2015b).

factors that are important to the research question. Exclusion criteria can include factors such as not reviewing publications that are printed in languages that the reviewers are not proficient in, certain populations based on gender or age, setting or health condition, certain study designs, and/or other factors.

A time frame needs to be determined for the literature period to be searched. If the subject area has not been researched earlier in the form of a systematic review, the reviewer must decide on the start date and justify the decision. For example, a review of the effectiveness of a procedure would need to include all studies after the date the procedure was implemented through an end date that is as current as possible. If a prior review using similar criteria is already published, the reviewer can begin from the end date of that prior review (Higgins & Green, 2011).

After study retrieval criteria have been identified and initially tested, the reviewer begins the process of the literature retrieval, searching the databases with the key words that were pre-identified. A record is maintained of the number of hits per database in relation to the specific keywords used. This record serves as documentation of the search pathway. After the database is searched, and the initial rounds of titles are yielded, two reviewers independently conduct a blinded review to determine whether the titles meet the inclusion or exclusion criteria of the study, maintaining a careful record of the process. Then, the reviewers discuss their decision regarding each title. If there is a difference of opinion, then both systematic reviewers determine together whether the title meets or does not meet the inclusion criteria. In the second step of this inclusion determination process, abstracts are pulled for the titles that are kept, and a similar process to title review occurs. After abstract review, full papers from all abstracts that are considered to have met inclusion criteria are pulled. The reviewers then work separately a third time, determining whether the full papers meet the inclusion criteria of the systematic review, following the same process as they did with the title. Finally, the reviewers conduct an abstract search. If the reviewers are unable to decide whether a study meets full inclusion criteria, a third reviewer can be asked to determine whether the publication will be included (Holly et al., 2012).

Reference lists of several different sources can also be searched to assess for any titles that may not have been present in the initial title review. Reviewers should search the publications that they decided to include in the review. In addition, searching similar systematic reviews is often a useful process to ensure that no titles are missed in the reviewer's topic area of study.

A summary of the literature search should be displayed as an algorithm to include the initial number of article titles found, the number remaining after title review, the number of abstracts reviewed and remaining, and the number of articles reviewed, resulting in the final number of articles to be used in the systematic review. This way, the reader sees the process documented for review and selection/exclusion. General reasons for abstract and article exclusions can be summarized in a box in the algorithm.

After the group of articles has been finalized for the review, the process of data extraction begins. Essential data are abstracted from each study. Commonly, reviewers use a table or matrix to organize the extracted data (Garrard, 2014). Column headings are decided by the reviewers; however, initial column headings often consist of paper identification information, including authors, year, title, and possibly country and journal origin. This allows for quick identification of publications in the organizational grid. The following columns include information about the study, including the research question or purpose of the study, design, sample, setting, measures, and what type of treatment the intervention and control groups received. Additional information is also included in the table depending on the needs of what the reviewers are trying to address with their research question.

Reviewers need to assess the quality of each paper that they are using in their systematic review. If the paper does not have sufficient quality, the reviewers may determine that the paper should not be used in their systematic review to avoid reaching faulty conclusions in their synthesis. Assessing for the risk of bias by using predefined criteria is important to reduce both the bias in the individual studies that contribute to the systematic review and the bias that can result from the studies selected for the systematic review (CRD, University of York, 2009; Stevens, 2014). Each aspect of individual studies needs to be initially assessed, including relevance of the population, the design chosen for the study, the intervention, the measures chosen to assess the outcome, and the fidelity of intervention implementation

(CRD, University of York, 2009; Eden et al., 2011). A funnel plot can be used to assess for publication bias (Stevens, 2014). A funnel plot is a scatter plot in which effect sizes of individual study results are presented on the X axis and study precision (generally sample size) on the Y axis. In the absence of bias, the resulting shape is a symmetrical inverted funnel shape with smaller studies showing greater variation in effect sizes and larger studies showing less variation. For qualitative systematic reviews, credibility can be determined as unequivocal, credible, or unsupported, allowing the reviewer to determine whether the study is rigorous enough to be synthesized within the context of a systematic review (Joanna Briggs Institute, 2014). Guidance on how to assess for methodological quality can be found in resources such as the 2014 Reviewer's Manual provided by the Joanna Briggs Institute.

To ensure consistency of data extraction, reviewers can use either an existing data extraction tool or a researcher-designed data tool that meets the specific needs of their study. Different methods can be used to extract data, including, but not limited to, paper and pencil, spreadsheet, or web-based software specifically designed for data extraction (Elamin et al., 2009; Penn Libraries, 2014). Three examples of web-based programs that will facilitate data extraction are RevMan from the Cochrane Collaboration (2014a), MASTARI data extraction tools with Joanna Briggs Institute (Joanna Briggs Institute, 2015), and the Systematic Review Data Repository (SRDR) with the Agency for Healthcare Research and Quality ([AHRQ], 2015).

The results of the study are synthesized using a number of different rigorous techniques, which are briefly discussed in this chapter. Generally, if it is a quantitative study, the results will be presented statistically, including using meta-analytic techniques. If a meta-analysis is not possible, then effect sizes may be presented. In addition, a narrative synthesis should be present, describing the results of the data extraction. Qualitative systematic reviews are conducted using different types of techniques.

In addition to reporting the data, whether the data is rooted in quantitative and/or qualitative origins, reviewers are responsible for carefully reporting the newly synthesized findings. Implications of the review findings for clinical use and to direct further research need to be clearly specified. Additionally, reviewers need to note how they managed heterogeneity if found within their review (Higgins & Thompson, 2002). As with any research, limitations of the study need to be addressed.

INTERPRETATION AND PRESENTATION OF SYSTEMATIC REVIEWS

The manner in which systematic reviews are interpreted and presented is dependent in part on the type of systematic review. Subsequently, the type of findings that resulted from the synthesis will drive the presentation of the results. In addition to a narrative presentation, data are often placed into a table, and a discussion is provided regarding similarities and differences, strengths and weaknesses, implications for health care, and other factors.

Description and Interpretation of Statistical Results Used in Quantitative Reviews

When conducting a systematic review of quantitative research studies, the process of summarizing results across the studies in the review presents unique challenges and opportunities. Because most clinicians are familiar with the design of the individual studies that are the building blocks of systematic reviews, it may be helpful to consider these studies as the unit of analysis for a systematic review in much the same way that researchers typically consider individual research subjects as the unit of analysis in an individual research study. In this sense, just as researchers select a sample of individual research subjects that represents a broader population of individuals, the goal of a systematic review is to collect a sample of studies that represents the population of all *possible* studies related to the phenomenon being reviewed. There is often inherent bias in what gets published. Researchers may be less likely to submit null or negative findings for publication; and, when submitted, journals may be less likely to publish null effects (Easterbrook, Berlin, Gopalan, & Matthews, 1991; McGauran et al., 2010). In the same way that a convenience sample or low participation rates may bias results in individual research studies, reliance on published findings may bias the results of systematic reviews toward stronger effects than actually found in the population. To help limit this bias, it is important to search for studies that may not have made it to press. Sources of such studies may be conference proceedings, online unpublished manuscripts, and reports to organizations that fund research.

Effect Size and Meta-Analysis

Once a sample has been determined, the next step is to gather the data. In quantitative reviews as in research studies, the goal is to ultimately collect the data in a way that allows the researcher to understand the patterns in the results. One of the benefits of conducting systematic reviews of quantitative studies is the ability to aggregate results across multiple studies into a small number of summary statistics (sometimes a single value) that represent the effect of interest across all studies included in the review. In individual research studies that analyze data from individual research subjects, all measures (i.e., for both independent/predictor variables and dependent/criterion variables) are almost always the same across all research subjects. Using the same measures across subjects makes it relatively straightforward to calculate measures of central tendency (e.g., mean), dispersion (e.g., standard deviation), and association (e.g., correlation coefficient, odds ratio, t test). Further, within intervention studies, the content of the treatment and the control interventions are generally consistent across all subjects such that the intervention received by Subject A is essentially the same intervention received by Subject B. In the case of systematic reviews, it becomes much more difficult to ensure that the same measures are used across all studies in a review or that the same interventions are used across all studies. Before aggregating data across studies, it is important to ensure that comparisons are "apples to apples" and not "apples to oranges." Although some degree of variation in measures and treatments is inevitable (and perhaps desirable), it is important to consider comparability of measures across studies. This issue can be particularly important when conducting a comparison across intervention studies. By having a clear definition for what is included in the target interventions (the "I" in PICO), one is ensuring that the range of interventions is included in the review.

In some instances, the same measures may be used across all studies included in a systematic review. For example, in a meta-analysis of the effects of empowerment-based self-management interventions for patients with chronic metabolic diseases,

Kuo, Lin, and Tsai (2014) examined effects on outcomes that used the same metrics across studies (HbA1C level, waist circumference, body weight, and body mass index [BMI]). Because all the studies included in the review used the same metrics, the results of the meta-analysis were presented in the original metrics. This has the advantage of presenting the results in a meaningful metric (e.g., change in body weight in kilograms) that can intuitively be understood by readers.

In most cases, when aggregating data across multiple studies, it is inevitable that there will be differences in the measures used for the outcome(s) of interest. For example, in studies of depression, some may use the Beck Depression Inventory (Beck, Steer, & Brown, 1996), whereas others may use the Center for Epidemiologic Studies Depression Scale (Radloff, 1977) or one of multiple other measures of depression. Because each of these scales uses a different metric, taking an average across the multiple studies would yield meaningless information. Instead, by converting results of all of the studies into a single common metric, one can directly compare the strength of effects across all studies in a review. An *effect size* is a measure of the strength of association between two variables (e.g., treatment condition and outcome, two correlates, change from pre- to post-test). Although effect sizes can be expressed in "raw" units of the measures (e.g., weight in kilograms), they are more often expressed in terms of standardized measures of effect. By converting results of the studies that are included in a systematic review into a single standardized effect size, one is able to make direct comparisons between studies and summarize across all studies in the review.

There are multiple types of standardized effect sizes depending on the nature of the independent/predictor variable and the dependent/outcome variable being described. Summarized in Table 3.3, the three most commonly used effect sizes are Cohen's d, the correlation coefficient (r), and the odds ratio. Cohen's d is a standardized mean difference between two groups and is used when comparing the means of two groups (e.g., treatment and control). Because the correlation coefficient is already a standardized measure of the relation between two continuous variables, it may be used to compare results of two studies without any alteration to the metric. Similarly, when comparing two groups based on a dichotomous outcome, the odds ratio can be directly used without further standardization.

Although journal editors are increasingly requesting that measures of effect size be included in published research papers, this is not uniformly the case (Wilkinson & APA Task Force on Statistical Inference, 1999). As a result, it is often necessary to calculate effect sizes based on the information available. For correlation coefficients, this is generally not necessary because the coefficient is already in standardized form and is almost always presented in papers that use correlations. For Cohen's d and odds ratio, some degree of calculation may be necessary. Lipsey and Wilson (2000) provide formulas for calculating effect sizes based on a variety of commonly presented data. Wilson (2013) has created an online calculator based on the formulas presented in the book. There are a number of other sources for managing data and calculating effect sizes for systematic reviews, including free software (e.g., Review Manager, Cochrane Collaboration, 2014c) and commercial software, such as Comprehensive Meta-Analysis (Borenstein, Hedges, Higgins, & Rothstein, 2007) or Mix 2.0 [Professional Version] (BiostatXL, 2011).

A single systematic review may include articles that rely on both binary and continuous variables, creating a situation in which multiple effect size measures may be the most appropriate to the articles being reviewed. Because d, r, and odds ratios

TABLE 3.3 Three Common Effect Sizes

Effect Size	Description	Formula	Interpretation
Cohen's d	The difference in means between two groups (e.g., treatment and control) expressed in standard deviation units. Ranges from $-\infty$ to ∞ though typically no larger than ± 2.	$d = \dfrac{M_1 - M_2}{s_{pooled}}$ $s_p^2 = \dfrac{(n_1 - 1)s_1^2 - (n_2 - 1)s_2^2}{n_1 - n_2 - 2}$	Small: 0.20 Medium: 0.50 Large: 0.80
Pearson's r	A standardized measure of association (covariance) between two variables. Ranges from -1 to 1.	$r = \dfrac{\Sigma(X - M_X)(Y - M_Y)}{\sqrt{\Sigma(X - M_X)^2}\sqrt{\Sigma(Y - M_Y)^2}}$	Small: 0.10 Medium: 0.30 Large: 0.50
Odds ratio (OR)	The ratio of the odds of an occurrence in one group to the odds of an occurrence in another group. Important to keep in mind that there is a reference group. If the odds ratio = 1, then there is no difference in odds between the comparison group and the reference group. Ranges from 0 to ∞ though more extreme than .01 to 100 is very rare.	$OR = \dfrac{\dfrac{p(X_{Group\,1})}{1 - p(X_{Group\,1})}}{\dfrac{p(X_{Group\,2})}{1 - p(X_{Group\,2})}}$	If OR >1 Small: 1.44 Medium: 2.47 Large: 4.25 If OR < 1 Small: 0.69 Medium: 0.40 Large: 0.24

are not comparable from one to another, it becomes necessary to convert these measures of effect size into a single, common measure. For example, if reviewing intervention effects on physical fitness, it is likely that most effect sizes will be ds, but odds ratios may be presented for a subset of studies with binary outcomes. Fortunately, along with formulas for calculating effect sizes from information available, there are formulas for converting between each of these three effect size measures.

In the case of quantitative analyses, once the results from a set of studies have been converted into one of the standard effect sizes, the next step is to explore patterns of results across the studies. Most often, this is accomplished using a meta-analysis. *Meta-analysis* broadly refers to a set of statistical methods for pooling the results (effect sizes) across multiple studies to identify (a) a mean standardized effect across all studies, and (b) factors that may relate to variation in effect sizes (e.g., interventions that include a group component have stronger effects than those without a group component). An example of a meta-analysis summarizing correlational data is an examination of the relation between psychosocial risk factors and musculoskeletal disorders in nurses and aides. Among the findings of this meta-analysis were that the incidence of low back pain was higher among those with high psychosocial demands but with low job control (OR = 1.52; 95% CI = 1.07–4.54). An example of a meta-analysis summarizing intervention effects is a review of nursing interventions for smoking cessation (Rice, Hartmann-Boyce, & Stead, 2013). Rice and colleagues completed a meta-analysis of 35 studies that included more than

17,000 participants. The results of the meta-analysis of 35 studies compared those in the control/usual care groups with those who received nursing interventions and found that those who received an intervention were significantly more likely to stop smoking (RR [respiration rate] = 1.29; 95% CI = 1.20–1.39).

Variation in effect size (heterogeneity) is an important consideration in a meta-analysis. Similar to an analysis of individual subjects, large variability in outcomes often creates concerns about the suitability of measures of central tendency (e.g., the mean) to serve as an appropriate summary of the data available. When there is a large amount of variation in a sample of individuals, the result is a large area of uncertainty (confidence interval) around the mean. Similarly, in the case of a meta-analysis, high heterogeneity of effect sizes should be evaluated and meta-analytic methods should be reconsidered if heterogeneity is excessive.

The mean effect size for a set of studies is calculated to represent the single best estimate of the individual-level effect size in a population. Because studies that are included in a meta-analysis generally have a range of different sample sizes, the calculation of the mean effect size is weighted by sample size in which larger studies are given more influence. In addition to the mean effect size, an associated standard error is calculated based on the variation in the effect sizes entered into the analysis. Using the mean effect size and the standard error, the analyst is then able to assign a probability to the likelihood that the mean effect size is equal to zero. As with other forms of inferential statistics, a low probability (generally less than .05) is interpreted to mean that the effect is significant.

In addition to the weighted mean effect size, which provides a single summary estimate of effect, meta-analyses often include forest plots to summarize the individual studies as well as the overall mean effect size. An example of a forest plot is presented in Figure 3.2.

In a forest plot, the effect size is represented on the horizontal axis with the point of null effect generally at the midpoint of the axis. The null effect will typically be either 0 (mean difference or correlation) or 1 (odds ratio or risk ratio). The individual

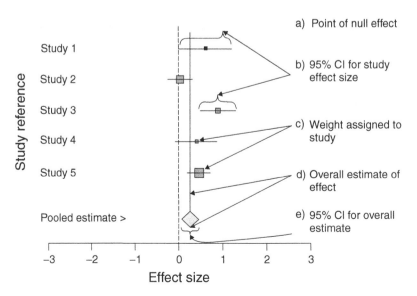

Figure 3.2 Sample forest plot.
CI, confidence interval.

studies are represented on the vertical axis and are generally labeled using the study citation (authors and year). Each study is marked with three pieces of information: (a) the effect size for the study (the vertical midpoint of the box for the study), (b) the weight assigned to the study (the size of the box), and (c) the 95% confidence interval for the effect size (the horizontal line passing through the box). Sometimes for small sample sizes, the effect size is presented as a small vertical line so that the midpoint is clear. In addition to data for each individual study, information about the pooled estimate for the effect size across all studies is represented by the diamond shape at the bottom of the forest plot. The vertical midpoint represents the mean effect size, and the width of the diamond represents the 95% confidence interval. A vertical line extends upward from the diamond at the mean effect size. This allows an easy comparison of the individual studies to the overall mean. For the individual studies as well as for the pooled estimates, lines/shapes that cross the point of null effect indicate nonsignificant findings at the level of alpha selected for the meta-analysis (5% in sample forest plot). Often, forest plots also contain information about the significance testing for the pooled estimate as well as about other statistical copies that are relevant to the meta-analysis being presented.

When statistical analysis is not possible, most likely due to large heterogeneity, and therefore the inability to measure similar variables is present, then results can be presented in a tabular and/or narrative format. In a tabular format, column headings depict information about each individual study, including design, setting, sample, and measure information. In the narrative format, the reviewer can give a summary of the findings, assessing for similarities and differences among the study variables.

Description and Interpretation of Results Used in Qualitative Reviews

Qualitative systematic reviews are an important part of systematic review science. They offer insight into aspects of patient care that quantitative systematic reviews, alone, are not able to explore. Qualitative systematic reviews allow for examination of the experiences that people have in health care (Joanna Briggs Institute, 2014). Qualitative methodologies seek to understand people typically within in their natural setting, exploring the phenomena that shape their health and the health care that they seek out and receive (Eden et al., 2011; Joanna Briggs Institute, 2014). There are many qualitative methodologies, including phenomenology, ethnography, grounded theory, action research, feminist research, and discourse analysis (Joanna Briggs Institute, 2014). These methodologies can use a number of different data collection methods, including, but not limited to, observation, interviews, focus groups, textual analysis, and reflective journals (Joanna Briggs Institute, 2014).

There are multiple approaches to conducting a qualitative systematic review. Debate continues about how and when to combine various qualitative studies for a systematic review, and if, indeed, it is appropriate to do so at all, since findings are not meant to be generalizable (CRD, University of York, 2009). Also, qualitative methodologies are derived from different theoretical underpinnings (CRD, University of York, 2009). Regardless of this, the qualitative systematic review process takes place and uses a variety of different approaches in the review process. A qualitative systematic review may only use studies from one particular methodology, for example, ethnography, but it is quite common for researchers to review studies that use different qualitative methodologies as they seek to answer a research question. In addition, researchers are now combining qualitative and quantitative research studies in the same review to answer complex research questions that are best studied by exploring a large spectrum of research studies available on the specific topic (Sandelowski, Barroso, & Voils, 2007).

Different methods for synthesizing qualitative studies include, but are not limited to, qualitative meta-synthesis, qualitative meta-summary, narrative synthesis, meta-ethnography, thematic analysis, content analysis, and critical interpretive synthesis (Barnett-Page & Thomas, 2009; CRD, University of York, 2009; Joanna Briggs Institute, 2014; Noyes & Lewin, 2011; Sandelowski et al., 2007). Regardless of the type of method that is used, qualitative systematic reviews follow the same rigor that quantitative systematic reviews do, preferably using a review protocol process as well. The qualitative review type and process is determined by the research question and methodologies of the studies that are being reviewed. Generally, data are reviewed and coded for key concepts and differences, or recurrent themes. Actual case descriptions, statements, or participant data are extracted and used to support the key concepts or themes. In the final step of the process, findings are subjected to meta-aggregation or a similar process to create a through set of synthesized findings. These findings generally provide a new representation in understanding the research question posed at the beginning of the systematic review process.

APPRAISAL OF SYSTEMATIC REVIEWS

When critically appraising a systematic review to be used for clinical decision making, essentially the clinician is seeking to determine whether a clearly focused question was addressed, if valid methods were used in the review, what are the results of the review, and, finally, whether the results are useful for clinical decision making. There are many tools that already exist and are available for clinicians to use when appraising systematic reviews. For example, these tools include a "Systematic Review Appraisal Sheet" from the Centre for Evidence-Based Medicine (2005), which asks five questions to determine whether the results of the review are valid and one question that examines how the results are presented. The Critical Appraisal Skills Programme (2013) has a "10 questions to help you make sense of a review" sheet. Eleven questions are used to assess the methodological quality of systematic

---

TABLE 3.4 Critical Appraisal Questions

1. Is there a clear question that guided the systematic review?
2. Is an a priori study protocol used?
3. What are the inclusion and exclusion criteria in the systematic review?
4. Is the literature search comprehensive and described in detail?
5. Are there at least two reviewers working independently to determine study inclusion and data extraction?
6. Is the scientific quality of individual studies assessed using specific criteria?
7. Are the statistical methods used appropriate and precise?
8. Is heterogeneity between studies assessed?
9. Is the synthesis of the studies appropriately conducted?
10. Are limitations of the review provided?
11. Are the results presented clearly?
12. Are the results of the study applicable to guide clinical decisions?

reviews with the AMSTAR tool. Ressing, Blettner, and Klug (2009) provide a seven-step checklist to analyze systematic reviews. An eight-step table titled "Critical Appraisal of a Systematic Review" is available in a Joanna Briggs Institute "Appraising Systematic Reviews" information sheet. These tools, as well as others, provide different approaches to critical appraisal, using very specific to broad questions. However, a critical appraisal of a systematic review for clinical decision making is generally guided by asking the 12 questions found in Table 3.4. Knowing which questions to ask to appraise systematic reviews gives clinicians the ability to make a scientifically sound decision to either use or not use the systematic review results when they are making clinical decisions.

SUMMARY

In summary, carefully conducted systematic reviews provide essential knowledge for clinical practice in a way not previously available. A systematic, rigorous process used by researchers to locate, appraise, and synthesize data to answer a clinical question is critical. The systematic review embodies this process and can make a high-level contribution to the evidence used in practice. In fact, the systematic review and the meta-analysis provide the highest levels of evidence available (Mantzoukas, 2008). All clinicians must understand what a systematic review is, the basics of how it is conducted, and its power to inform practice. They must actively search the literature to find systematic reviews that can have a bearing on their clinical interventions. Many readers of this chapter will hopefully not only fully embrace the use of systematic reviews in practice but also join or lead teams to design and conduct systematic reviews.

REFERENCES

Agency for Healthcare Research and Quality. (2015). *SDR systematic review data repository.* Retrieved from http://srdr.ahrq.gov

Alliance for Health Policy and Systems Research. (2015). *Centres for systematic reviews of health policy and systems research in low- and middle-income countries.* Retrieved from http://www.who.int/alliance-hpsr/projects/unicatolica_srccrosscutting/en/

American Diabetes Association. (2015). *Standards of medical care in diabetes—2015.* Retrieved from http://professional.diabetes.org/admin/UserFiles/0%20-%20Sean/Documents/January%20 Supplement%20Combined_Final.pdf

Arksey, H., & O'Malley, L. (2005). Scoping studies: Towards a methodological framework. *International Journal of Social Research Methodology, 8,* 19–32.

Barnett-Page, E., & Thomas, J. (2009). Methods for the synthesis of qualitative research: A critical review. *BMC Medical Research Methodology, 9,* 59. doi:10.1186/1471-2288-9-59

Beck, A. T., Steer, R. A., & Brown, G. K. (1996). *Manual for the Beck Depression Inventory-II.* San Antonio, TX: Psychological Corporation.

Berryman, J. W. (2010). Exercise is medicine: A historical perspective. *Current Sports Medicine Reports, 9*(4), 195–201.

BiostatXL. (2011). *Professional software for meta-analysis in Excel. Version 2.0.1.4.* Retrieved from http://www.meta-analysis-made-easy.com

Borenstein, M., Hedges, L., Higgins, J., & Rothstein, H. (2007). *Comprehensive meta-analysis: A computer program for meta-analysis [computer software]*. Englewood, NJ: Biostat.

Buchholz, S. W., Wilbur, J., Halloway, S., McDevitt, J. H., & Schoeny, M. E. (2013). Physical activity intervention studies and their relationship to body composition in healthy women. *Annual Review of Nursing Research, 31*, 71–142.

Buchholz, S. W., Wilbur, J., Ingram, D., & Fogg, L. (2013). Physical activity text messaging interventions in adults: A systematic review. *Worldviews on Evidence-based Nursing, 10*(3), 163–173.

Centre for Evidence-Based Medicine. (2005). *Systematic review critical appraisal sheet*. Retrieved from http://www.cebm.net/critical-appraisal

Centre for Reviews and Dissemination, University of York. (2009). *Systematic reviews: CRD's guidance for undertaking reviews in health care*. Retrieved from http://www.york.ac.uk/inst/crd/pdf/Systematic_Reviews.pdf

Cheng, H. Y., Chair, S. Y., & Chau, J. P. (2014). The effectiveness of psychosocial interventions for stroke family caregivers and stroke survivors: A systematic review and meta-analysis. *Patient Education and Counseling, 95*(1), 30–44. doi:10.1016/j.pec.2014.01.005

Cochrane Collaboration. (2014a). *Cochrane informatics & knowledge management department: RevMan*. Retrieved from http://tech.cochrane.org/revman

Cochrane Collaboration. (2014b). *Cochrane qualitative and implementation methods group*. Retrieved from http://cqim.cochrane.org

Cochrane Collaboration. (2014c). *Review manager (RevMan) [computer program]. Version 5.3*. Copenhagen: Nordic Cochrane Centre.

Cochrane Collaboration. (2015). *About us*. Retrieved from http://www.cochrane.org/about-us

Conn, V. S., & Coon Sells, T. G. (2014a). Is it time to write a review article? *Western Journal of Nursing Research, 36*(4), 435–439. doi:10.1177/0193945913519060

Conn, V. S., & Coon Sells, T. G. (2014b). WJNR welcomes umbrella reviews. *Western Journal of Nursing Research, 36*(2), 147–151. doi:10.1177/0193945913506968

Conn, V. S., Hafdahl, A. R., & Mehr, D. R. (2011). Interventions to increase physical activity among healthy adults: Meta-analysis of outcomes. *American Journal of Public Health, 101*(4), 751–758.

Critical Appraisal Skills Programme. (2013). *CASP systematic review checklist*. Retrieved from http://media.wix.com/ugd/dded87_a02ff2e3445f4952992d5a96ca562576.pdf

Duke University Medical Center Library and the Health Sciences Library at the University of North Carolina at Chapel Hill. (2014). *What is evidence based practice?* Retrieved from http://guides.mclibrary.duke.edu/c.php?g=158201&p=1036021

Easterbrook, P. J., Berlin, J. A., Gopalan, R., & Matthews, D. R. (1991). Publication bias in clinical research. *Lancet, 337*(8746), 867–872. doi:0140-6736(91)90201-Y

Eden, J., Levit, L., Berg, A., & Morton, S. (Eds.). (2011). *Committee on Standards for Systematic Reviews of Comparative Effectiveness Research & Institute of Medicine. Finding what works in health care: Standards for systematic review*. Washington, DC: National Academies Press.

Elamin, M. B., Flynn, D. N., Bassler, D., Briel, M., Alonso-Coello, P., Karanicolas, P. J., . . . Montori, V. M. (2009). Choice of data extraction tools for systematic reviews depends on resources and review complexity. *Journal of Clinical Epidemiology, 62*(5), 506–510. doi:10.1016/j.jclinepi.2008.10.016

Galbraith-Emami, S., & Lobstein, T. (2013). The impact of initiatives to limit the advertising of food and beverage products to children: A systematic review. *Obesity Reviews, 14*(12), 960–974. doi:10.1111/obr.12060

Garrard, J. (2014). *Health sciences literature review made easy: The matrix method* (4th ed.). Burlington, MA: Jones & Bartlett Learning.

Green, B. N., Johnson, C. D., & Adams, A. (2006). Writing narrative literature reviews for peer-reviewed journals: Secrets of the trade. *Journal of Chiropractic Medicine, 5*(3), 101–117. doi:10.1016/S0899-3467(07)60142-6

Greenwood, N., & Mackenzie, A. (2010). Informal caring for stroke survivors: Meta-ethnographic review of qualitative literature. *Maturitas, 66*(3), 268–276. doi:10.1016/j.maturitas.2010.03.017

Halloway, S., Buchholz, S. W., Wilbur, J., & Schoeny, M. E. (2015). Prehabilitation interventions for older adults: An integrative review. *Western Journal of Nursing Research, 37*(1), 103–123.

Higgins, J. P., & Thompson, S. G. (2002). Quantifying heterogeneity in a meta-analysis. *Statistics in Medicine, 21*(11), 1539–1558. doi:10.1002/sim.1186

Higgins, J. P. T., & Green, S. (2011). *Cochrane handbook for systematic review of interventions version 5.1.0*. Retrieved from http://handbook.cochrane.org

Holly, C., Salmond, S. W., & Saimbert, M. K. (2012). *Comprehensive systematic review for advanced practice*. New York, NY: Springer Publishing.

Joanna Briggs Institute. (2014). *Joanna Briggs reviewers' manual 2014 edition*. Retrieved from http://joannabriggs.org/assets/docs/sumari/ReviewersManual-2014.pdf

Joanna Briggs Institute. (2015). *Home page*. Retrieved from http://joannabriggs.org

Kreichauf, S., Wildgruber, A., Krombholz, H., Gibson, E. L., Vögele, C., Nixon, C. A., . . . Summerbell, C. D.; ToyBox-study group. (2012). Critical narrative review to identify educational strategies promoting physical activity in preschool. *Obesity Reviews, 13*(Suppl. 1), 96–105.

Kuo, C. C., Lin, C. C., & Tsai, F. M. (2014). Effectiveness of empowerment-based self-management interventions on patients with chronic metabolic diseases: A systematic review and meta-analysis. *Worldviews on Evidence-Based Nursing, 11*(5), 301–315. doi:10.1111/wvn.12066

Lipsey, M. W., & Wilson, D. (2000). *Practical meta-analysis (applied social research methods)*. Thousand Oaks, CA: SAGE Publications.

Mantzoukas, S. (2008). A review of evidence-based practice, nursing research and reflection: Levelling the hierarchy. *Journal of Clinical Nursing, 17*(2), 214–223. doi:JCN1912

Martin, A., Saunders, D. H., Shenkin, S. D., & Sproule, J. (2014). Lifestyle intervention for improving school achievement in overweight or obese children and adolescents. *Cochrane Database of Systematic Reviews, 3*, CD009728.

McGauran, N., Wieseler, B., Kreis, J., Schuler, Y. B., Kolsch, H., & Kaiser, T. (2010). Reporting bias in medical research—a narrative review. *Trials, 11*, 37. doi:10.1186/1745-6215-11-37

Melnyk, B. M., & Fineout-Overholt, E. (2011). *Evidence-based practice in nursing and healthcare: A guide to best practice* (2nd ed.). Philadelphia, PA: Wolters Kluwer Health/Lippincott, Williams & Wilkins.

National Center for Biotechnology Information & U.S. National Library of Medicine (NLM). (2015a). *Home—MeSH—NCBI*. Retrieved from http://www.ncbi.nlm.nih.gov/mesh

National Center for Biotechnology Information & U.S. National Library of Medicine (NLM). (2015b). *MeSH "intensive care units"*. Retrieved from http://www.ncbi.nlm.nih.gov/mesh/?term=intensive+care+unit

Noyes, J., & Lewin, S. (2011). Extracting qualitative evidence. In J. Noyes, A. Booth, K. Hannes, A. Harden, J. Harris, S. Lewin, & C. Lockwood (Eds.), *Supplementary guidance for inclusion of qualitative research in Cochrane systematic reviews of interventions. Version 1* (chapter 5). London, UK: Cochrane Collaboration Qualitative Methods Group. Retrieved from http://cqim.cochrane.org/supplemental-handbook-guidance

Penn Libraries. (2014). *Systematic reviews—tools for managing data*. Retrieved from http://guides.library.upenn.edu/content.php?pid=481656&sid=4177706

Petticrew, M., & Roberts, H. (2006). *Systematic reviews in the social sciences: A practical guide*. Malden, MA: Blackwell Publishing.

Radloff, L. S. (1977). The CES-D scale: A self-report depression scale for research in the general population. *Applied Psychological Measurement, 1*(3), 385–401.

Ressing, M., Blettner, M., & Klug, S. (2009). Systematic literature reviews and meta-analyses: Part 6 of a series on evaluation of scientific publications. *Deutsches Ärzteblatt International, 106*(27), 456–463. doi:10.3238/arztebl.2009.0456

Rice, V. H., Hartmann-Boyce, J., & Stead, L. F. (2013). Nursing interventions for smoking cessation. *Cochrane Database of Systematic Reviews, 8*, CD001188. doi:10.1002/14651858

Sackett, D. L., Rosenberg, W. M., Gray, J. A., Haynes, R. B., & Richardson, W. S. (1996). Evidence based medicine: What it is and what it isn't. *British Medical Journal (Clinical Research Ed.), 312*(7023), 71–72.

Sandelowski, M., Barroso, J., & Voils, C. (2007). Using qualitative metasummary to synthesize qualitative and quantitative descriptive findings. *Research in Nursing Health, 30*(1), 99–111. doi:10.1002/nur.20176

Spencer, R. A., Rehman, L., & Kirk, S. (2015). Understanding gender norms, nutrition, and physical activity in adolescent girls: A scoping review. *International Journal of Behavioral Nutrition and Physical Activity, 12*(1), 6. doi:10.1186/s12966-015-0166-8

Stankov, I., Olds, T., & Cargo, M. (2012). Overweight and obese adolescents: What turns them off physical activity? *International Journal of Behavioral Nutrition and Physical Activity, 9*, 53.

Stevens, K. R. (2014). Systematic reviews. In M. A. Mateo & M. D. Foreman (Ed.), *Research for advanced practice nurses: From evidence to practice* (2nd ed., pp. 267–282). New York, NY: Springer Publishing Company.

Stillwell, S. B., Fineout-Overholt, E., Melnyk, B. M., & Williamson, K. M. (2010). Evidence-based practice, step by step: Asking the clinical question: A key step in evidence-based practice. *American Journal of Nursing, 110*(3), 58–61. doi:10.1097/01.NAJ.0000368959.11129.79

Twyman, L., Bonevski, B., Paul, C., & Bryant, J. (2014). Perceived barriers to smoking cessation in selected vulnerable groups: A systematic review of the qualitative and quantitative literature. *BMJ Open, 4*(12), e006414. doi:10.1136/bmjopen-2014-006414

U.S. National Library of Medicine (NLM). (2013a). *Building blocks.* Retrieved from http://www.nlm.nih.gov/bsd/disted/pubmedtutorial/020_340.html

U.S. National Library of Medicine (NLM). (2013b). *Introduction to Boolean logic.* Retrieved from http://www.nlm.nih.gov/bsd/disted/pubmedtutorial/020_350.html

U.S. National Library of Medicine (NLM). (2015). *PubMed.* Retrieved from http://www.ncbi.nlm.nih.gov/pubmed

U.S. Preventive Services Task Force. (2014). *The guide to clinical preventative services 2014.* Retrieved from http://www.uspreventiveservicestaskforce.org/Page/Name/tools-and-resources-for-better-preventive-care

Walker, D. G., Wilson, R. F., Sharma, R., Bridges, J., Niessen, L., Bass, E. B., & Frick, K. (2012). *Best practices for conducting economic evaluations in health care: A systematic review of quality assessment tools.* Retrieved from http://www.ncbi.nlm.nih.gov/books/NBK114545/pdf/TOC.pdf

Whalen, K. J., & Buchholz, S. W. (2009). *The reliability, validity and feasibility of tools used to screen for caregiver burden: A systematic review.* Retrieved from http://works.bepress.com/cgi/viewcontent.cgi?article=1011&context=kimberly_whalen

Whittemore, R., & Knafl, K. (2005). The integrative review: Updated methodology. *Journal of Advanced Nursing, 52*(5), 546–553. doi:JAN3621

Wilkinson, L., & APA Task Force on Statistical Inference. (1999). Statistical methods in psychology journals: Guidelines and explanations. *American Psychologist, 54*(8), 594.

Wilson, D. B. (2013). *Practical meta-analysis effect size calculator.* Retrieved from http://cebcp.org/practical-meta-analysis-effect-size-calculator

Windle, P. E. (2010). The systematic review process: An overview. *Journal of Perianesthesia Nursing*, 25(1), 40–42. doi:10.1016/j.jopan.2009.12.001

Wolfenstetter, S. B., & Wenig, C. M. (2011). Costing of physical activity programmes in primary prevention: A review of the literature. *Health Economics Review*, 1(1), 17.

World Health Organization. (2011). *Use of glycated haemoglobin (HbA1c) in the diagnosis of diabetes mellitus*. Retrieved from http://www.who.int/diabetes/publications/report-hba1c_2011.pdf?ua=1

APPENDIX 3.1 SYSTEMATIC REVIEW RESOURCES

Name of Resource Internet Address of Resource Description of Resource
• Center for Evidence-Based Medicine Resources • www.cebm.net/category/ebm-resources • Provides resources that are useful when conducting systematic reviews
• Centers for Systematic Reviews of Health Policy and Systems Research in Low- and Middle-Income Countries • http://who.int/alliance-hpsr/projects/unicatolica_srccrosscutting/en • Provides resources for conducting systematic reviews in low- and middle-income countries
• Cochrane Handbook for Systematic Reviews of Interventions Version 5.1.0 • www.cochrane.org • Provides resources for clinicians who are reviewing and preparing to conduct Cochrane Intervention reviews
• Finding What Works in Health Care (Institute of Medicine [IOM]) • www.iom.edu/Reports/2011/Finding-What-Works-in-Health-Care-Standards-for-Systematic-Reviews.aspx • Provides recommendations for standards for scientifically valid systematic reviews
• Joanna Briggs Institute • http://joannabriggs.org • Provides resources for clinicians who are reviewing and preparing to conduct various types of systematic reviews
• The Campbell Collaboration • www.campbellcollaboration.org • Provides resources for clinicians who are reviewing, preparing for, and disseminating systematic reviews
• The Evidence for Policy and Practice Information and Coordinating Center (EPPI-Center) • http://eppi.ioe.ac.uk/cms • Provides resources on developing methods for systematic reviews and research syntheses
• University of York Center for Reviews and Dissemination • www.crd.york.ac.uk/prospero • Provides resources for reviewing, preparing for, and writing systematic reviews

APPENDIX 3.2 EXAMPLES OF SYSTEMATIC REVIEW ABSTRACTS FROM THE PUBLISHED LITERATURE

Because of the high prevalence of tobacco use worldwide, as well as associated pulmonary diseases like lung cancer, knowing when and how to screen for lung cancer continue to be important questions for clinicians. Here are links to abstracts of two systematic reviews. A link to a third abstract is provided, which is referenced earlier in the chapter, and it reviews nursing interventions for smoking cessation. Last of all, there is a link to guidance on lung cancer screening.

A. SCREENING FOR LUNG CANCER

By Renée Manser, Anne Lethaby, Louis B. Irving, Christine Stone, Graham Byrnes, Michael J. Abramson, and Don Campbell

Cochrane Database of Systematic Reviews, Issue 6

http://onlinelibrary.wiley.com/doi/10.1002/14651858.CD001991.pub3/abstract

Authors' Conclusions

The current evidence does not support screening for lung cancer with chest radiography or sputum cytology. Annual low-dose CT screening is associated with a reduction in lung cancer mortality in high-risk smokers but further data are required on the cost effectiveness of screening and the relative harms and benefits of screening across a range of different risk groups and settings.

B. SCREENING FOR LUNG CANCER: SYSTEMATIC REVIEW TO UPDATE THE U.S. PREVENTIVE SERVICES TASK FORCE RECOMMENDATION

Evidence Syntheses, No. 105

Investigators: Linda Humphrey, MD, MPH, Mark Deffebach, MD, Miranda Pappas, MA, Christina Baumann, MD, MPH, Katie Artis, MD, MPH, Jennifer Priest Mitchell, BA, Bernadette Zakher, MBBS, Rongwei Fu, PhD, and Christopher Slatore, MD, MS.

Pacific Northwest Evidence-Based Practice Center
Rockville (MD): AHRQ (U.S.); July 2013

Report No.: 13-05188-EF-1

www.ncbi.nlm.nih.gov/pubmedhealth/PMH0060145/pdf/TOC.pdf

Authors' Conclusions

Good evidence shows low dose computed tomography can significantly reduce mortality from lung cancer. However, there are significant harms associated with screening that must be balanced with the benefits. More efforts to reduce false-positive examinations are of paramount importance and smoking cessation remains the most important approach to reducing lung cancer mortality.

C. NURSING INTERVENTIONS FOR SMOKING CESSATION

By Virginia Hill Rice, Jamie Hartmann-Boyce, and Lindsay F. Stead
Editorial Group: Cochrane Tobacco Addiction Group
Assessed as up to date: June 27, 2013

http://onlinelibrary.wiley.com/doi/10.1002/14651858.CD001188.pub4/abstract

Authors' Conclusions

The results indicate the potential benefits of smoking cessation advice and/or counselling given by nurses, with reasonable evidence that intervention is effective. The evidence for an effect is weaker when interventions are brief and are provided by nurses whose main role is not health promotion or smoking cessation. The challenge will be to incorporate smoking behaviour monitoring and smoking cessation interventions as part of standard practice so that all patients are given an opportunity to be asked about their tobacco use and to be given advice and/or counselling to quit along with reinforcement and follow-up.

D. AMERICAN CANCER SOCIETY—LUNG CANCER PREVENTION AND EARLY DETECTION

By the American Cancer Society.

http://www.cancer.org/cancer/lungcancer-non-smallcell/moreinformation/lung cancerpreventionandearlydetection/lung-cancer-prevention-and-early-detection-guidelines

Authors' Conclusions

The American Cancer Society has thoroughly reviewed the subject of lung cancer screening and issued guidelines.

CHAPTER FOUR

QUALITY IMPROVEMENT RESEARCH

CATHERINE JOHNSON, MARY ELLEN SMITH GLASGOW,
AND MARY ELIZABETH "BETSY" GUIMOND

OBJECTIVES

After reading this chapter, readers will be able to:

1. Describe the national initiatives supporting expanded quality improvement research
2. Discuss foundational concepts of quality improvement research
3. Identify sources of clinical performance standards and their influence on quality improvement in health care
4. Describe the formative quality improvement research methods plan, do, study, act (PDSA) and the Toyota Production System (TPS)
5. Describe summative quality improvement research methods—epidemiological approach
6. Discuss approaches to program evaluation, including formative and summative research approaches
7. Discuss a framework for increasing collaboration between PhD researchers and Doctor of Nursing Practice (DNP) scholars to achieve health care system and patient outcome improvements

THE IMPORTANCE OF QUALITY IMPROVEMENT

"Measurement and accountability for quality and cost are the foundations for health care improvement. Implementation and system redesign are essential for changing the health care system and changing health care outcomes" (Dougherty & Conway, 2008, p. 2319). Federal agencies and health care organizations have been increasing and broadening their efforts to build a stronger internal capacity to evaluate their health care programs. Since early in the 20th century, reliable quality improvement methods and consistent quality outcomes have emerged as one of the most important, yet illusive, elements of successful organizations. Health care quality improvement approaches were slow to emerge as a priority for individual providers or organizations, and most often they moved forward in response to federal mandates.

In this chapter we provide a foundation for understanding the current federal mandate and the ways that it has developed to support the importance of quality improvement policy and procedures in our health care system. Quality improvement approaches have long been used in the business world prior to their import to health care. Included here are descriptions of the PDSA and TPS experiences in developing their quality improvement approaches. Next, we describe the application of quality improvement research approaches currently available for use in the health care system. The nursing profession has an opportunity to make significant contributions to quality improvement in the health care system. We have available skilled PhD researchers and DNP leaders who, as a collaborative team, can apply their expertise to the design and implementation of quality improvement approaches.

National Mandate for Quality Health Care

Nearly two decades ago, the Institute of Medicine's (IOM's) publication *To Err Is Human* (Institute of Medicine [IOM], 1999) incited both public and regulatory agencies' demand for change in the U.S. health care system to address the safety concerns pointed out in the report. The IOM followed this report with *Crossing the Quality Chasm: A New Health System for the 21st Century* (2001) and *Health Professions Education: A Bridge to Quality* (2003), with both reports making recommendations for sweeping reform in the structure and process of health care provisions in the United States. These reports identified significant gaps between health care research and practice; these gaps supported their recommendations to redesign the educational processes for all clinical practitioners to improve quality and safety. In addition, they recommended development of health care leaders who could create and implement effective and safe clinical systems committed to safety and reliability. This demand for reform based on increasing quality health care outcomes focused the redesign effort on the development and use of evidence gathered through health care research and expanded quality improvement measures. Since that time, external regulatory standards for patient and system outcomes have been expanded and implemented within all patient care settings. However, health care system performance continues to fall below acceptable outcomes standards when compared with other industrialized nations, despite significant efforts and financial support put forth by the U.S. Department of Health and Human Services (HHS, 2010; IOM, 2001).

In 2010, enactment of the Patient Protection and Affordable Care Act (PPACA) brought about a significant focus on the expansion of health care quality improvement methods through the infusion of billions of dollars intended to stimulate health care financing and service delivery innovation (HHS, 2010). This legislation also established the National Quality Strategy (NQS), which provided leadership guidance for this development (HHS, 2011). This guidance focused on three aims and six strategies that were designed to stimulate health care innovation and associated quality research and program evaluation. In 2012, HHS submitted a progress report to Congress regarding its agencies' response to these strategies. This report described several innovative approaches designed to address the triple aims of: (a) better patient care; (b) better health outcomes; and (c) lower health care cost (HHS, 2012). Through this national consensus building process, effective quality measurement approaches continue to be built to achieve these ubiquitous health care reform aims.

This national framework of triple aims as applied to quality measurement and analysis has provided a common language for researchers, educators, and administrators. They could now engage in the development of new and innovative approaches to health care delivery and measurement with the hope that at last quality improvement research and programs would finally gain the respect and support they have long needed. As an outcome of the NQS, clinical performance standards for specific patient populations were needed that: (a) prioritized areas for program development, alignment training, and role development across disciplines; and (b) identified focus areas for quality improvement research and evaluation (HHS, 2012). National Quality Forum (NQF, 2014), a not-for-profit, nonpartisan, membership-based organization, has emerged as a reliable source of evidence-based clinical performance standards developed through a rigorous consensus development process. This formal consensus development process is used to evaluate and endorse consensus standards, including performance measures, best practices, frameworks, and reporting guidelines. This organization's process now serves as a model for standards development and quality improvement practices nationally.

The Centers for Medicare and Medicaid Innovation (CMMI) was established to provide incentives to administrators, providers, and quality improvement researchers to work together to develop innovative approaches to health care that would improve health care outcomes and at a lower overall cost. Central to the development of these proposals was the need to develop measurement approaches for patient outcomes, the health care process, and cost of care. The Agency for Healthcare Research and Quality (AHRQ) *Working for Quality* program has supported this development through funding for development of: (a) quality improvement processes and outcomes measures; and (b) tools (AHRQ, 2014b). Furthermore, AHRQ has also provided forums to assist health care providers, researchers, and administrators who would be involved in program innovation and measurement. Examples of these quality improvement innovations are listed in Table 4.1.

Coordinating National Quality Improvement Research

AHRQ priorities include support for the availability of clinical information on evidence-based practice (EBP), clinical guidelines, medical effectiveness, pharmaceutical

---

TABLE 4.1 The National Quality Strategy's* Six Priorities to Guide Efforts to Improve Health and Health Care Quality

1. Making care safer by reducing harm caused in the delivery of care
2. Ensuring that each person and family is engaged as partners in their care
3. Promoting effective communication and coordination of care
4. Promoting the most effective prevention and treatment practices for the leading causes of mortality, starting with cardiovascular disease (CVD)
5. Working with communities to promote wide use of the best practices to enable healthy living
6. Making quality care more affordable for individuals, families, employers, and governments by developing and spreading new health care delivery models

*Led by the Agency for Healthcare Research and Quality.

Source: Retrieved from www.ahrq.gov/workingforquality/about.htm#priorities.

therapy, new technology, screening and preventive services, and outcomes research. This is evidenced by AHRQ's mission to produce clinical evidence to improve the quality, safety, equitability, accessibility, and affordability of health care in the United States. Working with other HHS departments and partners and with universities, research centers, and health care organizations across the country, AHRQ has created the Effective Health Care (EHC) Program, which is focused on producing comparative effectiveness research and translating research findings into summaries (AHRQ, 2014a). These summaries assist both clinicians and patients, helping them become more knowledgeable about health concerns and aiding them in making more informed decisions. AHRQ's Library of Resources provides updated research summaries and standards for a variety of conditions, including cancer, diabetes, heart disease, mental illness, women's health, men's health, and other chronic conditions. These can be found on AHRQ's website (www.ahrq.gov/profes sionals/clinicians-providers/ehclibrary/index.html).

Health care providers need assistance not only in staying on top of the volumes of clinical research findings but also in being aware of standardized clinical practice standards that provide guidance in care provision incorporating evidence-based research. AHRQ developed the National Guidelines Clearinghouse, which includes more than 2,389 clinical practice guidelines on a specialized website (www.guide-line.gov). These standards include management of diseases and conditions, treatment and interventions, and health services administration standards. Health care providers and organizations need support in developing quality improvement activities within their organization to meet regulatory standards for practice. The Health Resources and Services Administration (HRSA) has been providing support to these important endeavors by sharing practical tools that have been compiled by a variety of HRSA organizations. These tools include systematic approaches for performance measurement techniques and guidance in integrating quality improvement activities in all aspects of their practice. Identifying care processes that are common within their practice and relevant to the population served is a first step in identifying the measurement approach. Each performance measure must include specific data that would be required to inform the organization and provider of the scope and methods of clinical documentation necessary to meet the data demands. Standardized performance measures have been increasingly used throughout the health care system, which has allowed for comparisons between providers and promoted identification of the best practices. This quality improvement toolbox can be found on HRSA's website (www.hrsa.gov/quality/toolbox/introduction/index.html).

REASONS WHY NURSE SCHOLARS SHOULD USE QUALITY IMPROVEMENT RESEARCH APPROACHES

The Nursing Profession's Response to the National Quality Improvement Mandate

The IOM's 2010 *The Future of Nursing* report called on the nursing profession to respond to this demand for increased standardization of practice. In order to meet the national mandate for improved quality of health care, the nursing profession is called on to: (a) increase the preparation of doctoral-level nurse scientists, clinical leaders, and executives; and (b) broaden its graduate nursing programs to include quality improvement research methods. Translational research and implementation and evaluation research methods have been added to PhD nursing programs. These topics already exist in many DNP programs. Program evaluation, quality improvement, and epidemiology curricula have been added to strengthen DNP programs for clinicians and executives. These foundational steps are critical and must be expanded to reduce the gap between research and practice and to bring about reliable and sustainable practice improvement. This preparation has strengthened the nursing profession's response to this national focus on improving health care through innovation and quality measurement; however, more engagement in these opportunities is needed. This increased focus and engagement must begin with practicing clinical nurses at all levels of preparation. Nurses must join together in their commitment to provide EBP and to broaden their knowledge of clinical performance standards in their practice area. This engagement must also include increasing their participation in measurement of their own patient and process outcomes and measurements within the organization and communities where they practice.

Practicing nurses are generally not involved in reading the latest research as soon as it is published. In fact, nurses are very busy with their day-to-day clinical practices; thus, they often rely on others for information about the latest clinical findings. Although many nurses read journals and attend conferences to learn about current practices with respect to EBP and the best practice models, it remains very challenging for nurse clinicians to know what new research should be applied to practice and how it is to be applied. It is estimated that it takes anywhere between 10 and 30 years for research to be implemented into clinical practice (Fitzpatrick, 2008). The Robert Wood Johnson Foundation's (2007) "Author in the Room" initiative is one such example intended to speed the translation of nursing research "from the ivory tower to the bedside." The Author in the Room initiative convened researchers of recently published articles and practitioners for the sole purpose of accelerating the time spent in implementing new clinical findings into the clinical setting. A total of 3,517 individuals participated in the 15 conference calls conducted monthly from March 2005 through May 2006. The number of participants varied per call—1,061 participants also participated to provide input for an article on health care performance. Of the 119 participants who completed a 3-month follow-up survey, 43% said that they had made a change in professional practice based on the Author in the Room discussion. The Author in the Room is a critical link to promoting dissemination of clinical research findings and their implementation into the practice setting (Robert Wood Johnson Foundation, 2007). Scaling and diffusion of effective interventions via learning and social networks are necessary to implement quality improvement and system redesign strategies (Dougherty & Conway, 2008). See Chapters 7 and 8 in this book for more information on dissemination and implementation approaches.

The American Association of Colleges of Nursing (AACN, 1990) noted the importance of increasing academic–clinical partnerships. Achieving a high level of engagement in the dissemination of pertinent research can also be strengthened through regional and national academic–clinical partnerships to bring nurse researchers and clinicians together to develop and implement new innovative interventions and care models. This academic–clinical partnership would involve collaborations among nurse academics, clinicians, and executives with the goal to create systems that support high-quality clinical experiences for all stakeholders. By creating and sustaining strong partnerships, there is an energetic, reflective environment focused on continuous learning and development among nursing professionals. In essence, these academic–clinical partnerships are strategic relationships between educational and clinical practice settings that are established to advance their mutual interests related to practice, education, and research (AACN, 1990). Therefore, academic–clinical partnerships can be expanded to share clinical research findings and to accelerate the implementation of high-impact interventions and care models (Beal, 2012).

The stage has been set by the enactment of the PPACA and its related national health care quality improvement mandates for nursing researchers and practice scholars to join together and contribute to the development of high-quality, evidence-based clinical practice standards and quality improvement methods and measurements that will assist in meeting the triple aim through improved health care. Although academic nurse researchers, by the nature of their role, are the best positioned to know the latest research in their respective fields when it is published, the implementation of these new findings into practice is a more problematic, complex, and even sometimes political process (Rycroft-Malone, 2006). The introduction of new interventions or practice models will require a thoughtful, collaborative, and focused dialogue between PhD-prepared nurse researchers and DNP-prepared clinical leaders with the intent to improve quality. The DNP-prepared nurse is in an ideal position to effect change in the practice setting (Dreher & Smith Glasgow, 2011). Innovations on how new knowledge is rapidly and reliably incorporated into clinical practice is an urgent priority (Dougherty & Conway, 2008). The opportunity to build new models of quality improvement that incorporate nursing research methods with program evaluation methods will strengthen quality improvement efforts. These models must clearly define the roles for all nursing stakeholders, including the roles of nursing scientists, clinical leaders, and executives. Models are needed to give support for consistent academic curricula that demonstrate the coordinated effort of PhD- and DNP-prepared nurses to meet health care needs for clinical and research leadership.

METHODS FOR QUALITY IMPROVEMENT RESEARCH

Sustainable practice improvements require deliberate redesign of practices and processes grounded in EBP research findings and knowledge of human factors. With the increasing awareness of the complexity of health care systems as well as of the dynamics of health beliefs and behaviors of individuals, families, and communities, health service researchers have called into question the reliability of quality improvement approaches and methods of the past. It is now widely acknowledged that multiple quality improvement research and evaluation approaches are necessary to measure various quality aspects of health care delivery. Currently, one of the most critical and creative areas of health services research is evolving research methods and models of past quality improvement research. Several theoretical approaches to health care quality have been developed over the past 50 years; however, their commonality is based on using systematic approaches targeted at decreasing waste in health care systems by decreasing error rates, improving efficiency, and reducing costs.

Formative and Summative Approaches

The methodologies of formative and summative research have significantly different approaches. Formative research approaches involve iterative techniques for evaluation of conditions that affect project execution and implementation. Challenges to progress and effectiveness can be mitigated through analysis of and response to information gathered during the execution of a project. In contrast, summative research approaches require control over procedures and methods. Traditional experimental or quasi-experimental designs are used to test the degree of success of outcomes from quality improvement projects (Stetler et al., 2006).

The formative nature of the quality improvement process introduces great variability and systematic approaches to data analysis that challenge traditional research and evaluation methods. In addition, the interpretation of quality improvement data, especially those related to impact and reliability, have lagged behind the development of other research measurements compared with other forms of research. Because the process of improvement is iterative, there is a need to continually revise and evaluate; this iterative process makes this research approach substantively different from traditional research methods. Despite these challenges, nurses engaged in quality improvement research must employ the most effective means and methods to collect and evaluate new and diverse sets of data to enhance understanding of the quality of health care processes and their outcomes.

It has been proposed that the use of both formative and summative research and evaluation methods is the most effective approach to building comprehensive quality improvement programs (AHRQ, 2013). Together, these two basic approaches to research and evaluation provide a rigorous assessment process designed to identify actual and potential influences in the quality and effectiveness of health care programs. This process also provides for more timely feedback regarding the implementation of interventions while they are taking place, allowing for essential practice and policy changes. This purposely contrasts with the traditional unidirectional implementation research studies in which data are not available for many years after the implementation of the intervention. Within the national mandate for strengthening quality improvement activities is the expectation that quality information will be accessible to clinicians and staff working with patients. This dissemination of "real-time" results can make health care more effective and safe.

Rapid Cycle Evaluation

In 2010, when the PPACA established the CMMI, the center was charged to test innovative payment and service delivery models designed to improve the coordination, quality, and efficiency of health care in the United States. The CMMI created the Rapid Cycle Evaluation Group, a new rapid cycle evaluation approach that combined use of both summative and formative methods. Recognizing that there is not one "best" evaluation method that works in all circumstances, the Rapid Cycle Evaluation approach addresses the specific goals and processes of the program being evaluated. When using this approach, data are gathered both from organization and system processes and from patient outcomes. Findings from analyses of these data provide comprehensive and effective evaluation of change from multiple vantage points. In the next section, the TPS model is discussed. This approach is a form of rapid cycle formative and summative evaluation process from which DNPs and PhDs can learn as they develop their collaborative relationships to create effective quality improvement models.

TPS and Lean Models Inform Quality Improvement in Health Care

There are quality improvement models used in nursing practice and health care with the intention of reviewing retrospective data via health information technologies (e.g., electronic health records [EHRs], administrative practice management systems) or prospective interventional strategies to improve productivity, efficiency, and cost-effectiveness of health care. An explanation of some innovative models and their impact is provided next.

The TPS

The use of TPS has demonstrated superior results in organizations seeking to increase efficiency and effectiveness, reduce cost, and enhance achievement of stated goals. TPS principles, derived from one of the leading automobile manufacturing companies and developed in post–World War II Japan, have been proposed as a model to address significant quality and safety concerns. Nurses, who comprise the largest group of health professionals caring for patients, have the greatest impact on patient outcomes and are a vital link between access to care and quality outcomes (IOM, 2010). In addition, nurses play a vital role in preventing medical errors, increasing patient safety, reducing infection, decreasing fragmentation of services, and providing culturally sensitive, ethical, and compassionate care (Campbell, Gantt, & Congdon, 2009; Thompson, Wolf, & Spear, 2003).

When the Toyota Motor Company faced financial ruin, Sakichi Toyoda led the development of the company's core philosophy and principles by using a process-oriented systems model that focused on respect for people, teamwork, mutual trust and commitment, elimination of waste, and continuous quality improvement (CQI). TPS is the best known in health care for its dramatic results in quality improvement while also decreasing costs at Virginia Mason Medical Center (VMMC) in Seattle, Washington. In 2003, Gary Kaplan (president and chief executive officer), Charlene Tachabani (chief nursing officer), and other executives at VMMC implemented TPS throughout the organization to address serious patient safety concerns and diminishing financial resources (Kenny, 2011; Ziskovsky & Ziskovsky, 2007). At VMMC, Dr. Kaplan recognized the need for system-level change. Through his chance meeting with a former Boeing executive, he was introduced to the accomplishments achieved at Boeing through the application of TPS principles in the aviation industry. Dr. Kaplan then embarked on a mission to transform patient care by introducing TPS at VMMC (Blackmore, Mecklenburg, & Kaplan, 2011; Kenny, 2011). By 2010, after successful implementation of TPS, VMMC was a financially prosperous health care institution that had saved $15 million in revenues over 6 years. In addition, the Leapfrog Group (2010) named VMMC the *hospital of the decade* for its improvement of quality and safety while decreasing the cost of health care.

A key organizational practice is the expectation for supervisors to practice *Genchi-Genbutsu*, which is translated as going to the source to find the facts, making informed decisions, consensus building, and shared problem solving. Genchi-Genbutsu provides the basis for a culture that supports stopping to fix problems and getting quality right the first time to deliver a value-added service to customers (Liker & Hoseus,

2008; Liker & Meier, 2007). VMMC's senior leadership understood the importance of incorporating system-level thinking where the philosophy and mission of the organization goes beyond an isolated focus of quality dashboards and benchmarking.

The emphasis is to grow leaders among bedside nurses and other health care professionals who understand the work of patient care, live the philosophy, and can teach it to others (Serembus, Meloy, & Posmontier, 2012). The analyses of workflow and standardization of work are critical to TPS application. Systems are carefully scrutinized, step by step, to eliminate extra steps to improve efficiency with the goal of "zero" defects. The TPS application complements a patient-first philosophy: Waiting is bad, whereas defect-free medicine, rigorous accountability, judicious resource allocation, real-time quality assurance, management on site, and an urgency to intervene are good. The VMMC hyperbaric department is a clear example of the impact of TPS on its department's operations and outcomes:

- Patient wait time disappeared
- Financial margins per patient increased 145%
- Hours of operation were reduced to 8-hour days, a 42% reduction
- Patient satisfaction increased
- Staff satisfaction increased (Kenny, 2011)

There are numerous examples of TPS's impact across the United States. For example, in Pennsylvania, the Veterans Administration Pittsburgh Healthcare System (VAPHS), a 629-bed hospital serving a veteran population of more than 360,000 veterans, reduced the incidence of methicillin-resistant *Staphylococcus aureus* (MRSA) infections in surgical units through the "Getting to Zero" Campaign. Initially, TPS was fully implemented on acute care surgical units applying TPS principles; MRSA infections were reduced 82% after 2 years. MRSA-related infections decreased from 1.40 per 1,000 bed days to 0.27 (Richmond, Bernstein, Creen, Cunningham, & Rudy, 2007).

Lean Methodology

Lean is a modified methodology created from TPS design and is aimed at the elimination of non-value-added operations in the workplace to create flow and a quick response to customer demand. Lean is a process improvement strategy that focuses on identifying the waste (non-value-added work) in a process and then applying various tools to eliminate the waste and achieve flow; therefore, it is termed *lean*. When applied to the health care setting, Lean can enhance the patient experience by cutting out waste and providing a streamlined, safer patient visit. The Lean methodology is a principle that is used in a number of health care organizations to increase the value of the patient experience while decreasing waste. Lean methodology identifies areas of waste that are prevalent in any system process (Belter et al., 2012; Lean Enterprise Institute, 2011). Based on a review of the literature, there have been increased applications of the Lean transformation process.

Van Lent, Goedbloed, and van Harten (2009) published the results of a Lean methodology intervention to improve efficiency in a hospital-based chemotherapy day unit. Due to increased demand for services, the unit was experiencing bottlenecks that increased patient wait times and staff work pressure. The goal of the intervention was to provide a 20% increase in patient care and to maintain high-quality services and patient satisfaction without adding resources. This included a multipronged approach: alterations in scheduling; limiting interruptions; receiving chemotherapy orders on the day before service if not dependent on laboratory results; preparing specific medications in advance; and performing laboratory analyses on the day before service for patients receiving long treatments.

Belter et al. (2012) also used the Lean Model in an outpatient chemotherapy unit to increase productivity and to decrease patients' waiting time. After the Lean methodology workflow analysis and intervention was implemented, the average overall patient wait time from arrival to chemotherapy infusion decreased from 88 minutes to 68 minutes (6-month average). Applying Lean methodology to the oncology infusion center's workflow subsequently enhanced productivity. Therefore, more patients were able to receive chemotherapy due to the time saved in performing the treatment process. The overall value of the Lean Model to the oncology patient and organization was that the Lean process enabled shorter waiting periods, eliminated waste, and administered chemotherapy in a safe, efficient manner.

MODELS FOR QUALITY IMPROVEMENT DEVELOPED IN HEALTH CARE

Hybrid models for quality improvement approaches blend formative and summative research methods. These hybrid models integrate effectiveness, implementation, and associated evaluation methods to enhance knowledge and strategy development in "real-world settings" (Bernet, Willens, & Bauer, 2013). Aspects of comparative effectiveness research (Chapter 6) are integrated with quality improvement approaches that study process, structure, and outcomes. In this section, the PDSA cycle is discussed, which is a formative evaluation approach that nurse scholars can use in their quality improvement efforts. Furthermore, study designs can be developed that integrate formative measurement with summative evaluation enhancements. The next section explores epidemiological research methods that can increase the value of conducting multi-method approaches for quality improvement research.

The Institute of Healthcare Improvement (IHI) was founded with the goal of improving the quality of health care by applying quality improvement methods to health care. IHI's mission is "to improve health and health care worldwide." To this end, IHI has supported quality improvement initiatives and disseminated findings from quality improvement science. Initial projects focused on incremental change at the microsystem level that led to identifying the best practices that were disseminated at the local level. Projects evolved and became larger, leading to the dissemination of the best practices focused on system-wide change. More recently, IHI quality improvement initiatives have developed larger scale practice-based projects targeting entire systems through their "100,000 Lives Campaign," "5 Million Lives Campaign," and "Triple Aim Initiative." These accomplishments are model examples for systematic dissemination of incremental success (IHI, 2015).

IHI's Model for Improvement

The Associates in Process Improvement developed the IHI approach to quality improvement and uses the Model for Improvement as a core element in the process of quality improvement (Scoville & Little, 2014). Because the IHI quality improvement process is grounded in the work of early quality improvement innovators in

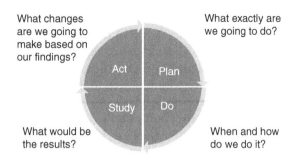

Figure 4.1 Plan, do, study, act cycle.
Source: Centers for Medicare and Medicaid Services (2014).

industrial settings, some background is necessary to fully appreciate its application to nursing and health care. William Shewart is credited as the "father of statistical quality control" (Best & Neuhauser, 2006, p. 142). His efforts to study and eliminate variation resulted in the development of the PDSA cycle or Shewart cycle. The iterative nature of the cycle (Figure 4.1) is the underlying principle for CQI (Best & Neuhauser, 2006).

Shewart became a mentor for William Deming, a statistician and quality innovator in his own right, who developed a management philosophical approach to quality improvement, which is called the System of Profound Knowledge. The elements of the System of Profound Knowledge are as follows:

● Appreciation for a system
● Understanding variation
● A theory of knowledge
● Understanding psychology and human behavior (Best & Neuhauser, 2005, p. 311)

Central to Deming's philosophy is the belief that *leadership* is the key element to quality improvement. The PDSA cycle and the System of Profound Knowledge combine to provide the underlying concepts for the Model for Improvement. IHI's leadership supported the quality improvement initiatives that promoted adaptation of this model for use in the health care industry through close collaboration with the group, the Associates in Process Improvement.

The PDSA Cycle

The PDSA cycle is an excellent example of formative evaluation. It provides formative data and is data driven by key questions (Langley et al., 2009). These quality improvement initiatives provide excellent opportunities for collaborative nursing scholarship among PhD researchers and DNP practice leaders.

The key questions are the same regardless of the quality improvement context. They drive the PDSA cycle and are shown in Figure 4.2. The key questions are as follows:

● *What are we trying to accomplish?* The aim statement or question directs the entire process. The responses to this question define the purpose, rationale, population, and end goal for the improvement process. Measurable, achievable goals must be included in the statement.

● *How will we know that a change is an improvement?* The response to this question is the mandate to develop measures for goals that can be easily quantified and visually communicated to line personnel, for example, through the use of run charts.

● *What change can we make that will result in improvement?* The response to this question requires the description and documentation of changes to the system that could alter how work is accomplished, produce observable change, and could be sustainable.

The PDSA cycle might be thought of as generating pilot data and may require multiple iterations before improvement is achieved. If the improvements are successful at the bedside or in the unit, can they be generalized to the larger system? The PDSA model is geared toward "rapid cycle" testing, which can reliably produce improved outcomes and is an essential component of the Model for Improvement.

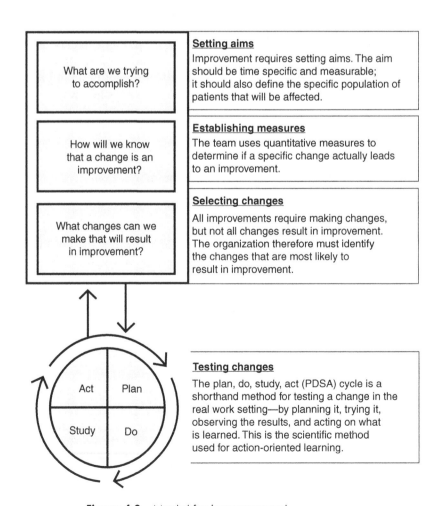

Figure 4.2 Model for improvement.
Source: Health Resources and Services Administration (2011).

The advantage of PDSA is that the complexity of the system and problem do not affect the process. The PDSA cycle provides a systematic way to test ideas that have worked in other settings for consideration of the institution's culture, goals, and resources. PDSA is infinitely scalable to adaptation, and it provides a framework for facilitating and measuring change (Scoville & Little, 2014).

The problem with the classical approach to statistical evaluation is that it applies strict rules to control variability. In contrast, the iterative nature of the PDSA cycle resists control, as it is designed to be flexible and to allow for real-world changes when evidence shows the intervention is not working. There are situations where PDSA can involve statistical evaluation. Data points can be identified and gathered through an electronic documentation system. In addition, when modified experimental designs can be employed system wide, changes could be launched after adequate rounds of micro-system testing have been completed. Speroff, James, Nelson, Headrick, and Brommels (2004) proposed several study designs that were compatible with PDSA quality improvement research. For example, for study designs that involve continuous data collection, a case-control design could be used; this approach is discussed in the next section. This approach relies on repeated measures over time with baseline data used for historical control. Data are examined for random variability prior to PDSA improvement commencement. After the intervention, data collection continues to identify changes, and marked change is attributed to the intervention. Continued use of the intervention should produce stable data that document the effects of the intervention. Criteria that indicate effectiveness are: (a) immediate change, (b) clearly defined measurable magnitude of change, and (c) stability of the pattern.

Unobtrusive measures (e.g., chart data) improve the measurement process and address challenges related to blinding (e.g., subjects are often the observers in this design). A major weakness in the design is failure to control history. A careful consideration of extraneous factors that might confound results must be performed. This is done frequently when there are benchmarks and stretch goals. The control chart is posted documenting a benchmark goal, and as iterations continue, the relationship between more frequent and consistent applications of the intervention influences the process as higher levels of performance are attained. When the performance greatly exceeds the criterion, the relationship between the intervention and performance is suspect. Other factors should be considered as potential contributors to the change. The design can be strengthened with use of annotated control charts to implement and document process improvement and to evaluate for the link between performance and criterion shifts. Carefully documenting the replication of findings can overcome the issue of internal validity, demonstrating the need for scrupulous data collection and clear protocol implementation (Speroff et al., 2004).

PhD and DNP collaboration in quality improvement program development can lead to expansion of traditional CQI methods by using innovative approaches. CQI has been seen as a process-based approach that depends on the best sources of data for improving quality, based on the belief that there is always an opportunity to improve the quality of a service. Through the inclusion of the specific processes and programs in the CQI approach, the PhD/DNP team can identify appropriate stable programs as candidates for quasi-experimental designs. Expanded tools such as control charts for measuring the effect of the intervention can also be developed. This expansion of traditional quality improvement can also include case-control design, appropriate baseline measures, stability of the baseline, use of replication, and measurement of constancy of the intervention effect.

There is a need for an increased appreciation of the difference in the knowledge, skills, and competencies of PhD and DNP nursing professionals. These nurse scholars offer significant expertise to quality improvement initiatives when matched with the needs of creating innovative approaches to health care service delivery and the associated quality measurements of process, structure, and outcome effectiveness and efficiency. Clearly, this opportunity sets the stage for increasing the nursing profession's leadership in answering the national mandate for health care reform.

Applying Epidemiological Methods to Enhance Quality Improvement Research

Relevance of epidemiological methods to quality improvement research has been increasingly recognized as a means to provide both formative and summative data to the analysis of quality in health care. Epidemiological methods contribute understanding to the etiology and prevention of disease and provide tools for the proper evaluation of interventions and treatment outcomes for the individual, group, community, and population. Epidemiologic studies have traditionally been used for demonstrating associations and deriving causal inferences. These studies have traditionally been the primary approach to evaluation of public health interventions and provide assistance with development of reports intended to generate public policy. Focused on the domain of outcomes measures in health outcomes research, epidemiology has gained increased attention with a recent shift toward broader evaluations of health care interventions and programs. This has been emphasized through the Affordable Care Act's (ACA) implementation of its Triple Aims Initiative of improved patient outcomes, health care processes, and efficiency. In the past, epidemiology focused on measures of morbidity and mortality outcomes research; however, these new demands have expanded to include outcome measures of patient satisfaction, quality of life, degrees of dependence and disability, and other similar measures (Gordis, 2014).

The classical approach to epidemiological studies of disease etiology examines possible relationships between putative causes (independent variable) and adverse health effects (dependent variables; Gordis, 2014). In quality improvement research, health care programs or interventions are the independent variables and reductions in adverse health effects are the anticipated outcomes or dependent variables (Gordis, 2014). Epidemiological studies focus on measures of efficacy, effectiveness, and efficiency. If a health care program has demonstrated efficacy (works under ideal conditions), it can then be implemented in real-life situations for evaluation of effectiveness and efficiency. Selection of appropriate, well-defined, and measureable outcomes that can be standardized outcomes are critical to advancing quality improvement research. Clarity regarding the specific outcomes being measured is considered a major influence in a study's acceptability and its use in practice. Efficiency is also being looked at broadly, including not only financial but also human factors such as pain, absenteeism, disability, and social stigma. These lessons learned from epidemiological studies can greatly inform quality improvement research related to specificity and care in identifying outcomes and their applicability to clinical practice.

Epidemiology Research Designs Applied to Quality Improvement Research

Based on the recent shift toward outcomes research, both epidemiology and quality improvement researchers can use many of the same study designs and measurements. Case-control research design is increasingly used as a quality improvement research method, particularly in evaluation of prevention and screening programs (Gordis, 2014). Case-control design is efficiently used in etiology studies once the outcome of interest occurs. Then, a retrospective assessment of many antecedent factors can be conducted. This design requires careful specification of cases and suitable controls, which makes it the most useful for studies about evaluations of prevention of specific diseases or adverse outcomes. Challenges exist with stratification of severity and other prognostic factors; however, this approach can be considered when evaluating appropriate clinical programs.

Epidemiologists, by their training, are familiar with how to use large data sets for clinical and public health research. With the expansion of available clinical data through the broad implementation of EHRs, quality improvement researchers and evaluators are faced with how to make use of these large data sets to expand the range and effectiveness of quality improvement studies. Much can be learned, and rigor of analyses strengthened, when employing epidemiological approaches to large aggregated-level data as well as to individual-level data sets in evaluating health care outcomes.

Program evaluation spans both epidemiology and quality improvement science. Within epidemiology there is widespread acceptance of the valuable role of research and evaluation in understanding the efficacy, effectiveness, and efficiency of clinical programs through answers to different questions. The primary questions for researchers focus on exposures, predictors, and adverse outcomes in often randomly assigned study participants. The primary purpose of evaluation is to assess similar types of exposures within the context of participation in programs that already exist (Magnus, 2016). The evaluation paradigm stresses the inclusion of evaluation findings into overall program design and the use of these findings to improve program design. In addition, feedback loops are built into program development to support continuous evaluation of programs throughout the change process. These feedback loops mirror the CQI process. Within the context of health care, clinical research is frequently conducted, though evaluation is much more common. In many situations, however, program evaluation and clinical research can coexist within the same program using the same data in order to answer their different questions. Through PhD/DNP collaboration, these coexisting designs can be created to broaden quality improvement opportunities as well as to conduct clinical research.

Centers for Disease Control and Prevention's Framework for Program Evaluation for Public Health

Nurse scholars need to know that various methods for program evaluation exist (see Chapter 1). An example of an evaluation framework that can be used to build evaluation studies as well as quality improvement programs is the Centers for Disease Control and Prevention's (CDC, 1999) framework for Program Evaluation for Public Health. This framework is particularly useful in that it engages stakeholders throughout the process, is circular in nature, and reflects the nonlinear, iterative, and feedback qualities of evaluation (Magnus, 2016), based on the CDC's (1999, p. 11) definition of *evaluation* as a "systematic investigation of the merit, worth or significance of an object." The values or merits of program components and activities were critically analyzed based on the following questions:

- What will be evaluated? (i.e., What is the program and in what context does it exist?)
- What aspects of the program will be considered when judging program performance?
- What standards (i.e., type or level of performance) must be reached for the program to be considered successful?
- What evidence will be used to indicate how the program has performed?
- What conclusions regarding program performance are justified by comparing the available evidence to the selected standards?
- How will the lessons learned from the inquiry be used to improve public health effectiveness? (CDC, 1999, pp. 13–14)

Through this analysis, key steps were identified as critical in the program evaluation process and four standards were described to guide the study. Table 4.2 provides a brief description of the six steps of the program evaluation process that are applicable to quality improvement research.

As previously discussed, a variety of epidemiological study designs can be used to evaluate how a program is working. Using this comprehensive framework to determine the most appropriate methods and designs based on unique characteristics of the program will serve as the foundation for an effective program evaluation process. An additional critical element in the program evaluation process is the role of the evaluator. Ongoing supervision, management of data collection and analysis, and interpretation of findings fall on the skills and abilities of the evaluator or team. If all of the elements outlined in the CDC framework are fully considered and the design process is implemented as directed, then the evaluation results in a credible process. Outcome data collection, analysis, and interpretation stages of the program evaluation process can not only be used to improve the specific program under review but also be generalized to support expansion of programming to wider audiences. See Chapter 1 for more information on program evaluation, especially if submitting a grant application that includes program evaluation.

PhD/DNP MODEL OF COLLABORATION FOR QUALITY IMPROVEMENT IN HEALTH CARE

Through PhD/DNP collaboration, rigorous program evaluations can be implemented that meet the specific needs of both new and existing clinical programs. As described throughout this chapter, national mandates and new sources of funding are in place to build teams focused on innovation in health care service delivery and quality improvement. These opportunities will only add to the exponential growth in evidence-based research knowledge that needs to influence clinical practice as quickly as possible. Nurse scientists often focus on their area of research interest within a narrow context outside of clinical programs. DNP-prepared advance

TABLE 4.2   Applying CDC's Program Evaluation Framework to Quality Improvement Research: Steps in Program Evaluation

Step 1. Engage Stakeholders Prior to Starting the Evaluation

The benefits of engaging stakeholders (those who use, provide, implement, or research the program under review) include increased awareness and support of the program by these stakeholders, provision of unique information regarding elements of the program otherwise missed, and the inclusion of community needs from multiple perspectives.

Step 2. Describe the Program

Formative and summative methods are used to identify elements of the program under study. These include observations, interviews, comprehensive reviews of standard operating procedures, and previous quality improvement data.

Step 3. Focus on the Evaluation Design

After the evaluation of the program through the previous two steps, the evaluator identifies research questions, null and alternative hypotheses, and available data sources prior to determining the specific evaluation study design. A variety of possible designs are considered; however, ranging from process to outcomes evaluation, all are driven by the research questions. In evaluation studies, research questions may be redefined throughout the process, making the process iterative in nature.

Step 4. Gather Credible Evidence

The quality of the data source directly impacts the quality of the program evaluation. Most often, the database being used is developed for other purposes (e.g., ICD-10 diagnostic coding or CPT billing codes). Inherent limitations of data sources must be acknowledged when evaluating the findings. If necessary, new data sources are developed to investigate new programs and innovations.

Step 5. Justify Conclusions

Quality data analysis is within the complete control of the evaluator who must create a well-executed analysis that is inclusive of any limitations of the data sources. Interpretation follows data analysis with conclusions drawn and justified directly from data.

Step 6. Ensure Use and Share Lessons Learned

One of the differences between research and evaluation is that evaluation studies must improve programs. Findings must be acknowledged, provided as feedback, and used to improve program efficiency and effectiveness. This cycle ensures that quality data are shared and used for program improvements.

Critical Standards

Four critical standards have been developed for the program evaluation process. They are utility, feasibility, propriety, and accuracy. Together, these standards guide the six-step program evaluation process throughout, assuring consistency and comparability between program evaluation cycles and sites.

CDC, Centers for Disease Control and Prevention; CPT, Current Procedural Terminology; ICD, International Classification of Diseases.

Source: CDC (1999).

practice clinicians and executives may focus on their area of clinical or leadership expertise outside of the world of research. This lack of collaboration between PhDs and DNPs often results in few of the multidimensional program evaluations that are now in demand. Few structured collaborative educational or research programs exist between PhD and DNP students. Models that describe this collaborative process are even fewer.

The authors propose consideration of a model based on innovation as the means to describe the collaborative roles of the two doctoral-prepared nurse leaders. The Diffusion of Innovations Model has benefited over the past 50 years from broad application to research in many settings, including agriculture, business, medicine, and, recently, health care (Dearing, 2009). As described in the preceding sections, health care is one of the few industries that is overwhelmed with innovations coming in the form of groundbreaking research, broad dissemination of research findings, industry-wide incentives to create clinical practice standards, and organization-wide quality improvement initiatives that impact every process of care. The widespread agreement of the aims of this coordinated approach underscores the need for improvement of the means and methods of implementation of these innovations.

"Health care is rich in evidence-based innovations, yet even when such innovations are implemented successfully in one location, they often disseminate slowly or not at all" (Berwick, 2003, p. 19). Berwick (2003) went on to identify the usefulness of the Diffusion of Innovations Model and made recommendations to health care providers and administrators to identify and support innovation through: (a) supporting innovators and early adopters; (b) trusting and enabling innovation; and (c) creating an environment that is open to change. The nursing profession has responded to this invigorating time with the development of pathways for doctorate programs: research (PhD) and practice (DNP). It has also broadly identified the roles of these two programs; however, it has stopped short in explicating a model that would support these two groups of potential innovators collaborating to bring about the needed changes in the health care system. The Diffusion of Innovations approach provides well-developed methods of creating the innovation, supporting the change, and supporting the individuals and organizations undergoing the needed change. The nursing profession can lead the needed diffusion of EBP research, guidelines, and standards into each nurse's practice through the coordinated efforts of PhD researchers and DNP nursing practice leaders.

SUMMARY

Implementation and system redesign science, as in the case exemplars of TPS and IHI, have the potential to transform health care (Berwick, 2008). For the nursing discipline to have impactful, timely, system-wide interventions and practice change, nurses will need to implement innovative approaches to care, assess the promise of quality improvement strategies, and create evidence-based quality enhancing policies (Dougherty & Conway, 2008). The acceleration of innovative research findings to the bedside will require a commitment from PhD- and DNP-prepared nurses to lead this transformation. The PhD-prepared nurse is primarily focused on the generation of rigorous research/external evidence, including translational research, to inform practice and policy. The DNP-prepared nurse is primarily focused on providing leadership for implementation of EBP. This requires competence in translating research into practice, evaluating evidence, applying research in decision making, and implementing viable clinical innovations to change practice. PhD-prepared nurses should know how to work with health care systems and clinicians on the translation of their research findings into practice to improve quality of care and patient outcomes to reduce the long research–practice time gap. DNP-prepared nurses should be the best translators of research evidence and evidence-based guidelines into real-world settings to improve health care quality and patient outcomes, and to reduce costs. PhD- and DNP-prepared nurses must collaborate in meaningful ways to improve health and health care through knowledge translation (AACN, 2014; Auerbach et al., 2014). The Diffusion of Innovations Model provides a framework from which to consider the needs of the complex health care organizations in which nursing takes place and how each role can contribute to meeting the aims of improving patient care outcomes and health care systems, as well as reducing the cost of care.

REFERENCES

Agency for Healthcare Research and Quality. (2014a). *Effective health care.* Retrieved from http://effectivehealthcare.ahrq.gov

Agency for Healthcare Research and Quality. (2014b). *Working for quality.* Retrieved from http://www.ahrq.gov/workingforquality

American Association of Colleges of Nursing. (1990). *Resolution: Need for collaborative relationships between nursing education and practice.* Washington, DC: Author.

American Association of Colleges of Nursing. (2014). *The doctor of nursing practice (DNP).* Retrieved from http://www.aacn.nche.edu/media-relations/fact-sheets/dnp

Auerbach, D. I., Martsolf, G., Pearson, M. L., Taylor, E. A., Zaydman, M., Muchow, A., . . . Dower, C. (2014). *The DNP by 2015: A study of the institutional, political, and professional issues that facilitate or impede establishing a post-baccalaureate doctor of nursing practice program.* Retrieved from http://www.aacn.nche.edu/dnp/DNP-Study.pdf

Beal, J. (2012). Academic-service partnerships in nursing: An integrative review. *Nursing Research and Practice, 9.* doi:10.1155/2012/501564

Belter, D., Halsey, J., Severtson, H., Fix, A., Michelfelder, L., Michalak, K., . . . Ianni, A. (2012). Evaluation of outpatient oncology services using Lean methodology. *Oncology Nursing Forum, 39*(2), 136–140.

Bernet, A. C., Willens, D. E., & Bauer, M. S. (2013). Effectiveness-implementation hybrid designs: Implications for quality improvement science. *Implementation Science, 8*(Suppl. 1), S2.

Berwick, D. M. (2003). Disseminating innovations in health care. *Journal of the American Medical Association, 298*(15), 1969–1975.

Berwick, D. M. (2008). The science of improvement. *Journal of the American Medical Association, 299*(10), 1182–1184.

Best, M., & Neuhauser, D. (2005). W. Edwards Deming: Father of quality management, patient and composer. *Quality and Safety in Health Care, 14*(4), 310–312.

Best, M., & Neuhauser, D. (2006). Walter A. Shewhart, 1924, and the Hawthorne factory. *Quality and Safety in Health Care, 15*(2), 142–143.

Blackmore, C. C., Mecklenburg, R. S., & Kaplan, G. S. (2011). At Virginia Mason, collaboration among providers, employers, and health plans to transform care, cut costs, and improved quality. *Health Affairs, 30*(9) 1680–1687.

Campbell, R. J., Gantt, L., & Congdon, T. (2009). Teaching workflow analysis and Lean thinking via simulation: A formative evaluation. *Perspectives in Health Information Management, 6*, 3.

Centers for Disease Control and Prevention (CDC). (1999). Framework for program evaluation in public health. *Morbidity and Mortality Weekly Report, 48.*

Centers for Medicare and Medicaid Services. (2014). *PDSA cycle template.* Retrieved from http://www.cms.gov/Medicare/Provider-Enrollment-and-Certification/QAPI/downloads/PDSACycle debedits.pdf

Dearing, J. (2009). Applying the theory of innovation to intervention development. *Research on Social Work Practice, 19*(5), 503–518.

Department of Health and Human Services. (2010). *The Affordable Care Act, section by section.* Retrieved from http://www.hhs.gov/healthcare/rights/law/index.html

Department of Health and Human Services. (2011). *National strategy for quality improvement in health care.* Retrieved from http://www.ahrq.gov/workingforquality/nqs/nqs2011annlrpt.htm

Department of Health and Human Services. (2012). 2012 Annual Progress Report to Congress National Strategy for Quality Improvement in Health Care. Retrieved from http://www.ahrq.gov/workingforquality/reports/annual-reports/nqs2012annlrpt.htm

Dougherty, D., & Conway, P. H. (2008). The "3T's" road map to tranform US health care: The "how" of high quality care. *Journal of the American Medical Association, 299*(19), 2319–2321.

Dreher, H. M., & Smith Glasgow, M. E. (2011). *Role development for doctoral advanced nursing practice.* New York, NY: Springer.

Fitzpatrick, J. (2008). Lag time in research to practice: Are we reducing or increasing the gap? *Applied Nursing Research, 21*, 1.

Geonnotti, K., Peikes, D., Wang, W., & Smith, J. (2013). *Formative evaluation: Fostering real-time adaptations and refinements to improve the effectiveness of patient-centered medical home models.* Rockville, MD: Agency for Healthcare Research and Quality (AHRQ Publication No. 13-0025-EF).

Gordis, L. (2014). *Epidemiology* (5th ed.). Philadelphia, PA: Elsevier.

Health Resources and Services Administration. (2011). Model of improvement. *Quality Improvement.* Retrieved from http://www.hrsa.gov/quality/toolbox/508pdfs/qualityimprovement.pdf

Institute for Healthcare Improvement. (2015). History, 2015. Retrieved from http://www.ihi.org/about/Pages/History.aspx

Institute of Medicine. (1999). *To err is human.* Washington, DC.: National Academy of Science Press.

Institute of Medicine. (2001). *Crossing the quality chasm: A new health system for the 21st century.* Washington, DC: National Academy of Science Press.

Institute of Medicine. (2003). *Health profession education: A bridge to quality.* Washington, DC: National Academy of Science Press.

Institute of Medicine. (2010). *The future of nursing: Leading change, advancing health.* Retrieved from http://www.nap.edu/read/12956/chapter/1#xvii

Kenny, C. (2011). *Transforming healthcare Virginia Mason Medical Center's pursuit of the perfect patient experience.* New York, NY: Productivity Press.

Langley, G. J., Moen, R. D., Nolan, K. M., Nolan, T. W., Norman, C. L., & Provost, L. P. (2009). *The improvement guide: A practical approach to enhancing organizational performance* (2nd ed.). San Francisco, CA: Jossey-Bass.

Lean Enterprise Institute. (2011). *Principles of Lean.* Retrieved from http://www.lean.org/whatslean/principles.cfm

Leapfrog Group. (2010). *The leapfrog group announces top hospitals of the decade.* Retrieved from http://www.leapfroggroup.org/news/leapfrog_news/4784721

Liker, J. K., & Hoseus, M. (2008). *Toyota culture: The heart and soul of the Toyota way*. New York, NY: McGraw Hill.

Liker, J. K., & Meier, M. (2007). *Toyota talent: Developing your people the Toyota way*. New York, NY: McGraw Hill.

Magnus, M. (2016). *Intermediate epidemiology*. Burlington, MA: Jones & Bartlett.

National Quality Forum. (2014). Retrieved from qualityforum.org/Home.aspx

Richmond, I., Bernstein, A., Creen, C., Cunningham, C., & Rudy, M. (2007). Best-practice protocols: Reducing harm from MRSA. *Nursing Management, 38*(8), 22–27.

Robert Wood Johnson Foundation. (2007). Cutting lag time in implementing findings, JAMA authors discuss research with healthcare practitioners during conference calls. Retrieved from http://www.rwjf.org/en/research-publications/find-rwjf-research/2007/06/cutting-lag-time-in-implementing-findings-jama-authors-discuss-r.html

Rycroft-Malone, J. (2006). The politics of evidence-based practice movements: Legacies and current challenges. *Journal of Research in Nursing, 11*, 95–108.

Scoville, R., & Little, K. (2014). Comparing Lean and quality improvement. *IHI white paper*. Retrieved from http://www.ihi.org/resources/Pages/IHIWhitePapers/ComparingLeanandQualityImprovement.aspx

Serembus, J. F., Meloy, F., & Posmontier, B. (2012). Learning from business: Incorporating the Toyota production system into nursing curricula. *Nursing Clinics of North America, 47*(4), 503–516.

Speroff, T., James, B. C., Nelson, E. C., Headrick, L. A., & Brommels, M. (2004). Guidelines for appraisal and publication of PDSA quality improvement. *Quality Management in Health Care, 13*(1), 33–39.

Stetler, C. B., Legro, M. W., Wallace, C. M., Bowman, C., Guihan, M., Hagedorn, H., . . . Smith, J. L. (2006). The role of formative evaluation in implementation research and the QUERI experience. *Journal of General Internal Medicine, 21*(Suppl. 2), S1–S8.

Thompson, D. N., Wolf, G. A., & Spear, S. J. (2003). Driving improvement in patient care: Lessons from Toyota. *Journal of Nursing Administration, 33*(11), 585–595.

van Lent, A. M. W., Goedbloed, N., & van Harten, W. H. (2009). Improving the efficiency of a chemotherapy day unit: Applying a business approach to oncology. *European Journal of Cancer, 45*, 800–806.

Ziskovsky, B., & Ziskovsky, J. (2007). *Doing more with less—going lean in education: A white paper on process improvement in education*. Shoreview, MN: Lean Education Enterprises.

PART II

EVOLVING PRACTICE-BASED
RESEARCH METHODS

CHAPTER FIVE

BIG DATA IN NURSING RESEARCH

PATRICIA ABBOTT AND BOQIN XIE

OBJECTIVES

After reading this chapter, readers will be able to:

1. Present a balanced argument of the pros and cons of big data analytics
2. Explain the concept of data liquidity and its relationship to big data science
3. Apply the concepts of veracity and provenance to a discussion of the results of a big data analysis
4. Debate the following point: "Success in big data science will come *not* just from advanced technical knowledge and skills"

Although collections of health and health care–related data have long been considered to be "big," in reality, this industry is a relative newcomer to the true big data science paradigm. As digitization and processing power expand, publicly available knowledge resources, large-scale shared data sets, and complex interdependencies between teams of scientists have moved health and health care into a deeper understanding of true big data science. This development parallels the progression of astronomers and physicists who decades earlier had adopted large-scale collaboration, sharing, and manipulation of massive data collections as the norm. Health care is somewhat late to the big data party.

At the same time, the complexity and heterogeneity of the data unique to humans and health systems add challenge and complexity that astronomy and physics have not faced. Therefore, although health care may be considered a latecomer by some, the use of big data in health and health care is considered a new frontier and one that provides new opportunities and novel challenges. Indeed, big data are giving rise to what many refer to as the emerging "fourth paradigm data-driven science, where the scientific method is enhanced by the integration of significant data" (Fox & Hendler, 2014, p. 68). Health and health care stand as the edge of a remarkable area of data-driven opportunity. Big data analytics in health has therefore become an area of intense interest and a fertile area for exploration and research. This is particularly so for scholars who are interested in understanding complex and often covert relationships present in the ever-growing data collections related to health.

It is important to note, at inception, that big data science is not just about the physical size or velocity of data collections. It is inherently interwoven with the deep science surrounding the analysis of longitudinal, complex, and uncertain data from disparate and often secondary sources of messy unstructured records. Furthermore, big data—and the science that brings it to life—can be disconcerting to many, particularly those in health care. Providers are accustomed to making decisions based on internal knowledge, experience, intuition, and personal judgment rather than relying on protocols that are derived from the analysis of big data. Therefore, big data analytics in health care also has emotional/behavioral components.

Considering all of these dimensions, researchers in the health sciences have plentiful opportunities for new discoveries. How can we conceptualize and apply big data within the realm of nursing, team, and health sciences? How may data science, big or small, impact our practice and the outcomes of care? How can we capitalize on the availability of big data to reduce harm and customize treatment to patients, families, and communities? What might the data that are present in untapped and noisy collections of nontraditional data (i.e., social media) have to tell us? What unexpected contributors to outcomes of interest are hiding in data sets that have yet to be considered or unearthed? How will we deal with the inherent uncertainty in big data? How can we adapt our beliefs and our practices to accept the fourth paradigm of data-driven science into our worlds?

To begin to answer some of these questions, this chapter is focused on helping the reader to deepen his or her understanding of big data science and the implications of its application in health-related domains. This will be accomplished by providing a broad overview of big data, its value and importance, and the benefits and challenges, and by reviewing several common approaches. In reality, however, a full discussion of big data analytics can fill volumes of text books, far exceeding the scope of this work. This chapter, therefore, provides a set of basic and common approaches used in big data science and introduces some of the vocabulary that underpins this area of research. Those who wish to learn more about these techniques are directed to a variety of books that cover the field in much greater depth. The overall goal of this chapter is to stimulate creative thinking by scholars and scientists, as well as to encourage proactive involvement and leadership in this emerging and lucrative area of inquiry.

DEFINING BIG DATA AND ANALYTICS

Big data have been defined as "large volumes of high velocity, complex, and variable data that require advanced techniques and technologies to enable the capture, storage, distribution, management and analysis of the information" (Cottle, Kanwal, Kohn, Strome, & Treister, 2013, p. 1). Ward and Barker (2013, n.p.) assert that "Big Data is defined by a high degree of permutations and interactions within a dataset . . . big data is intrinsically related to data analytics and the discovery of meaning from data." These descriptions illustrate what may be the biggest challenge that has thwarted us from harnessing big data to this point—it lies in the massive complexity, continual variation, and the "messiness" of secondary data. Ward and Barker (2013, n.p.), however, make an important additional point: "Complex data doesn't need to be big. If you are analyzing a terabyte of data to determine the correlation between two fields, I would question whether you are really doing

Big Data analytics. However, if you are mining the inter-relationship of 100 variables in a sparsely populated data set that is 50MB, then you will need to push the envelope of data science to extract a useful insight." Ward and Barker's distinction is critically important and can help to distinguish true big data analytics.

To enable readers to conceptualize the size of big data, we can use information provided by Hersh et al. (2011), who assert that by 2020, health care data sets will exceed 25,000 petabytes. To bring this into practical perspective, a single petabyte is 10^{15} bytes of data or 1 million gigabytes. One petabyte is enough to store the DNA of the "entire population of the US—and then clone them, twice" or ". . . . if the average MP3 encoding for mobile is around 1MB per minute, and the average song lasts about four minutes, then a petabyte of songs would last over 2,000 years playing continuously" (McKenna, 2014, n.p.).

In the sense of big data, *analytics* has been defined by the IBM Institute for Business Value as "the systematic use of data and related business insights developed through applied analytical disciplines to drive fact-based decision making for planning, management, measurement and learning. Analytics may be descriptive, predictive or prescriptive" (Cortada, Gordon, & Lenihan, 2014, p. 2). Examples in which big data analytics are brought to bear on massive data collections are commonplace in many business sectors. Macy's (a large retail department store in the United States) uses big data analytics to process incoming data streams from inventory and point-of-sale systems, in near real time, to update prices for 73 million items at one time. United Healthcare uses very large collections of audio data from call center recordings to better predict customer dissatisfaction by using big data analytics to explore speech-to-text data (Laskowski, 2013). These brief examples may illustrate both the promises and the challenges inherent in big data, particularly when one considers the analytic and processing power that must be brought to bear on massive collections of data.

These definitions are not too far removed from traditional approaches, leaving one to question "what's new?" Data that are produced by health and health care–related sources are already known to be inherently big, complex, and challenging, and the analytic approaches used have always been fact based and used to drive improved decision making. Predictive, descriptive, or prescriptive analyses are not new. So one may ask, "What is different now?"

It is agreed that health-related data are considered by many to be big data already, particularly with the emergence of personalized medicine, genomics, sensor-based data collection, social networking for health, and the growth of the "Internet of Things" (IoT, a concept that is used to describe the massive digitization and interconnectedness of our lives). The goal of analytics, new or old, has always been for the purposes of discovering new things, finding areas for improvement or new development, and improving decision making. The difference arises when one considers the magnitude and availability of data that can influence the outcomes of any analysis or investigation. Traditional statistical techniques are unable to handle the size, complexity, multidimensionality, and uncertainty of big data. The manner in which data are represented, stored, and shared in health and health care is not sufficient for a world of big data. Therefore, not only is the size of data exponentially exploding, but so is the need to find new analytic techniques to wade through, and make sense of, nontraditional, error-prone, and frequently unstructured data. Data representation in digital sources is still suboptimal, and nursing data, in particular, is almost invisible (Keenan, 2014). New science will require an adjustment in the way we think about analysis and research, a point made clear in 2015 by various nursing leaders (Henly et al., 2015).

What Makes Data Big? Interest, Liquidity, and Boundaries

As alluded to earlier, the growth of the data sets is fueled partly due to large increases in data transparency, data accessibility, the "quantified self" movement, and the dawning awareness of the value hidden in disconnected and unconventional data sources. The term *data liquidity*, which is often used to describe this point, is defined as "data that is no longer confined to databases or data silos in supply chain management systems, financial systems, and health systems" (Courtney, 2011, p. 220). The federal government, payer systems, research and development firms, insurance companies, pharmaceutical companies, and many other industries are beginning to open large-scale databases, making the data liquid, accessible, and manipulable. This data liquidity has resulted in ever-growing digital collections of valuable information, recently referred to as a mother lode of opportunity for nurse researchers (Henly, 2014). In short, liquid data are data that are available for use "as is," no longer locked away in big data cemeteries.

The bigness of data is further enhanced as the boundaries that define the data of health and health care expand, and the new technologies and the data that originate from them become commonplace. For example, in the not-so-distant past, the use of social media data that arise from patient interactions (i.e., tweet streams, chat rooms, text messaging, etc.); sensor data collected from wearable or implantable devices such as FitBits, Apple Watch, and so forth; data from large-scale genomic, epigenomic, proteomic, and metabolic data collections; and information derived from point-of-sale systems in a local CVS were not necessarily viewed as data central to health and/or health care. The shift toward patient-centered care, patient self-management, and engagement combined with wearable sensors and social media has markedly accelerated health data generation. As the digitization of life continues to accelerate and the interconnectedness of these collections of data increases in value and density (the IoT), the power and appeal of big data becomes all the more apparent.

Big Data and the "Vs"

When would data be considered "big" and what are the characteristics of big data? One of the first conceptualizations associated with big data came from Laney (2001), who coined the three Vs of volume, velocity, and variety. Since that time, many others have added to the work of Laney. Hitzler and Janowicz (2013) speak to a compilation of five Vs: volume, velocity, variety, value, and veracity. Visualization and viability have been added recently, increasing the initial three Vs to seven, although many argue that visualization and viability are not sufficiently independent from the five suggested by Hitzler and Janowicz (2013). For the purposes of this chapter, the focus is on the five Vs of big data—volume, velocity, variety, value, and veracity—although visualization and viability should not be discounted.

Volume

Data volume, or the amount of data being stored, has increased markedly over time. Cheaper and faster ways to collect, store, and retrieve data has resulted in very large collections of highly dimensional data. The ability to exchange data across partners, customers, and stakeholders has also resulted in a "snowball effect," where in the process of data exchange and transmission, additional data are acquired along the way. For example, when claims data are merged with pharmacy records, drug codes may be persistently attached to the original claims data. Therefore, the data that *enter* may not be identical to the data that *exit*. As businesses and organizations begin to view data as a tangible asset, there is a growing hesitation to discard any of it. Therefore, the data volume continues to grow exponentially (Cortada et al., 2014).

Velocity

Data velocity, when used in the context of big data, has three dimensions: throughput, analysis, and rate of change. Primarily, velocity is most commonly associated with the speed or throughput of big data. Systems in which high-velocity data can be evidenced include monitoring systems in intensive care units (ICUs), streaming video, social media, sensors, and others. Such data are also referred to as *fast data*, *streaming data*, or *data in motion* and can comprise hundreds of thousands of events per second. Tweet streams, where users generate approximately 500,000 tweets every 10 minutes ("Internet Live Stats"), is a good example of high-velocity data, as they are collected by National Security Agency Signals Intelligence (SIGINT) Directorate. In 2012, SIGINT claimed to be taking in data at a rate of one terabyte of data per second—the equivalent of approximately 4.5 million 200-page books per second (Maass, 2015).

The second dimension of velocity refers to the real-time analytics and the powerful technology required to turn these rushing torrents of data into usable information. The speed and volume of data that originates from electro-physiological monitors 24 hours a day in an epilepsy monitoring unit illustrates analytic velocity. A continuous and rapid flow of dense data from a patient's EEG, EKG, pulse oximeter, other monitoring devices, and live video streams is routinely combined and processed in real time. The algorithms designed to extract, analyze, and convert the electrical signals into an interpretable visual representation are very challenging issues. Sampling and processing this type of data is challenging and likened to drinking from a fire hose (Abbott & Lee, 2005).

The third dimension of velocity involves the rate of constant change that is common in many very large collections of data. Values change, new collections of data are added and/or removed, pathways for connecting the data sources are altered, and the rate at which systems must respond to changes based on processing demands are in continual flux. The structures that must store, retrieve, and then process incoming high-velocity data, therefore, are also considered an element of velocity.

Variety

Variety, the third V of Laney's original conceptualization, reflects the increasing variety of data that is being tapped into for business intelligence and new knowledge discovery. Collections of previously unconnected data may illustrate relationships that were heretofore undetected. For example, combining point-of-sale data from the local Walgreens cash registers that show that the sales of antidiarrheal medication has spiked in the past 48 hours with the elementary school absentee data and with reports of increased sick leave from local employers can be used as an early indicator of a community outbreak of intestinal flu. In short, variety can be thought of as the combination of numerous, yet disparate, data collections to look for patterns and relationships between them. Variety in big data also refers, however, to how data in these collections are modeled, defined, and structured, as well as to the spatiotemporal dependencies that exist in those data. To illustrate this point, the large volumes of data generated by social networking and large collections of textual data are unstructured and nebulous in meaning. These types of data do not exist in neatly structured tables in which implications and relationships are generally understood, and the data have been collected for distinct purposes (such as research or billing). Instead, many large collections of big data are patient generated and plagued with quality issues such as incompleteness, error, faulty syntax, and misrepresentation. Variety, therefore, is more than just a consideration of the different assortments of sets that are joined not only in big data collections but also in the critical aspects of the underlying structure and meaning of big data.

Value

Value reflects the growing interest of big data as an organizational or practice asset, and the quest to extract insight and value from it. Because much of this data has been either too big or too inaccessible to analyze in the past, few organizations had the capacity to capitalize on it. As storage gets cheaper, processing power increases, and the perception of value increases, businesses are rapidly including big data analytics into short- and long-term planning. In a study titled "Industrial Internet Insights for 2015," from General Electric (GE) and Accenture (from the section of the analysis that dealt strictly with health care executives), the number one outcome from the use of big data analytics (44% of respondents) was the expectations of analytics to integrate a view of clinical, financial, and operational data (Accenture, 2014). Currently, these data are distributed across many disparate and disconnected systems that are internal and external to the organization, making a consolidated view nearly impossible. The second highest expectation of value to be gained cited by respondents was the ability to view integrated patient records (38%). The value in fully integrated collections of data that are needed to power high-quality, efficient, and personalized patient care is quite apparent.

As mentioned earlier, the number of Vs is expanding. The additional Vs of viability and visualization can be found in the current literature, although there is a degree of controversy in regards to continual additions and needless expansion. Anecdotally, blog postings seem to be discounting differentiation of viability and visualization, due to the beliefs of some that these dimensions are already contained within the other Vs. Other blog posts reflect a growing concern of the diffusion away from the initial core set of the three Vs posited by Laney in 2001. For scholars interested in conceptualization and model development around big data, the V discussion might be an interesting starting point for further inquiry.

Aside from the ongoing debate as to the number of Vs and their meaning, an additional perspective is worth mentioning. Interestingly, it appears that the intent of the analytics and the discipline applying it often dictate a focus on specific Vs.

For example, those involved in genomic data sets often describe their big data in terms of volume or size. People who are focused on live streaming data from a sensor-based system may be prone to describe big data in regards to the velocity (or throughput) of their data streams. Those in social sciences and humanities may be particularly focused on veracity, variety, and value. Why is this important? The rationale for including this is to emphasize the point that big data mean different things to different people, and that investigators often lose sight of the interconnectedness and "big picture" of the data and the methods used within it. Although it is true that different users and different applications may focus on a different "V," an important takeaway is that "at the end, all Vs have to be addressed in an interdisciplinary effort to substantially advance on the Big Data front" (Hitzler & Janowicz, 2013, p. 19). Likewise, knowledge of the language used in the field of big data is necessary. Table 5.1 lists some of the key terminology.

Veracity

The veracity of big data relates to the accuracy of the data and the degree of uncertainty that often accompanies it. As mentioned earlier, the variety and the velocity of the data create new challenges for real-time processing of the massive torrents of various types of "noisy" (also known as "dirty") data that become a part of big data collections. Veracity in big health-related data looms large in the minds of those who work to tame it. IBM (2015) asserts that poor data quality costs the U.S. economy $3.1 trillion a year, and that one in three business leaders do not trust the data based on which major organizational decisions are being made. Decisions made based on big data can drive life and death decisions, influence public policy, and drive clinical practice; therefore, accuracy and uncertainty are major areas of interest for those in the health sciences.

BIG DATA IN NURSING INQUIRY

Applying Classical Research Methods Versus New Innovative Methods

This area of inquiry is particularly valuable and important for nurse scholars, but it does require a willingness to embrace innovation and alternative, nontraditional methodologies. As many point out, such approaches challenge those who have been trained in classical scientific paradigms, and many graduate programs in U.S. schools of nursing are very slow in adapting to new science. Nursing Outlook contains several articles that make this point and call out for innovation in "e-science" for nurses (Henly, McCarthy, Wyman, Heitkemper, et al., 2015; Henly, McCarthy, Wyman, Stone, et al., 2015; Wyman & Henly, 2015). Wyman and Henly (2015), in particular, assert that nursing PhD programs are continuing to implement curricula better suited to the past, not the future, of nursing science. This may be related to the persistent focus of schools of nursing on *verification-based methods* compared with those that are considered *discovery driven*, both of which will be described later in this section.

How do big data threaten classical science paradigms? The answer is multifactorial; however, a primary issue relates to change, as big science challenges many of the foundational assumptions of traditional statistics. The complexity of health,

TABLE 5.1 Key Terminology

Association models	A method used to discover the probability of certain items co-occurring at a given time. Association modeling is commonly used in business to analyze purchasing patterns.
Big data	Defined by Cottle et al. (2013) as "large volumes of high velocity, complex, and variable data that require advanced techniques and technologies to enable the capture, storage, distribution, management and analysis of the information."
Big data life cycle	The life cycle of big data analytics consists of five general steps: (a) problem identification; (b) data extraction or acquisition; (c) data preprocessing [integration, cleaning, representation]; (d) analytics; and (e) interpretation and presentation.
Cluster analysis	An unsupervised approach to the analysis of big data, as the outcome is not known in advance and the algorithm is designed to find clusters of data that have some degree of similarity to one another.
Data liquidity	Data that have become "liquid" or accessible—no longer tied up in locked data warehouses or data cemeteries.
Data provenance	The process of tracing and recording the origins of data, how it was derived, and its movement between data sources.
Data visualization	Scientifically rigorous approaches to understanding and implementing visual representations that communicate information clearly and efficiently to users.
Descriptive analytics	A modeling approach often conducted post hoc that simply provides a description of the data, such as counts, percentages, averages, and sums, all of which can help convert massive data into understandable chunks of information.
Discovery-driven approaches	A term used to describe methods that sift through large collections of data to discover patterns and trends that may or may not be expected. Also referred to as a data-driven approach.
External model validation	When the prediction model derived from the internal model validation process is tested against unseen and novel data and performs accurately. The level of accuracy has various definitions.
Internal model validation	A measure of model accuracy related to its ability to discriminate between different outcomes and to illustrate the level of agreement (or calibration) between predicted and observed outcomes in groups with similar profiles.
IoT	A virtual network of fixed and mobile digitally interconnected devices and sensors that use machine-to-machine communication in the cloud. Massive data are being generated every second by the IoT.
Petabyte	A measurement of data size that equals 10^{15} bytes of data or 1 million gigabytes.
Predictive analytics	A method that creates probabilistic forecast models of what *may* happen in the future. A common example is a time series or trend model, in which data from the past are used to predict how data may behave in the future.

(*continued*)

TABLE 5.1 Key Terminology (*continued*)	
Semantic web	Defined by Berners-Lee to represent a futuristic, web-based, massive collection of information from disparate locations and formats integrated into one unified application.
Value	An estimation of the worth of big data as an organizational or practice asset.
Variety	A reflection of different types of data that may be utilized in big data analytics. The types can be in different formats and disconnected from each other. Interesting new findings may emerge, but there may be many spurious relationships.
Veracity	Relates to the accuracy of the data and the degree of uncertainty that often accompanies it.
Velocity	A measure of the speed of the data flow. It has three dimensions that can be measured: throughput, analysis, and rate of change.
Verification-based approaches	A term that generally refers to traditional analytic methods that are hypothesis driven. The goal is to "verify" the postulate.
Volume	A measure of the amount of data that are being stored. Often, this is not static due to the snowball effect.

IoT, Internet of Things.

the size and character of the data sets, and the impact from innumerable variables quickly overwhelm traditional methods, driving necessary innovation. Buchan, Winn, and Bishop (2009, p. 93) make the point that classical approaches are being increasingly challenged: "hypothesis-driven research and reductionist approaches to causality have served health science well in identifying the major independent determinants of health and the outcomes of individual health care interventions. But they do not reflect the complexity of health." Swan (2009, p. 492) adds further to this point:

> The ways of science are also changing, both in how it is being conducted and in who is conducting it. The historical notion of science consisted of investigating and enumerating physical phenomena and doing hypothesis-driven trial and error experimentation. An evolving notion of science adds additional steps to the traditional method to create a virtuous feedback loop.

Finally, and as mentioned at the very beginning of this chapter, big data is not just about size and speed—they are about innovation, uncertainty, change, and culture. Change is difficult, particularly among cultures that were trained in the traditional science paradigms and that have always relied heavily on personal judgment and expertise to drive practice.

What makes big data science so different? Why are these approaches seen as so disruptive? Prior to embarking on such a discussion, it is necessary to note that there is not a major line of demarcation where traditional approaches and big data approaches stop and start. In reality, there is some degree of intermixing, and a schooled understanding of research methods is critical to the outcome of either approach. As pointed out in a critically important paper by Kaplan, Chambers, and Glasgow (2014), large sample sizes do not automatically result in more meaningful results and caution is warranted in the interpretation of big data. Measurement error can be potentiated in big data in which veracity is unknown, and in which mathematical maximization can, and will, exaggerate effect sizes and correlations (Kaplan et al., 2014). Studies conducted under the auspices of big data analytics are also more prone to errors of measurement, aggregation, and sampling. Large amounts of missing data or data that have been abstracted or "rolled up" can lead to illusions of reality where none exists. Therefore, those who approach big data science without the requisite understanding of complex methodological processes that underpin it incur the risk of conducting and then potentiating bad science. This argument, based in the foundations of classic research methods, should not be taken as a reason to avoid innovative approaches to working with big data. Instead, it should be viewed as a way to parlay the basics of traditional methods into areas of pioneering research and discovery.

Verification Versus Discovery Approaches

How are the classical approaches conceptualized differently from those used in big data analytics? Traditional analytic methods are generally hypothesis driven or "verification-based approaches," whereas big data approaches are often said to be data or discovery driven. In general traditional approaches, the suspected contributors to the aspect being studied are isolated and analytic tools are used to either prove or refute the original postulate. Such approaches require that the investigator has a very deep understanding of the obvious and nonobvious characteristics in the data set that can affect the outcome. The investigator must be able to then interpret the outcome and understand enough about the data to pose iterative questions to further refine the analysis. The efficiency and effectiveness of such an approach is affected by the nature of the data, the ability of the investigator to fully grasp the implications of the data and to then reframe questions, to add or remove variables, and to compose complex queries in the attempt to answer the research question within the given data set. Many traditional approaches are structured to limit the dimensionality of the data, so as to prevent multicollinearity or variance inflation issues (the many variables small N issue). Data sets used with traditional approaches are often static in nature and clean. Finally, in most verification-based approaches, the focus is on the variables that are expected to emerge (those that were hypothesized). Outliers are frequently viewed as variables that invalidate the proposed model.

In contrast, a discovery-driven approach is one in which the unexpected is valued rather than frowned on and hypotheses are not explicitly stated. Using these types of discovery or data-driven approaches has been referred to as "letting the data speak," which is accomplished by using techniques that sift through very large collections of data, looking for patterns, correlations, and exceptions. These types of approaches are of great value when used in massive nonlinear and non-monotonic data collections. In discovery-driven approaches, the majority of the analytics are handled by machines, but directed by humans. As detailed earlier, however, discovery-based approaches can face serious challenges. It would seem as though the effort saved by automated data extraction, transformation, and analysis can exact a considerable price on human assessment, interpretation, and confidence in outcomes. Additionally, although the emergence of patterns and correlations may initially catch the investigator's eye, this is just the tip of the iceberg in regards to the analytic process of discovery. It is contingent on the investigator to also create the robust models that help us describe, interpose, and replicate the findings.

Finally, an interesting diversion that is occurring within the realm of big data deals with the prior assertions that the tools used in big data analytics were considered separate from the data on which they were used (Abbott & Lee, 2005). With the emergence of the fourth paradigm of research, this appears to be changing as data-intensive science permeates traditional computational science. Contemporary views are that data science is an inextricable weaving of massive data with tools, algorithms, and structures that facilitate the focus on the discovery of new knowledge instead of on the information technology that enables it. In short, big data science supports data federation and collaboration—automating the conversion of highly unstructured and noisy data into useable collections of analyzable variables. It would appear as though the boundaries between the data and the tools are becoming less certain, hence the divergence from prior beliefs. Big data science is quickly changing many tenets that were once considered true and unshakeable.

METHODS, TOOLS, AND PROCESSES USED WITH BIG DATA WITH RELEVANCE TO NURSING

Although it may be theoretically and conceptually interesting to debate the fourth paradigm of research and to consider focusing simply on collections of federated data that exist for the purpose of data-driven research, it is always advisable for any researcher to know where his or her data came from (provenance) and what a particular data element "means." This is not to imply that every nurse scholar must also become a data scientist. That would take years of focused study and application. However, a scholar who wants to interact in the world of big data science must understand the process of how data are captured, curated, and analyzed (Bell, 2009). National Institutes of Health (NIH), as part of their Big Data to Knowledge (BD2K) efforts in February 2013, addressed this matter by issuing a Request for Information (RFI; NIH, 2015). This RFI was targeted to gather information from the scientific community regarding the basic levels of understanding and skills needed for scientists to thrive in an era of big data. The results from that RFI were then used to create several big data boot camps, which were designed to provide the foundations of big data science to the research community.

The RFI also resulted in guiding principles for big data analytics in the health sciences. Of particular importance to the readers of this chapter, the following statement is central, calling for

> closely-collaborating scientists who are experts in their domain but also cross-trained, so that they can form high-functioning teams. There is a need to develop both human-focused and technical skills, the latter including skills in three basic categories: (1) statistics and math, (2) computation and informatics, and (3) a domain (e.g., biomedical, behavioral, clinical) science. (NIH, 2015, p. 1)

An important takeaway from the results of the RFI is the assertion that success in big data science will come *not* just from advanced technical knowledge and skills. The dimensions of human-based competencies such as collaboration, communication, domain knowledge, team-based cooperation, and ethics are given equal weight.

Therefore, as we begin to focus in on methods, techniques, and approaches, one should not lose the equally important aspects of human behavior in big data science and the major contributions that nurse scientists can bring. Indeed, Henly views big data science as a tremendous opportunity for nurse researchers to extend their reach in an era of big (and often personalized) data as domain experts, team collaborators, methodologists, and advocates of "a person-centered science of health" (Henly, 2014, p. 155). Snijders, Matzat, and Reips (2012, p. 1) sum this important point up quite eloquently in discussing big data science: "this stream of research has provided useful insights, but also suffers from some serious limitations. The interesting point is that these limitations can (and have to) be addressed by theory guided research that is typically conducted by social scientists. Accordingly, opportunities emerge for those social and behavioral scientists who are willing to collaborate with the Big Data researchers in the natural, engineering, and computer sciences."

Methods and Approaches

Foundational to discussions of methods and approaches is the discussion of the life cycle of big data. As detailed earlier in the discussion of the Vs, those involved in big data may describe their interest in this sphere of science as focused on the volume, the velocity, or the variability. Others think of big data analytics from the perspective of the analytic approach that will be used to digest reams of data into usable information. However, as alluded to earlier, good science is generated by those who understand the what, the where, the why, and the when—therefore, understanding the life cycle of the data used in the analysis is crucial. Complex analytic techniques are only as good as the data that they are used on, and a heavy reliance is placed on the knowledge of those conducting the analysis and interpreting the results. As mentioned earlier, big data are noisy, error prone, often incomplete, and often abstracted. An investigator who does not understand the domain relevance of the results, those with a blind focus on the analysis phase of big data, or a clinician who understands the relevancy but is not skilled in data acquisition or manipulation, or is ignorant of provenance creates a petri dish for spuriosity. Big data science requires a collaborative team with distributed expertise.

Understanding the Life Cycle of Big Data

The life cycle of big data analytics consists of five general steps: (a) problem identification; (b) data extraction or acquisition; (c) data preprocessing (integration, cleaning, representation); (d) analytics; and (e) interpretation and presentation (Abbott & Lee, 2005; Jagadish et al., 2014). During the entire process, it is possible to return to any of the previous steps for further iteration, as reflected in Figure 5.1.

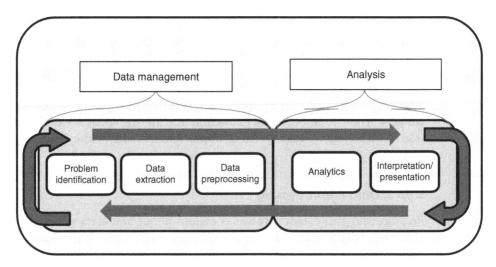

Figure 5.1 Big data life cycle.
Adapted from Abbott and Lee (2005) and Jagadish et al. (2014).

Step 1: Problem Identification

The initial step of working with big data entails the development of an *understanding of the domain problem*, the relevant prior knowledge, and the goals of the analysis. Big data appear at times to be all things to all people, whereas in reality, intense focus and domain understanding is crucial. For example, prior to drilling for oil or natural gas, drilling companies study the topography, history of prior successes, and failures in similar explorations; rely on experts in the field; and consider the costs and potential benefits of a given exploration before moving forward. This prevents a drilling rig from being set up in the middle of Grand Central Terminal. Due diligence is necessary to prevent "fishing," and a great deal of wasted time and effort in the hopes that something will emerge. This analogy is carried over to big data analytics in the health sciences as well. Blindly fishing for relationships or "data dredging" without requisite understanding of the domain is poor science. As data get bigger, the chances of mathematical maximization increase exponentially and patterns may emerge that are totally irrelevant to the problem under investigation. Case in point, Leinweber's (2009) work in big data illustrated that the production of butter in Bangladesh, combined with cheese production in the United States and the number of sheep in Bangladesh and the United States, was able to explain 99% of the variation in the S&P 500 over a 10-year period. Such ridiculous results are easily found if enough big data are combined and mined.

Step 2: Data Extraction

The *data extraction process* includes selecting data aggregations with variables focusing on the topic to be explored. Investigations will come up short if the variables of interest are not present in the data collections, or if they are so noisy, incomplete, or untrustworthy that the results are questionable. No analytic engine can find what does not exist, and dubious data can result in outcomes such as the widely discounted Google Flu Trends results of 2013 (Lazer, Kennedy, King, & Vespignani, 2014). Data exploration techniques are often used during this phase of the life cycle to examine the data prior to analysis—using techniques from simple histograms and frequencies to more complex, statistically oriented exploratory data analysis techniques for complex n-dimensional data. Such techniques may alert the researcher of data sparseness or error in a particular dimension that would warrant additional data extraction. Identifying adequacy of the data extraction result reemphasizes the critical importance of domain knowledge and research basics.

Step 3: Data Preprocessing

Preprocessing these data involves decisions about how data will be represented, cleaned, and integrated across collections. Preprocessing the data enables the investigators to study the impact of outliers and noise on the data set, and to decide on strategies for handling missing data fields and error. Also, in this step, dimension reduction or transformation methods are considered to reduce the effective number of variables under consideration. For example, if the focus of the inquiry is related to the presence or absence of hypertensive disease in general, then a researcher may want to compress all of the 50 ± International Classification of Diseases (ICD)-9 codes included in hypertensive disease categories 401 to 405 into a single variable that represents a simple presence or absence of hypertensive disease.

The process of data integration, particularly when considering the principles of the fourth research paradigm of big data, can be viewed as both a tremendous opportunity and a potential quagmire. As noted earlier, big data are not neat, and they are presented in a variety of formats. Audio files, image files, handwritten material, tweets, waveforms, and so forth require transformation to make them understandable and computable. Large contingents of scientists working in the big data space are developing data-cleaning algorithms, transformation engines, and various tools to eventually create a common framework in which both the rules for reasoning about the data and the data themselves can be shared and reused. Berners-Lee, Hendler, and Lassila (2001) coined the term *Semantic Web* to represent a futuristic web-based massive collection of information from disparate locations and formats integrated into one unified application. In 2015, 14 years after Berners-Lee et al.'s seminal work, we are seeing a markedly increased focus in this area. NIH's BD2K initiative and the building of the NIH Big Data Science "Commons" are two examples and they can be reviewed at https://datascience.nih.gov/bd2k. The take-away point in regards to data preprocessing is that big data science is moving toward the ambitious goal of having data sets that are open, available, and able to be preprocessed (or deconstructed) in a way that increases their rigor and reliability.

Step 4: Analytics

The analytics step includes choosing the modeling objective of the analysis (description, prediction, association, or clustering), selecting the algorithm to be used to best achieve the objective, and actively investigating the algorithm results for interesting patterns. Each of these modeling objectives will be briefly described next. The modeling objective dictates the algorithm, as different techniques and tools will produce different results, and it is not unusual for more than one model to be tested. The simplistic examples and explanations provided next are very limited in scope due to space considerations. Interested readers are referred to detailed analytic texts that provide deeper explanations, such as Maheshwari (2014).

Descriptive analytics is considered the most straightforward form of modeling, is generally conducted post hoc, and provides the investigator with a snapshot of the data. Descriptive analytics in health care may inform the researcher of how many visits to the emergency department (ED) occurred over a given period, how many posts came in on a given Twitter feed, the number of patients with a preserved ejection fraction of greater than 50% the age range of the sample, and so forth. In short, descriptive analytics are counts, percentages, averages, and sums, all of which can help convert massive data into some understandable chunks of information. Though a seemingly simplistic modeling objective, the compilations of data that are becoming available will allow researchers to access massive volumes of population-wide data for purposes of description. Gaining a deeper understanding of the characteristics of a given population opens new doors for intervention and further analysis.

Predictive analytics is used to create probabilistic forecast models of what *may* happen in the future. A common example is a time series or trend model in which data from the past are used to predict how data may behave in the future. Similar to weather forecasting, known data are used to project—given similar circumstances such as wind, humidity, temperature, and wind patterns—what the weather may be over the next 24 to 48 hours. As anyone who has planned an outside event based on a weather forecast has experienced, it is an imprecise science. Predictive analytics is, however, not constrained to time series data. Predictive analytics is also used to develop models of risk and probabilities; therefore, it can be applied prospectively. In general, prediction models are developed by analyzing a set of representative data in which the outcome of interest is already known. The chosen algorithm is applied to the data with the goal of identifying elements that have the strongest predictive value in relation to the known outcome, such as a diagnosis of cancer, the risk of a fall, participation in risk-taking behaviors, and so forth.

In a very simple example of predictive modeling in the analysis step, we can use the example of predicting admission from a long-term care (LTC) facility to an acute care facility. The data sets may include the LTC Minimum Data Set (MDS); the Online Survey, Certification, and Reporting (OSCAR) data set; and a set of inpatient claims files from potential acute care facilities. These sets combined could result in more than 2,000 variables per patient at a given moment in time and contain thousands of individual patients. The outcome variable of "admitted yes or no" can be obtained by matching a documented admission to an acute care facility from the local facility inpatient claims files to an LTC patient in the data set. The outcome variable for a given patient during a specific period is now known and can be used to train the prediction algorithm. The entire data set is then randomly divided equally into a training set and a testing set (also known as a holdout set). The holdout or testing set is specifically removed from the analysis altogether to test the model developed in the training set.

Using a supervised learning approach (called supervised because the outcome is known in advance and provided to the modeler), the predictive algorithm begins to sift through the training data set to look for underlying characteristics from the data sets that are associated with the outcome of "admission" across patients. The accuracy of the model is related to its ability to discriminate between patients with different outcomes (admitted vs. not admitted) and to illustrate the level of agreement (or calibration) between predicted and observed outcomes in groups of individuals with similar profiles. If the algorithm "converges" and is able therefore to produce a set of characteristics (or a "model") across all of the training data that accurately predict admission, the model is considered *internally validated*. However, internal validation in and of itself is insufficient.

A second step of *external validation* is required, in which the prediction model derived in the internal validation process is tested against the holdout set of the untouched data. If the internally validated prediction model is able to perform accurately on the holdout data set, then the model is considered externally validated. One can then use the validated model to prospectively (in similar data) predict admission or to quantify levels of risk for admission. Models such as this are used to intervene a priori in the goal to improve outcomes. Familiar prediction models in the health care domain include severity of illness (SOI) tools such as the Acute Physiology and Chronic Health Evaluation (APACHE) scoring system, the Simplified Acute Physiology Score (SAPS), and the Mortality Probability Model (MPM; Lee & Maslove, 2015).

Association models are used to discover the probability of certain items co-occurring at a given time. Association modeling was the method most commonly associated with the world of business and was often used to analyze purchasing patterns. Market basket analysis is an example of an association model in which point-of-sales data are analyzed to detect items that are frequently purchased at the same time. For example, an association model may detect that the purchase of a new suit is strongly associated with the purchase of a new tie. From a business perspective, this association factor may influence product placement (a rack of ties is located very close to the checkout counter), when associated items should be discounted (or not), and how to influence behaviors based on their association with other factors. In health care, an association model might detect that patients who visit the website affiliated with a weight management clinic are 60% likely to search for healthy diet plans. A practitioner may use that knowledge to ensure that an obvious and easy-to-use link exists on the website to direct patients to vetted healthy-eating sites. Business has already capitalized greatly with association analytics; one only needs to look at Amazon, where suggestions for other purchases based on a profile of buyers similar to oneself are offered to entice additional purchasing behaviors.

Cluster analysis is an example of an unsupervised approach to the analysis of big data, as the outcome is not known in advance and the algorithm is designed to find clusters of data that have some degree of similarity to one another. Although clustering may not perfectly describe groups or clusters, a measure of success in clustering is when members of a group or cluster have more in common with each other than with members of another cluster or group. A robust example of clustering analysis in pediatric asthmatic patients resulted in significant clinical implications (Fitzpatrick et al., 2011). This study identified four distinct clusters of asthmatic children with distinct phenotypes that did not fit within the current defined guidelines of asthma severity. Each cluster contained severely asthmatic children; however, the current guidelines for asthma severity determination based on lung function requirements (extrapolated from adult reference norms) were believed to be overly restrictive. The benefits of the clustering approach in this example allowed researchers to cluster patients based on phenotypical presentations, and to avoid the inherent bias introduced by using the current asthma severity scoring mechanism.

Step 5: Interpretation and Presentation

Interpreting and presenting the results is dependent on the intended user of the output. The results may be intended for immediate human consumption, for other automated systems, or for the use of the system that actually produced the results. In using the first case of immediate human consumption, interpretation and presentation may come in the form of visualizations, natural language outputs, decision support rules or suggestions, and others. If the result emerging from the analysis is an algorithm that is fed into another automated system, the output could be additional lines of a programming code. If the results are intended to be fed directly back into the system from which they emerged, they are considered domain knowledge (something that was learned and validated) and must be presented and structured as such. In the latter case, a system is said to be gaining intelligence—in short, it is making itself smarter. In essence, interpretation and presentation is highly dependent on the receiver.

Although it is easy to agree that humans cannot process and interpret high-velocity data streams, simply conducting a big data analysis does not guarantee that the output is automatically more interpretable or usable. Results that emerge can be nebulous, confusing, and sometimes contradictory. Therefore, many scientists interested in human perception and visualization find ample opportunity for study and work in this phase of analytics. Visualization, for example, focuses on techniques that can help people see patterns and effects that were not obvious to them earlier, even in overwhelming large collections of data. An excellent example of interpretation and presentation of big data using visualization techniques can be found on a commercial website called Name Voyager (www.babynamewizard.com/voyager). This site derives first names from Social Security records (beginning in 1900) and utilizes a unique visualization exploration method that allows individuals to explore U.S. naming trends (Wattenberg, 2005). Arcia and colleagues provide an excellent overview of how data visualizations can be used to present information to patients, families, and communities to influence health behavior (Arcia, Bales, Brown, & Manuel, 2013). In this study, specifically focused on low-literacy patients, specific visualizations were created and tested as a method of presenting usable and comprehendible information back to the target group. As is common to generalized statistical models, many other types of visualizations are used to explain results—cluster diagrams, scatterplots, tree maps, regression lines, heat maps, and so forth—all of which use visuals in order to aid interpretation.

Interpreting the results of a big data analysis can be challenging. An often cited concern of big data analytics is how to study and interpret without interjecting bias. Data that have been cleaned, processed, massaged, and manipulated are no longer a source of truth, if in reality they ever were. Data observations are subject to time and maturity threats, which, in turn, can affect the generalizability of the models developed during the process. Big data are dynamic and although some data remain constant over time (e.g., personal identifier, gender), much data either vary over time and place (e.g., weight, age, disease severity) or are influenced by surroundings (e.g., heart rate, lung function). Centers for Disease Control and Prevention (CDC) surveillance of flu trends will vary from month to month as new strains of virus ebb and flow; therefore, the models used and the interpretations of output are extremely temporal in nature.

Interpretation can also be impacted by data that have been abstracted. For example, repeated measurements can be clustered, averaged, and recorded as a summary score; therefore, the true data measurements are no longer available. The example provided earlier in the discussion of dimensionality reduction using hypertensive ICD-9 codes illustrates this point. Although the goal of the analysis under prior discussion regarding the ICD-9 codes was only interested in the presence or absence of hypertensive disease, once the data were "rolled-up" or summarized into a simple yes or no answer, the ability to delve deeper is lost (unless the raw data were retained). If the only data retained in the data set are the abstracted Yes or No, the next investigator cannot deconstruct the Yes or No variable to determine which ICD-9 codes were included.

In discussing data that emerge from electronic health records (EHRs), similar interpretation and presentation issues can be found. Parsons, McCullough, Wang, and Shih (2012) assessed the validity of quality measures and discovered disappointingly low levels of practice performance regarding mammography. Markedly few final reports of mammography findings were found after the data extraction and analysis. On closer examination, the issue was related to the structure of mammography results, which were in the form of a PDF file (an image) and therefore not a part of structured data stored in the EHR. Because image files are stored separately, they were not extracted during the data acquisition phase, and, therefore, appeared to be missing. This particular example emphasizes several points made earlier in this chapter that have a great impact on the interpretation of results from big data analytics. Domain expertise on the analytics team and the awareness of the varying standards of data representation resulted in a second look at the manner in which mammography results were recorded in the patient records. What could have been presented as a major failing by the medical staff to follow up on mammography results and poor adherence to practice standards was corrected by astute and thoughtful researchers who discovered the missing mammography results in appended PDF files.

EXAMPLES FROM THE PUBLISHED LITERATURE

Although nursing has not joined in on a large scale to big data analytics, there have been a series of nurses who were active in this space before big data was popular. Two current examples are provided next as examples of the application of this technique to nursing/health care research. A search of the literature will undoubtedly reveal many additional citations.

Example 1: Content Mining of Big Data Available Through Tweet Streams

Yoon, Elhadad, and Bakken (2013) described a method of content mining in big data to analyze tweet streams and to illustrate an application of this method to the study of physical activity. Understanding health behaviors such as physical activity in real-time life is difficult, because these behaviors are influenced by multiple factors and understanding the interactions is complex. According to Yoon et al., tweets can provide a source of real-time, real-word data about health behaviors, because Twitter users are able to, simultaneously and spontaneously, report their current activity and the characteristics of activity (e.g., location, social surroundings) in real time. Tweet streams are an example of big data, and they possess many of the "V" characteristics that make the analysis challenging.

To increase the understanding of physical activity, Yoon et al. (2013) conducted a content mining procedure, including these five steps: (a) selecting keywords; (b) importing data; (c) preparing data; (d) analyzing data; and (e) interpreting data. In the first step, they identified 17 diverse activities as the key terms for extraction of tweets to create the analytic corpus. A large collection of anonymized tweets were imported, and by searching the selected keywords and a data corpus, the tweet data set was created. In the next time-consuming step, the researchers supervised the text cleaning (automated), which removed all nonstandard characters and symbols. In the preparation step, the researchers also supervised the generation of attributes as text was transformed, and they reduced the dimensionality of a data set through attribute selection. At this point, the tweets' text corpus was ready for data analyses.

The frequencies of terms in tweets related to physical activity were obtained. Two-dimensional graphs about the frequently occurring terms and three-dimensional motion charts about the data trends over time were created. A clustering algorithm was used to summarize physical activity tweet content, and a sentiment analysis (which reflects any emotion associated with a variable) was conducted to categorize tweets as positive or negative in nature. The last step was to interpret data and make the decision regarding the sufficiency of the model. The content-mining process was repeated until the model converged (determined to be sufficient), and the results were interpreted.

Through these content-mining steps, Yoon et al. (2013) reduced the corpus from 174,394 to 31,489 tweeted terms related to physical activity. The researchers found the tweet content varied by specific physical activity, changed over time, and was mostly reflective of positive attitudes toward exercise. The tweet data set was very rich. In addition to the data of interest, the researchers also found data related to specific physical activities such as the duration of exercise, miles run, and intensity of activity. These additional findings added extra and unexpected depth to the findings. Yoon et al.'s study supported the applicability of tweets as a useful source of timely health behavior data, and it led them to believe that the data, patterns, and sentiments detected from tweets can be used to develop stronger and more targeted health behavior interventions as a longer term goal.

Example 2: Applying Big Data Analytics to the Outcome and Assessment Information Set Data Set

Westra, Bliss, Savik, Hou, and Borchert (2013) conducted a study to evaluate the prevalence, incidence, and effectiveness of home health care (HHC) agencies' services with and without wound, ostomy, and continence (WOC) nurses. Although the effectiveness of advanced practice nurses (APNs) with formal advanced degrees was known, few studies examined the effectiveness of nurses with specialty certifications that required additional certified education but not an advanced degree (such as WOC nurses). The research team evaluated the prevalence and incidence of six conditions (pressure ulcers, stasis ulcers, surgical wounds, urinary incontinence, bowel incontinence, and urinary tract infections [UTIs]) in 785 HHC agencies, examining whether the presence or absence of a WOC nurse could serve as a predictor of the prevalence or incidence of any of these six conditions. The team also used the presence or absence of a WOC as a predictor of improvement and/or stabilization of these six conditions. Using the Outcome and Assessment Information Set (OASIS) data set and a short Internet survey, the research team analyzed approximately 450,000 episodes of care across the participating Health and Human Services (HHS). The researchers then used various methods to preprocess the data, run exploratory data analysis, and, eventually, transform the data set into a reasonable collection of material for final analysis (Westra et al., 2013).

This study, using a large set of data, is an example of a descriptive analysis, in that the characteristics of the patients that emerged illuminated the prevalence and incidence of the six conditions and painted an interesting picture of the patient population overall. The second part of the study resulted in a model that illustrated that most of the HHC agencies with WOC nurses had lower levels of incidence of incontinence, wounds, and UTIs than those without WOC nurses. Significant improvements in outcomes and stabilization outcomes for pressure ulcers, surgical wounds, urinary incontinence, bowel incontinence, and UTIs were also found in HHC agencies with WOC nurses as a result of this analysis (Westra et al., 2013).

This study is an excellent real-world example of the difficulties that can be encountered when working with big data and is also reflective of the current state of nursing research with big data. A critical appraisal of this study will illustrate the intense amount of manual manipulation and error checking that was required, the need for physical effort to transform variables into usable data, and overlapping and conflicting measurements that confounded the model building.

Comparison of Approaches Used in the Two Examples

In comparison with the Yoon study, the Westra study is more reflective of a blended approach in which traditional and more manual techniques combined with elements of big data analytics were used. A further area of discrimination between the two studies exists in the methods used and in the results of the studies. With its focus on descriptive analytics, the Westra et al. (2013) study describes the data and provides the implications for use of the findings in a more traditional sense. Yoon et al. (2013) provided deeper meaning and modeling expertise that can be replicated and reapplied for those interested in this technique.

In regards to the analytic approaches used, Yoon et al. (2013) utilized content-mining techniques that, though still requiring manual manipulation to some degree, can be handled by specific tools that are designed to directly work with textual data. For example, Yoon et al. used "find and replace" functions to remove punctuation; they used N-gram approaches to transform text into features. The selection of attributes for the analysis was handled by automated routines for removing "stop words" (those that bring no value to an analysis such as "to," "and," "it," etc.) and stemming control (i.e., removing "ing" from the word "exercising," so that the attribute is simply "exercise"). Approaches of this sort are an indicator of the direction in which big data analytics will move. As discussed much earlier in this chapter, although the human cannot be replaced in analysis and interpretation of big data, there is a large push to automate and remove the burden of requiring researchers to immerse themselves in massive data collections to manually manipulate them. Manual approaches do not scale, a point realized some time ago by some data scientists.

SUMMARY

This chapter focuses on introducing the concepts and techniques of big data science and on illustrating its application in health-related domains. An overview of several key data science terms were provided to assist with gaining a deeper understanding of this rapidly expanding field. The case is made regarding the opportunities for scholars interested in capitalizing on the emerging fourth paradigm of data-driven science. Finally, the point was made that the complexity of big data science requires a team approach, where domain science, statistics, computation, and informatics must work together to discover reliable relationships in large, messy, and often secondary collections of data.

Returning to the beginning of this chapter, the following questions were posed: How can we conceptualize and apply big data within the realm of nursing, team, and health sciences? How may data science, big or small, impact our practice and the outcomes of care? How can we capitalize on the availability of big data to reduce harm and customize treatment to patients, families, and communities? What might the data that are present in untapped and noisy collections of non-traditional data (i.e., social media) have to tell us? What unexpected contributors to outcomes of interest are hiding in data sets that have yet to be considered or unearthed? How will we deal with the inherent uncertainty in big data? How can we adapt our beliefs and our practices to accept the fourth paradigm of data-driven science into our worlds? Each of these questions awaits concerted effort to be answered. Today's scholars stand at incredible opportunity intersections or as Henly (2014) says, "the mother lode of opportunity for nurse researchers."

Answering these questions will require that we begin to think differently, adopt new approaches to research, and open our minds and educational structures to critically prepare for our digitally transforming health industry. Of vital importance is a deep understanding of the pros and cons of big data and fully acknowledging the caveats and limitations of big, disparate, and noisy collections of data. The literature is replete with examples of spurious and silly findings that have emerged from big data analyses—emphasizing the criticality of rigor and distributed expertise within teams. We know from the literature that large samples do not necessarily result in more meaningful results, and woe will come to those who do not understand this fundamental truth. Provenance matters. At the same time, this cannot and should not dissuade nurse researchers from engaging directly and immediately in big data science. Instead, investigators should parlay theory-guided, known, and traditional approaches into pioneering, rigorous research. Ultimately, the contributions of clinical scholars are vital to the emerging fourth paradigm of data-driven science. This author is convinced that the hidden data can be used to change the life of a single patient, a village, a region, or the world. It requires awareness, expertise, and understanding. This calls to mind the statement of Louis Pasteur (1854), who said, "Dans les champs de l'observation le hasard ne favorise que les esprits prepares" or "Chance favors only the prepared mind." Be prepared, capitalize, excel, and use your knowledge to change our world.

REFERENCES

Abbott, P. A., & Lee, S. (2005). Data mining & knowledge discovery. In V. M. K. Saba (Ed.), *Essentials of nursing informatics* (pp. 469–479). New York, NY: McGraw Hill.

Accenture. (2014). Industrial Internet Insights for 2015. Retrieved from http://www.ge.com/digital/sites/default/files/industrial-internet-insights-report.pdf

Arcia, A., Bales, M., Brown, I., & Manuel, C. (2013). *Method for the development of data visualizations for community members with varying levels of health literacy.* Paper presented at the AMIA Annual Symposium Proceedings.

Bell, G. (2009). Forward. In T. Hey, S. Tansley, & K. Tolle (Eds.), *The fourth paradigm: Data intensive scientific discovery* (pp. xi–xvii). Redmond, WA: Microsoft Research.

Berners-Lee, T., Hendler, J., & Lassila, O. (2001). The semantic web. *Scientific American, 284,* 34–43. doi:10.1038/scientificamerican0501-34

Buchan, I., Winn, J., & Bishop, C. (2009). A unified modeling approach to data-intensive healthcare. In T. Hey, S. Tansley, & K. Tolle (Eds.), *The fourth paradigm: Data-intensive scientific discovery* (pp. 91–98). Redmond, WA: Microsoft Research.

Cortada, J. W., Gordon, D., & Lenihan, B. (2014). *The value of analytics in healthcare: From insights to outcomes.* IBM. Retrieved from http://www.ibm.com/smarterplanet/global/files/the_value_of_analytics_in_healthcare.pdf

Cottle, M., Kanwal, S., Kohn, M., Strome, T., & Treister, N. (2013). *Transforming health care through big data strategies for leveraging big data in the health care industry.* Institute for Health Technology Transformation. Retrieved from http://ihealthtran.com/big-data-in-healthcare

Courtney, P. K. (2011). Data liquidity in health information systems. *Cancer Journal, 17*(4), 219–221. doi:10.1097/PPO.0b013e3182270c83

Fitzpatrick, A. M., Teague, W. G., Meyers, D. A., Peters, S. P., Li, X., Li, H., . . . Moore, W. C. (2011). Heterogeneity of severe asthma in childhood: Confirmation by cluster analysis of children in the NIH/NHLBI Severe Asthma Research Program (SARP). *Journal of Allergy and Clinical Immunology, 127*(2), 382–389. e381–313. doi:10.1016/j.jaci.2010.11.015

Fox, P., & Hendler, J. (2014). The science of data science. *Big Data, 2*(2), 68–70.

Henly, S. J. (2014). Mother lodes and mining tools: Big data for nursing science. *Nursing Research, 63*(3), 155.

Henly, S. J., McCarthy, D. O., Wyman, J. F., Heitkemper, M. M., Redeker, N. S., Titler, M. G., . . . Dunbar-Jacob, J. (2015). Emerging areas of science: Recommendations for nursing science education from the CANS idea festival. *Nursing Outlook, 63*(4), 398–407.

Henly, S. J., McCarthy, D. O., Wyman, J. F., Stone, P. W., Redeker, N. S., McCarthy, A. M., . . . Moore, S. M. (2015). Integrating emerging areas of nursing science into PhD programs. *Nursing Outlook, 63*(4), 408–416.

Hersh, W., Jacko, J. A., Greenes, R., Tan, J., Janies, D., Embi, P. J., & Payne, P. R. (2011). Health care: Hit or miss? *Nature, 470*(7334), 327–329.

Hitzler, P., & Janowicz, K. (2013). Linked data, big data, and the 4th paradigm. *Semantic Web.* http://corescholar.libraries.wright.edu/cse/161

IBM. (2015). *The four V's of big data.* Retrieved from http://www.ibmbigdatahub.com/infographic/four-vs-big-data

Internet Live Stats. (2015). Retrieved from http://www.internetlivestats.com

Jagadish, H. V., Gehrke, J., Labrinidis, A., Papakonstantinou, Y., Patel, J. M., Ramakrishnan, R., & Shahabi, C. (2014). Big data and its technical challenges. *Communications of the ACM, 57*(7), 86–94.

Kaplan, R. M., Chambers, D. A., & Glasgow, R. E. (2014). Big data and large sample size: A cautionary note on the potential for bias. *Clinical and Translational Science*, *7*(4), 342–346. doi:10.1111/cts.12178

Keenan, G. (2014). Big data in health care: An urgent mandate to CHANGE nursing EHRs! *Online Journal of Nursing Informatics*, *18*(1), Retrieved from http://ojni.org/issues/?p=3081

Laney, D. (2001). 3-D Data Management: Controlling Data Volume, Velocity and Variety. *META Group Research Brief; File* 949. Retrieved from http://blogs.gartner.com/doug-laney/files/2012/01/ad949-3D-Data-Management-Controlling-Data-Volume-Velocity-and-Variety.pdf

Laskowski, N. (2013). *Ten big data case studies in a nutshell.* Retrieved from http://bigdata-madesimple.com/ten-big-data-case-studies-in-a-nutshell

Lazer, D. M., Kennedy, R., King, G., & Vespignani, A. (2014). The parable of Google Flu: Traps in big data analysis. *Science*, *343*(6176), 1203–1205.

Lee, J., & Maslove, D. M. (2015). Customization of a severity of illness score using local electronic medical record data. *Journal of Intensive Care Medicine.* doi:0885066615585951

Leinweber, D. J. (2009). *Nerds on Wall Street: Math, machines and wired markets.* Hoboken, NJ: John Wiley and Sons.

Maass, P. (2015). Inside NSA, officials privately criticize "collect it all" surveillance. *The Intercept.* Retrieved from https://firstlook.org/theintercept/2015/05/28/nsa-officials-privately-criticize-collect-it-all-surveillance

Maheshwari, A. (2014). *Business intelligence and data mining made accessible: create space independent publishing platform.* E-book. Retrieved from http://www.ebooks.com/1911815/business-intelligence-and-data-mining/maheshwari-anil/

McKenna, B. (2014). What does a petabyte look like? *Computer Weekly.com.* Retrieved from http://www.computerweekly.com/feature/What-does-a-petabyte-look-like

National Institutes of Health (NIH). (2015). *Data science at NIH: BD2K.* Retrieved from https://datascience.nih.gov/sites/default/files/bd2k/docs/July29%20RFI%20summary.pdf

Parsons, A., McCullough, C., Wang, J., & Shih, S. (2012). Validity of electronic health record-derived quality measurement for performance monitoring. *Journal of the Medical Informatics Association*, *19*(4), 604–609.

Pasteur, L. (1854). Lecture, University of Lille (7 December 1854). In M. Martinussen & D. Hunter (Eds.), *Aviation psychology and human factors* (p. xi). Boca Raton, FL: CRC Press, Taylor & Francis Publishing.

Snijders, C., Matzat, U., & Reips, U. D. (2012). Big data: Big gaps of knowledge in the field of Internet science. *International Journal of Internet Science*, *7*(1), 1–5.

Swan, M. (2009). Emerging patient-driven health care models: An examination of health social networks, consumer personalized medicine and quantified self-tracking. *International Journal of Environmental Research and Public Health*, *6*(2), 492–525.

Ward, J. S., & Barker, A. (2013). *Undefined by data: A survey of big data definitions: Cornell library.* Open Source Library. Retrieved from http://arxiv.org/abs/1309.5821

Wattenberg, M. (2005). *Baby Name Voyager.* Retrieved from http://www.bewitched.com/namevoyager.html

Westra, B., Bliss, D., Savik, K., Hou, Y., & Borchert, A. (2013). Effectiveness of wound, ostomy, and continence nurses on agency-level wound and incontinence outcomes in home care. *Journal of Wound Ostomy and Continence Nursing*, *40*(1), 25–53.

Wyman, J. F., & Henly, S. J. (2015). PhD programs in nursing in the United States: Visibility of AACN core curricular elements and emerging areas of science. *Nursing Outlook*, *63*(4), 390–397.

Yoon, S., Elhadad, N., & Bakken, S. (2013). A practical approach for content mining of tweets. *American Journal of Preventive Medicine*, *45*(1), 122–129.

CHAPTER SIX

COMPARATIVE EFFECTIVENESS RESEARCH

GEORGIA L. NARSAVAGE

OBJECTIVES

After reading this chapter, readers will be able to:

1. Define comparative effectiveness research (CER) with reasons for using CER methods
2. Discuss the methods involved in creating CER
3. Contrast the objectives and distinctive features of CER
4. Interpret findings from CER

The use of comparative effectiveness methods in practice-based clinical inquiry has inspired a new era of research. The Patient Protection and Affordable Care Act of 2010 founded the Patient-Centered Outcomes Research Institute (PCORI) to "assist patients, clinicians, purchaser, and policy-makers in making informed health decisions . . ." (PCORI, 2010, p. 665). To achieve informed decision making, the focus of patient-centered research had to move beyond whether an intervention was better than placebo treatment (efficacy studies) to direct a comparison of treatments in practice settings, that is, comparative effectiveness. CER, as defined by the U.S. Federal Coordinating Council for CER (2009, p. 16), is

> . . . the conduct and synthesis of research comparing the benefits and harms of different interventions and strategies to prevent, diagnose, treat and monitor health conditions in "real world" settings. The purpose of this research is to improve health outcomes by developing and disseminating evidence-based information to patients, clinicians, and other decision-makers, responding to their expressed needs, about which interventions are most effective for which patients under specific circumstances.

The development of CER, a fairly new field of investigation, has been an exemplar of interprofessional work across many disciplines, including health information technology (HIT), pragmatic clinical research, epidemiology, health economics, and health services research.

To support improved patient outcomes, and thus CER, the U.S. Congress authorized development of the PCORI as an independent, nonprofit organization

(PCORI, 2012). From December 2012, PCORI spurred the development and funding of CER studies needed to identify evidence to improve patient-centered health outcomes and to disseminate the results in ways that patients, doctors, nurses, and others would find useful and valuable. PCORI engages patients and the broader health care community in the process of evaluation and funding of CER proposals. In partnership with the Agency for Healthcare Research and Quality (AHRQ), PCORI has been involved in generating critical data about the comparative benefits and risks of treatments in practice settings. PCORI and AHRQ are especially interested in research that helps patients make informed decisions. More information about funding opportunities may be found at the website www.pcori.org.

DESCRIPTION OF CER

The definitions of CER given by PCORI (2012) and the U.S. Federal Coordinating Council for CER (2009), compared with the definitions of CER from other organizations such as the Institute of Medicine (IOM) and the American Nurses Association (ANA), incorporate four key areas to be considered in developing CER studies:

1. Comparison of interventions and strategies must be feasible in "real world" settings.
2. A wide range of study designs using multiple data sources can be applied, including quasi-experimental evaluations and observational studies using existing databases/data. Randomized controlled trial (RCT) designs that use an alternative treatment rather than placebo may also be applicable to CER.
3. Data should include a variety of sources, both quantitative and qualitative findings, as well as electronic records and large data sets in order to detect and explain differences.
4. CER outcome assessments should focus on those that are important to patients, clinicians, and funders (Glascow & Steiner, 2012).

As with other outcomes research, CER studies are critical for development of the body of evidence about priority populations and subgroups to address health disparities, as well as to help identify how groups respond differently.

Outcomes Research Related to CER

Outcomes research is an umbrella term used in multiple ways in the literature and is difficult to define. The U.S. AHRQ website (www.ahrq.gov/research) is a good source for identifying outcomes-related research and links to CER. Clancy and Eisenberg's (1998, p. 245) classic article stated that "Outcomes research—the study of the end results of health services that takes patients' experiences, preferences, and values into account—is intended to provide scientific evidence relating to decisions made by all who participate in health care." With the introduction of PCORI, patient-centered outcomes research (PCOR) focused on outcomes research that:

- Assesses the benefits and harms of preventive, diagnostic, therapeutic, palliative, or health delivery system interventions to inform decision making, highlighting comparisons and outcomes that matter to people

- Is inclusive of an individual's preferences, autonomy, and needs, focusing on outcomes that people notice and care about, such as survival, function, symptoms, and health-related quality of life
- Incorporates a wide variety of settings and diversity of participants to address individual differences and barriers to implementation and dissemination
- Investigates (or may investigate) optimizing outcomes while addressing burden to individuals, availability of services, technology, personnel, and other stakeholder perspectives (PCORI, 2012)

Some, although not all, CER is PCOR. Not all CER will meet PCORI's definition of being patient centered; for example, addressing questions that are important to patients and other health care stakeholders or studying outcomes that are meaningful to patients and other stakeholders. Nevertheless, CER is a valuable methodology to approach outcomes research that can be used in patient/clinician decision making, and PCORI has become a valuable resource for funding CER practice-based studies.

To be useful as practice-based clinical inquiries, CER studies must be relevant and appropriate to the issue, objective, and use rigorous scientific methods, with clear links to the issues that face major stakeholders—patients, clinicians, and the public. Three primary features of research that are designed to compare the effectiveness of interventions are: (a) assessment of an all-inclusive review of patient outcomes for diverse populations in typical practice settings—synthesis CER studies; (b) comparison of distinct treatments (e.g., medications, medical devices, behavioral-change strategies, procedures, delivery systems)—pragmatic CER studies; and (c) systematically exploring a variety of data sources and methods to be able to predict clinical responses—observational CER studies. CER studies are limited neither to RCTs nor to any one specific kind of study, although development of CER research should be based within what is currently known. The goal is to first complete a research review of multiple relevant outcome studies and keep them in the context of who, what, when, and where the intervention was studied. The approach for CER studies, synthesis, pragmatic/practice based, or observational, will be based on the research review.

Many different types of CER studies can be developed by applying the "four essential attributes of CER (feasible implementation, flexible research designs, rich data sources, and relevant outcomes)" as described by Glascow and Steiner (2012, p. 73). In CER, researchers explore all evidence about the benefits and harms of alternatives for varied groups of people from existing RCTs, pragmatic clinical studies, and other research. The research review thus leads to the three approaches or categories of CER research that are used throughout this chapter: (a) Systematic reviews of existing evidence can be an end in themselves as "Synthesis CER studies," often with cost analyses; (b) A review of existing research can be used to identify the comparators to be studied in a practice (pragmatic) setting to generate new evidence of effectiveness or comparative effectiveness of a test, treatment, procedure, or healthcare service, referred to as "Pragmatic CER studies"; and (c) A third type of CER, categorized as "Observational CER studies," uses existing data to compare patient outcomes at multiple sites and to predict clinical response. Examples of published articles of CER research placed within these categories may be found in Table 6.1.

TABLE 6.1 Examples of Published Articles of CER Research, Listed in Categories Related to Observational, Pragmatic, and Synthesis Review CER

CER Category	Author (year)	CER Study Description
Observational CER studies	Walker et al. (2014)	The CER Hub informatics platform developed a quality assurance process using tools and data formats available to study smoking cessation services in primary care. Specifically, they used the "emrAdapter" tool programmed with a set of quality checks to query large samples of primary care encounter records.
	Schalet et al. (2015)	The study's goal was to establish a common reporting metric of physical function so scores on commonly used physical function measures can be comparable for CER. Main measures of PROMIS PF, SF-36 PF, and the HAQ-DI were compared and found to measure the same concept.
	Root, Thomas, Campagna, and Morrato (2014)	Because geographic variation in health care delivery is ubiquitous, it could be the best practice of CER to test for possible geographic confounding in observational data. This paper demonstrates how to use exploratory spatial data analysis and spatial statistical methods to investigate and control for these potential biases. (Note that methods to address geographic analysis are discussed in Chapter 9.)
Pragmatic CER studies	Levsky et al. (2014)	Study design described for comparing treadmill stress echocardiography and coronary computed tomography angiography in chest pain patients in emergency departments (EDs). Key outcomes include hospital admissions, length of stay in the ED/hospital, and cost of care. Safety outcomes include subsequent visits to the ED, hospitalizations, and major adverse cardiovascular events at 30 days and 1 year.
	Taveras et al. (2013)	The STAR is a three-arm, cluster RCT in 14 pediatric offices in Massachusetts. The study examines computerized decision support tools in the EHR delivered to primary care providers at the point of care to enhance adoption of CER evidence for management of obese children. Point-of-care outcomes include obesity diagnosis, nutrition and physical activity counseling, and referral to weight management. One-year child-level outcomes include changes in BMI and improvements in diet, physical activity, screen time, and sleep behaviors, as well as cost and cost-effectiveness.
	Xian, Hammill, and Curtis (2013)	The Federal Coordinating Council for CER recommends further efforts on longitudinal linking of administrative or EHR-based databases, patient registries, private sector databases (particularly those with commercially insured populations that are not covered under federal and state databases), and other relevant data sources containing pharmacy, laboratory, adverse events, and mortality information. Advancing the infrastructure to provide robust, scientific data resources for patient-centered CER must remain a priority.

(continued)

TABLE 6.1 Examples of Published Articles of CER Research, Listed in Categories Related to Observational, Pragmatic, and Synthesis Review CER (*continued*)

CER Category	Author (year)	CER Study Description
Synthesis review CER studies (cost analyses)	Chao et al. (2014)	This systematic review and analysis of cost-effectiveness identified 584 studies with 26 studies meeting full inclusion criteria to assess surgical interventions in low-income and middle-income countries to help quantify the potential value of surgery. The findings showed that many essential surgical interventions are cost-effective in resource-poor countries. Quantification of the economic value of surgery provides a strong argument for the expansion of global surgery's role in the global health movement.
	Timbie et al. (2012)	This systematic review considered 5,716 reports for this CER. The aim was to identify the best available evidence regarding strategies for allocating scarce resources during mass casualty events. Although the final review included 170 studies, no one approach was superior than the others. The authors noted the importance of a broad, inclusive, and systematic engagement process.

Note: This table is not meant to be exhaustive. These articles were retrieved on the federal website titled NLM Resources for Informing Comparative Effectiveness (www.nlm.nih.gov/nichsr/cer/cerqueries.html) retrieved June 4, 2015. The total number of CER-published articles retrieved through this website that link to PubMed on June 4, 2015 was 572.

BMI, body mass index; CER, comparative effectiveness research; EHR, electronic health record; HAQ-DI, HAQ-Disability Index; RCT, randomized controlled trial; STAR, Study of Technology to Accelerate Research.

REASONS FOR USING CER

Reasons for using CER are numerous and include its applicability to:

- Develop clinical guidelines
- Propose reimbursement policies
- Compare costs to control health spending with improved care outcomes
- Support informed decision making by clinicians, patients, agencies, and payers to improve health care for individuals and populations
- Promote the use of the safest and most effective treatments
- Decrease use of ineffective treatments or those for which an equivalent, but less expensive treatment exists

CER methods starting with research reviews include systematic reviews of existing evidence (AHRQ, 2014). CER methods incorporate a type of systematic review and may include meta-analysis, expanding the review focus from evaluating one individual intervention to comparing alternative interventions for a specified clinical problem or disorder. For example, CER researchers at Johns Hopkins University (Wang et al., 2013) collected all the published studies that explored school-based interventions for childhood obesity prevention. They found 131 articles describing 124 interventional studies, of which 104 studies were school based. They synthesized the results of these studies in a CER review using systematic review methods to compare school-based with home-based interventions. They included a meta-analysis with quantitative pooling of data to calculate the separate effects of the interventions on changes in body mass index (BMI, an obesity indicator) in the findings. The outcome of this work found moderate evidence regarding the effectiveness of school-based interventions in preventing childhood obesity. "Physical activity interventions in a school-based setting with a family component or diet and physical activity interventions in a school-based setting with home and community components had the most evidence for effectiveness" (Wang et al., 2013, p. vii). CER thus has a foundation in systematic review methods (Chapter 3).

Efficacy to Effectiveness Research

In addition to Synthesis CER studies appraising intervention research, a continuum evolves from research methods initially focused on *efficacy*, which is defined as the evaluation of an intervention under ideal, controlled circumstances in a homogenous sample of a population. When an intervention can be seen to work under ideal circumstances, research can move toward studying its effectiveness or its ability to be implemented under real-world conditions. Thus, the difference between efficacy and effectiveness can be described in that efficacy measures the ability of the intervention to produce a desired outcome in a controlled environment (e.g., an RCT), whereas effectiveness is the actual effect of the intervention in a clinical practice setting. The focus of CER is not safety and efficacy alone—it is the relative benefits and harm that occur in using the different interventions that could be applied in a real-world clinical setting.

In moving on the continuum from efficacy to effectiveness research, a careful analysis of the varying levels of available evidence using a format such as the Oxford 2011 Levels of Evidence Table (Oxford Centre for Evidence-Based Medicine [OCEBM] Levels of Evidence Working Group, 2011) is critical to understanding research data. In any review, there will be limitations that must be identified and robust conclusions may not be possible, especially for population subgroups. Nevertheless, building on what is known—the existing evidence—is an essential starting point to CER for more informed clinical decision making, to determine what additional evidence is needed to support improved quality and safety, and to achieve lower costs and higher patient satisfaction.

METHODS OF CREATING CER

CER has several dimensions: A basic two-dimensional diagram (see Figure 6.1) can help display the relationship of comparing treatments for cost and effectiveness without increased harm. CER may include many of the same methods as cost-effectiveness analyses, such as a ratio of the change in costs of an intervention compared with the alternative (incremental cost-effectiveness ratios [ICERs]) or quality-adjusted life years (QALYs). In Figure 6.1, an intervention that is a category four (IV), which increased effectiveness without increased harm at lower cost, would be the most desirable for policy makers. An example of findings approaching a category IV recommendation and their use for policy development can be seen in the American Urological Association's Guideline for *Early Detection of Prostate Cancer* (Carter et al., 2013). They proposed a prostate-specific antigen (PSA) screening interval of 2 years for

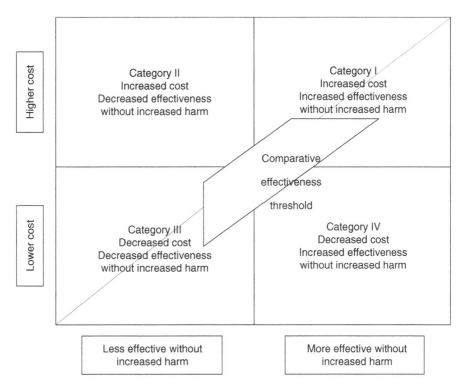

Figure 6.1 Comparing treatments for cost and effectiveness.
CER, comparative effectiveness research.

specific groups of men, instead of annual screening, based on research outcomes indicating that "as compared to annual screening, it is expected that screening intervals of two years preserve the majority of the benefits and reduce over-diagnosis and false positives" (Carter et al., 2013, p. 2). However, there are also points along the comparative–effectiveness threshold where an intervention in category one (I) or category three (III) could be considered applicable for some patients if no interventions fell within category IV. CER does not provide one answer in most situations; rather, it provides an analysis that can be applied to inform clinical decision making.

Clinical Inquiry Questions Guide CER

In selecting a question to address while conducting a CER review study, consider the following format based on the AHRQ Methods Guide (AHRQ, 2014).

- The question should be central to patient care with a body of literature or large data sets available for review. Longitudinal research data have been more informative than cross-sectional research findings when examining the risks versus benefits of interventions.
- The evidence needed will be determined by the question. For example, if the intervention is new, observational data may be the best available evidence (Observational CER studies using existing data sets), whereas pharmaceutical studies of drug efficacy will include RCTs as well as cost data.

● Generalizability of data may be limited—especially if the population for which the decision is desired has not represented a proportionately large sample in the available studies. Clearly describing the characteristics of patients, clinicians, and setting in research studies allows judgments about the generalizability of findings and helps in determining the ability of the intervention to make a change in a specific study (efficacy) for the question being asked.

● The manner in which benefits versus harms of the findings will be determined in studying comparative effectiveness should be clearly stated. For example, if urinary tract infections (UTIs) in the intensive care unit (ICU) are a negative outcome under study, it may be more meaningful to say a treatment results in fewer UTIs per patient days in a specific setting (e.g., ICU) rather than per patient or per patient days in hospital.

These methods for selection of a clinical inquiry question to address a problem can then be placed into a format to guide CER.

Using PICOTS Questions to Guide CER

In framing the study, consider using a format such as a population, intervention, comparison, outcome (PICO) question, as seen in Chapter 3 on systematic reviews and expanded to include the timing and setting (PICOTS) for CER, as shown in Table 6.2.

TABLE 6.2 PICOTS Research Questions as Basis for CER

Terminology	Applicable Questions
Population	What is the population group of interest? Do they usually receive the interventions? What subgroups will be considered in terms of age, gender, ethnicity, economic status, etc.?
Intervention	What is the area of interest (e.g., drug, devices, procedure, or tests)? Have the interventions to be compared been shown to work in research settings? Are they being used in practice settings? Can they be used with the population of interest in the setting of interest?
Comparison	What two or three alternatives are to be studied? Is there support for their effectiveness? Will they be studied related to observation using available data? Will RCT-tested interventions be used? Will a systematic review of literature with cost analysis be used?
Outcome	What are the outcomes and end points of interest? How will they be measured? Will benefits and possible harms be identifiable?
Timing	What is the time frame of interest for assessing outcomes? Are clinicians, patients, policy makers, and others interested in short- or long-term outcomes?
Setting	What is the "real world" setting of interest (e.g., hospital, primary care, community center, etc.)? Can multiple settings be compared in different areas? How will the settings be selected?

CER, comparative effectiveness research; PICOTS, population, intervention, comparison, outcome, timing, setting; RCT, randomized controlled trial.

Adapted from "PICOTS typology for developing research questions," p. 13 in *Developing a Protocol for Observational Comparative Effectiveness Research: A User's Guide.* www.effectivehealthcare.ahrq.gov/Methods-OCER.cfm

Similar to a systematic review, CER requires a clear, clinically informed question regarding alternative interventions and strategies to improve health outcomes. PICO questions provide a framework for formulating focused clinical questions as a foundational component of evidence-based practice (Stillwell, Fineout-Overholt, Melnyk, & Williamson, 2010). Comparative effectiveness methods suggest that the PICO question then be stated in an expanded format identified as PICOTS (population, intervention, comparator, outcome, timing, setting) format. The PICOTS question can be used to frame the analysis. For example, CER can be a next step to test the outcomes of a systematic review on methods of screening for lung cancer. A sample draft question for CER would be: In adults with a history of smoking and dyspnea, how reliable is a chest x-ray versus a CT scan in detecting lung cancer?

Once preliminary data are reviewed, the researcher could find that most of the studies examined were focused on patients in primary care settings who were not hospitalized and findings were different for early stage lung cancer. The outcome effectiveness of the chest x-ray versus CT scan as a screening intervention thus could vary based on when the screening occurs (timing) and based on types of primary care settings—the S of the PICOTS question. Those settings are the places where most patients experiencing lung cancer symptoms are initially seen. For CER, it is important to clarify the outcomes that will be of interest, as well as the timing and setting where the intervention alternatives will be studied, and to examine differences in findings that could relate to the disease/condition, patient characteristics, intervention, or treatment regimen. The PICOTS question could thus be further focused for CER: In primary care of community-dwelling adult patients with a history of smoking and dyspnea, how reliable is a chest x-ray in comparison to a CT scan in detecting lung cancer in stages I to III?

Analytical Frameworks to Guide CER

The next step would be to prepare an analytic framework that identifies the variables and processes that will be examined—this framework will guide the CER based on the PICOTS question. Using a visual representation of the analytic framework for a comparative analysis will show corresponding links with the model of care to direct the research team. A draft analytic framework could be used to focus attention on the components of the system of care (interventions) that could have the potential to improve individual-level outcomes for people. As the question is refined with key informant input and targeted literature reviews, a provisional analytic framework can be developed from the draft framework. See Figure 6.2 for a provisional analytic framework. Clarifying the PICOTS question and the analytic framework sets the stage for the CER study.

Finding evidence for comparing interventions will use multiple sources of evidence. The search strategies and sources should be examined to identify work coming from the same study and reported differently, or work that indicated an outcome in the protocol without reporting the findings on that outcome. Selection analysis and reporting bias may be identified by a marked difference in results between articles written from the same database or clinical trials. Inconsistencies can suggest selective outcome and analysis recording biases. For example, mortality might be indicated as an outcome that can be changed by an intervention, whereas the report of outcomes may indicate only quality of life—perhaps because mortality did not change. Nevertheless, negative findings can be as important as significant

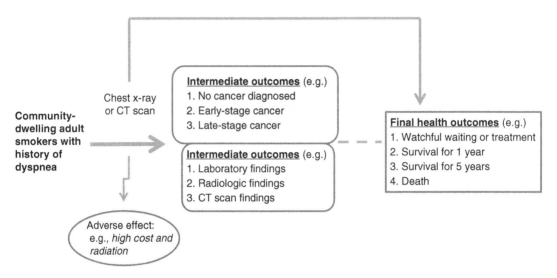

Figure 6.2 Analytic framework for comparison of chest x-ray to CT scan in diagnosing lung cancer.

changes. Another example can be seen in a report by Dwan, Kirkham, Williamson, and Gamble (2013), who found that 18 of 46 studies in Cochrane reviews of cystic fibrosis research had a discrepancy between the protocol and reported outcomes (Dwan et al., 2013). They noted a need to follow up directly with the investigators. Another obvious area in which bias can be inferred is when mortality is an indicator of treatment failure, so those data must have been collected but are not reported in the analyses. A framework for assessing selective reporting should be detailed in the research reviews; further information and samples of structuring a search for evidence can be found in an article by Relevo and Balshem (2011), "Finding Evidence for Comparing Medical Interventions" with an update in the AHRQ Methods Guide, Chapter 5 (AHRQ, 2014). This is a must read if conducting CER, because detailed search strategies are explained to minimize bias, such as a failure to disseminate negative findings (publication bias).

Conference abstracts and other non-published data should usually not be used for assessment of outcomes, as they inform our understanding and interpretation without being considered "evidence." Nevertheless, these may need to be included if clinical trial data are not sufficiently available. Using a decision-making process for determining whether to include observational and other studies with a level of evidence lower than RCTs is recommended.

In a CER review, RCTs are always considered first, as they are the highest level of evidence. Then, one needs to consider whether there are gaps in the RCT evidence—if not, then one should restrict the review to RCTs; if there are gaps, then one should consider other types of well-designed studies, particularly cohort and case-control studies. The question to ask is whether nonexperimental methods will provide valid and useful information to compare the interventions under study. The reviewer should identify the gaps and the suitability of the nonrandomized studies available to address the gaps in terms of the natural history of the condition and potential for biases in interpretation. Analytic rigor is a key criterion when evaluating whether these observational studies are suitable. After the additional non-randomized study data are collected and synthesized, the results will be added to RCT data with strengths and limitations explained for all the data.

CER can develop conclusions (Synthesis CER study) based on the research review and appropriate meta-analysis if there are sufficient data available from RCTs. The knowledge gained from a synthesized review that focuses on a comparison of alternative interventions/treatments currently in use can provide decision-making support—the purpose of CER. However, if the research review has identified alternatives that need further study, the CER research can move into observational or quasi-experimental, or even an RCT (non-placebo), by studying two alternative treatments in practice settings. Velentgas, Dreyer, Nourjah, Smith, and Torchia (2013) provide a user's guide to develop these protocols for CER. Table 6.3 compares the method/design components for a systematic review, an

TABLE 6.3 Comparison of Study Methods: Systematic Reviews, Efficacy Studies, and Comparative Effectiveness Studies

Method/ Design	Systematic Review	Efficacy Studies (e.g., RCT) (Intervention vs. placebo)	Effectiveness Studies (Intervention A vs. B)
Sites Where will data be collected?	Electronic database and published articles or other reports	Research sites that are motivated and interested in the study	Random/varied to reflect the "real world" of practice
Clinicians How will they be involved?	May be specified as to nurse/doctor and others for literature reviews	Interested and able to do criteria-based patient recruitment	All employees who usually use treatments included in CER study
Patients How will they be selected?	Often specified by diagnosis	Minimal comorbidity/ meet inclusion and exclusion criteria	All patients who have diagnosis and potential intervention decision at included sites
Intervention(s) How will it be implemented?	Key word search used to specify topic of study	Ideal conditions with rigorous protocol consistency	Real conditions—vary related only to alternatives in study
Training Who will be trained? How?	Literature retrieved by trained people using standard coding	Specific people limited to IRB-approved and IRR-approved staff	Many have usual training and specific training on intervention basics
Protocol format What will guide the study?	Review format for literature based on standards	Specific steps clearly listed with written and approved protocol	General guidelines for comparison and for treatments
Monitoring How and what standards are tested?	Often, at least blinded dual decisions on meaning; reliability checked	Frequent on-site checks for fidelity—IRR with training at specific time points	Qualitative/observed Staff/patient observed interactions; team input into process

(continued)

TABLE 6.3 Comparison of Study Methods: Systematic Reviews, Efficacy Studies, and Comparative Effectiveness Studies (*continued*)

Method/ Design	Systematic Review	Efficacy Studies (e.g., RCT) (Intervention vs. placebo)	Effectiveness Studies (Intervention A vs. B)
Outcome measure What findings are expected?	Data extraction on selected studies; standardized tools	Specific measures/ accurate Tested for reliability and validity	Routine practice assessed by usual data collected; interviews/patient or other records
Subgroup analysis What if there are differences?	Organization of data can address heterogeneity	Exclusion criteria often limit variation between groups; data analysis usually excludes outliers	Diverse—prespecified multiple variables that could be different are studied
Duration How long will the study last?	Predetermined by literature review for specified years of interest	Usually short (months) within protocol for treatment and follow-up	Longer time impact based on expected impact time/ maintenance of effect
Application How will findings be applied?	Synthesize/interpret and report major conclusions	Next study can be based on findings of gaps and expanded to other sites	Adapted to practice in real settings as indicated by outcomes
Effects on sites Does participation in the research impact the site?	May be qualitative data identified in studies reviewed— could be focus	Not usually applicable as study in selected controlled settings	Qualitative assessment, for example, staff interviews and differences in records
Cost analysis Is there a cost benefit?	May be in studies— cannot control	Not usually applicable— may be in studies	Cost measures usually important for decisions

CER, comparative effectiveness research; IRB, institutional review board; IRR, inter-rater reliability; RCT, randomized controlled trial.

efficacy study, and an effectiveness study to show similarities and differences in these related methods.

Outcome Measures

Selection of outcome measures is another critical component of CER. Outcome measures can be selected and classified according to the AHRQ definitions of clinical, humanistic, and economic and utilization outcomes (AHRQ, 2000). Clinical outcomes represent the clinician perspective. Humanistic outcomes represent the patient perspective. Economic/utilization outcomes represent the payer and societal perspective. Clinical/clinician, humanistic/patient, and economic/utilization outcomes can also be categorized within a study as of primary or secondary importance, or as composite data combination outcomes. Primary outcomes are those that are the most important to answer the question. Related factors or secondary outcomes and a combination of the outcomes or composite outcomes can provide meaningful interpretations to answer the question; these may be assessed in addition to the primary outcome. Examples of these outcomes within categories for a CER study of interventions for patients experiencing a myocardial infarction are shown in Table 6.4. As outcome decisions are made, it is critical that they are clearly defined and consistently applied in reviewing the studies included in the CER process.

Cost cannot be ignored in CER outcome measurement, even with multiple challenges in quantifying costs and effectiveness. Pearson and Bach (2010) outlined a range of questions related to cost: (a) Is effectiveness measured in terms of survival, surrogate outcome measures, quality of life, or events averted (e.g., failed to rescue)? (b) How do we assess the meaning of time and relative health to those who know they are nearing the end of life? (c) Unit costs and utilization rates represent the basic building blocks of CER analyses. However, how are they best quantified?

Finding reliable cost data is a challenge, and then using these cost data to express value in ways that make sense to patients and other stakeholders must be addressed. Although cost literature includes cost utility metrics, such as cost per QALY, these measures may not be understood or appropriately interpreted by

TABLE 6.4 Outcome Examples, Definitions, and Measurement Classification

Outcome	Definition	Outcome Examples Using AHRQ Classification		
		Clinical Outcome	Humanistic Outcome	Economic and Utilization Outcome
		Clinician perspective	Clinically meaningful and based on patient perspectives	Payor and society perspectives as measures of cost/ cost-effectiveness
Primary	Outcome of greatest importance to answer the question	Cardiovascular death from myocardial infarction	HQoL	QALYs
Secondary	Data used to evaluate other effects of the intervention	Disability from myocardial infarction	FS that impacts HQoL	Cost of treatment
Composite	Multiple data combined to answer the question	All cause cardiovascular deaths	HQoL + FS	Cost of treatment per QALYs

AHRQ, Agency for Healthcare Research and Quality; FS, functional status; HQoL, health-related quality of life; QALYs, quality-adjusted life years.

TABLE 6.5 Online Sites for Cost Data

Website	Type of Cost Data
www.ahrq.gov/research/data/hcup	Hospital data available through the AHRQ Healthcare Cost and Utilization Project
www.medicare.gov/hospital compare/search.html	Medicare data available by hospital name or zip code
http://engage.changehealth care.com/hcti	HCTI is a measure of costs and cost variability of services that health care consumers purchase on a recurring basis from aggregated medical claims
www.newchoicehealth.com	Costs for common medical procedures by insurance and zip code
https://healthcarebluebook .com/page_ConsumerFront .aspx	Searchable database for cost of health care services, including medications, by zip code
www.healthdata.gov/dataset	Health data from government sources, including health care cost sources
www.ama-assn.org/ama	Search term "The Medicare Physician Payment Schedule" provides updated payment information

AHRQ, Agency for Healthcare Research and Quality; HCTI, health care transparency index.

clinicians and patients. Reports using cost consequences such as "cost per adverse event avoided" may be more meaningful. Nevertheless, costs that do not provide a final effectiveness measure may not help quantify a budget impact for a treatment. Although it is difficult to identify cost data from individual studies, there are general resources such as Medicare data available through the national Centers for Medicare and Medicaid Services (CMS) website www.medicare.gov/hospitalcompare/search .html. The American Medical Association (AMA) website has been used to find what Medicare pays physicians for services. The AHRQ Healthcare Cost and Utilization Project (HCUP; AHRQ, 2015) website is currently the most comprehensive source of hospital data (www.ahrq.gov/research/data/hcup) These and other sources of cost data may be found in Table 6.5.

INTERPRETATION OF CER

Consider Possible Biases When Interpreting CER Evidence

As in research reviews, considering biases in interpretation of CER is important. Similar to preparing a systematic review, CER methods should incorporate assessment of the risk of bias in interpreting evidence, including the following as identified by Higgins and Green (2011):

1. Selection bias includes differences in baseline group characteristics arising from systematic likelihood of selection or treatment (e.g., RCT participants have higher educational levels)

2. Performance bias where intervention and control group exposures are similar (e.g., control participants interact with trial participants and receive the same educational information)
3. Attrition bias where participants drop out or are lost to follow-up related to systematic differences (e.g., control group realizes it is not getting monitored and drops out)
4. Detection bias related to measurement techniques or other outcome assessment errors (e.g., scales in two clinics are not calibrated)
5. Recording bias where selected findings are reported (e.g., only positive findings related to funders are reported)

Perceptive or knowledge-based biases play an important role in interpretation of CER evidence and may be a challenging barrier in all phases of translation of CER into application of findings. For example, biases in perception of findings may influence the way clinicians interpret the CER evidence. Confirmation bias is a tendency for an individual to welcome evidence that confirms preconceived ideas of treatment effectiveness and to reject evidence that supports a contrary position— often reinforcing established practice patterns, such as use of antibiotics for sinus infections in previous years. Additionally, perceptive bias can be a belief that an aggressive intervention such as cancer treatment, even with low benefit, is better than not doing anything. A third bias, often seen in the United States, is the common tendency to perceive new technologies as better than older ones (Schneider, Timbie, Fox, Van Busum, & Caloyeras, 2013).

Publication bias is also a consideration in interpreting CER data, because results of a majority of clinical trials are never published. The potential for pharmaceutical funders, for example, to withhold negative findings resulted in the strict Research Conflict of Interest guidelines that we have today. Studies with positive or statistically significant results tend to report greater treatment effect, and they are published sooner within higher impact journals than those with negative or nonsignificant effects (Riveros et al., 2013). Searches that exclude non–English language literature may bias understanding of treatment effects as well (Riveros et al., 2013).

Evaluating CER for Translation Into Clinical Practice

Clinical decision support systems along with patient decision aids designed for patients with specific conditions can help inform clinical practice with CER evidence, but may not be used for multiple reasons. Clinical decision support systems in many health care settings are limited, and patient decision aids could be much more widely used to inform decision making within CER (Benner, 2009). A structure for Comparative Effectiveness Research Dissemination (CERD) that addresses bias in interpretations can be found in the Schneider et al. (2013) report for the U.S. Department of Health and Human Services (Figure 5.1) on page 15: the "Conceptual Framework for Translation of CER Into Clinical Practice," available at http://aspe .hhs.gov/health/reports/2013/CERDissemination/rpt_RANDFinal.pdf.

Quality CER must also include the assessment of risk or increased harm as well as benefits for informed decision making. If harm is increased, then the diagram in Figure 6.1 regarding cost and effectiveness will not apply, and additional data are needed. Santaguida and Raina (2008) developed a form (McHarm) for evaluating studies reporting harms that is published as the "McMaster Quality Assessment

Scale of Harms." This tool guides a reviewer to determine for each study whether harms were predefined within a specified time frame and provides a specific checklist for identifying harms: Were they serious or severe, resulting in deaths? Were harms found using active or passive collection of data? Who collected the data on harms and what was the training provided? Were specified attrition data collected? Were number and type of harm recorded by study groups? What analyses were used to identify harms data? The answers are yes (less bias risk), no (high bias risk), or unsure.

Finally, further guidance for comparing interventions using quantitative synthesis, often including meta-analyses, is important (see Chapter 3). Completing a CER must be a well thought-out process, and multiple analyses are essential to rigorously summarize information from multiple studies—either to complete the research as a Synthesis CER study or to lay the foundation for an Observational CER study of existing data or a pragmatic CER study conducted in clinical settings. Chapter 12 in the AHRQ (2014), *Methods Guide for Effectiveness and Comparative Effectiveness Reviews*, is a helpful resource for preparing a quantitative synthesis. Chapters are available at www.effectivehealthcare.ahrq.gov.

The decision to use quantitative synthesis should be based on appraisal of similarity among identified studies, assessing the potential of each to provide meaningful responses to the question under study. Both clinical and methodological similarities and differences in the studies should be considered, including the impact of missing data that may need to be deleted. If multiple study results list similar effect sizes (the strength or likelihood of the intervention to have an impact), they could be quantitatively synthesized. However, if there appear to be differences in selected variables in each study, analyzing subgroups is recommended prior to a quantitative synthesis. The logic behind making a decision to combine studies for analyses should be clearly described, and explanations of findings should address any limitations. Reporting the methods for quantitative synthesis of studies should include the rationale behind combining the studies, the outcome selection criteria, the types of studies combined, an explanation of the outcome measure (effect), methods used for combining the study estimates of population outcomes, statistical methods used for analysis of differences (statistical heterogeneity), and sensitivity analyses.

THE PRESENTATION OF CER

A CER review must include decisions about whether the accessible research evidence is based on real-world situations. There should be an understanding of which patients under what circumstances will be needed to inform clinical or policy decisions. All studies of comparative effectiveness should be conducted and reported in a fashion that makes the methods and practices clear. There are multiple sources of findings from CER in the literature—Academy Health, a group committed to using health services research to improve health care, published a summary (Holve & Pittman, 2009) that may be found at www.academyhealth.org/files/publications/CERMonograph09.pdf.

The process of CER requires investigators to make decisions and assumptions that may affect the final outcome recommendations. Therefore, "sensitivity analysis" should be conducted early if a meta-analysis will be used to examine the robustness of results related to decisions and assumptions. A simple sensitivity analysis can be done by changing one decision/assumption at a time and examining the impact on the estimate/conclusion (Fu et al., 2011). Results are considered robust if changing decisions and assumptions does not result in large changes in the statistical estimates (judgments about the population based on sampling characteristics) and conclusions. Robust estimates increase confidence in findings of the CER. If the estimates are not robust when studies are combined, one should report all estimates, carefully interpreting why studies of lesser quality are included or excluded (Fu et al., 2011). Reporting the results should include descriptive data for each study, the study's quality and level of evidence, and tables or graphs illustrating individual and combined estimates followed by narrative interpretation.

To enhance quality presentation of findings in an Observational CER study using existing data and to facilitate CER's use in decision making of therapeutic options, the Good ReseArch for Comparative Effectiveness (GRACE) initiative was created (Dreyer et al., 2010). GRACE principles provide guidance on the presentation of CER that should follow the identified question. Examples of presentation of CER findings using the GRACE principles may be found in Table 6.6 and are categorized as diseases/conditions, interventions, treatment regimens, and characteristics of patient populations.

As in interpretation of CER, it is critical that the presentation of CER results should not be selective of only those areas that support a preconceived or expected

TABLE 6.6 Examples of Information to Include When Presenting CER Findings

Item	Presenting CER Findings
Diseases/ conditions	How diagnostic certainty was attained Severity of disease/condition Time since diagnosis Significant comorbidities Treatment history Additional factors that might affect the interpretation of the outcomes

Interventions	Identify what will be compared—one treatment or multiple areas
	Complexity should address interventions' use in practice settings
	  (Comparing multiple real-world alternatives that are usually desirable)
	  Identify extent to which treatment alternatives are used in practice
	Support adequate numbers for meaningful analyses and interpretation

Treatment regimens	Delineate applicable brand names/dosage and delivery method Describe extent of actual use Indicate if off-label or labeled indications applied Describe other therapeutic alternatives currently used Determine how data are accurately recorded and accessible Other factors that could impact understanding final recommendations
Patient characteristics	Age, gender, ethnicity, geographical location, socioeconomic status, accessibility of medical care (e.g., health insurance, distance), opportunity for all alternatives if a clinician wanted to use them, and any cultural or other related factors that could impact the outcomes

CER, comparative effectiveness research.

outcome. Variety and richness of data sources are essential. Causative assumptions should be avoided. Presenting findings objectively, including clear explanations of decisions made in the selection of data and analyses, will best support the decision making desired from CER for policy decisions and in practice.

A 10-Step Practical Approach to Using Real-World Data for CER

CER will likely be of use to clinicians who want to make practice decisions based on real-world data found in medical records and electronic databases that capture clinical interventions and outcomes. Based on the publication by Wilke and Mullins (2011), 10 CER steps can be delineated:

1. Identify a topic that will address the three key areas for applying CER—a specific treatment choice, an appropriate patient population, and meaningful outcome measures.
2. Develop a well-designed research question using PICOTS format, with a design and set of data that can be expected to answer the question.
3. Explore the data in terms of how they were created, the limitations and potential biases, and how bias can be addressed in analyses.
4. Design a provisional analytic framework (Figure 6.2) that focuses on the state of existing knowledge and the gap in evidence.
5. Complete data exploration, statistical analyses, and review each possibly significant variable for its impact on the outcome under study; then, explore relationships between and among variables that impact the outcome under study. If data are missing, examine whether they are random or not, and how they can be addressed (e.g., deleted, calculated imputations).
6. In analyzing the outcomes, control for observed factors (e.g., gender) that impact both the intervention and the outcome (confounders) and consider the impact of potentially unobserved confounders, applying and analyzing multiple methods via a "sensitivity analysis."
7. Select statistical methods applicable to the question and the available data so results are meaningful and can be interpreted in terms of the three key areas: treatment, population, and outcome.
8. Report the resulting outcomes, including/excluding poorer quality data and carefully interpreting the benefits and risks of either including or completely excluding such data. Knowing the needs of decision makers can be helpful in providing a complete report.
9. Remain objective and avoid causal conclusions in discussing the outcomes; place results in context of the data available on the treatment and population.
10. Be certain that human subjects are protected and institutional guidelines are followed throughout the process of data access and analysis.

Using real-world data for CER should be guided by a methodological approach that includes the structured processes described in this chapter. If outcome data are bivariate (e.g., life vs. death; less than 5 years of survival vs. 5 or more years of survival), outcomes can usually be clearly stated. However, outcomes are often continuous data such as functional levels or blood pressure measures. Continuous data require analyses that explore the average (mean) differences; multiple statistical tests are available, and a full description is beyond the scope of this chapter. The researcher is encouraged to obtain guidance from a statistician in designing the analytic plan; that way, relevant analyses can be identified a priori, before the study begins. (More details on how to choose and work with statisticians are described in Chapter 10.)

SUMMARY

CER provides information for clinicians and patients to make informed decisions about health care, and for policy makers to structure improved systems of care. This chapter is designed to help the reader develop the skills needed to study the effectiveness of practice in the real world in which we and our patients live. Preparing for CER requires a detailed approach, which is far beyond the scope of this chapter. A good methods guide with detailed information on conducting CER has been prepared by AHRQ (Publication No. 10 (14)-EHC063-EF) and is available at: www.effectivehealthcare.ahrq.gov/ehc/products/60/318/CER-Methods-Guide-140109.pdf. Appendix 6.1 includes web links to multiple comparative effectiveness resources, and Appendix 6.2 includes examples of CER abstracts from the published literature. CER is clearly an innovative interprofessional translational approach that can improve the health of our people, and it is conducted by informed practitioners and researchers, thus involving multiple professions.

REFERENCES

Agency for Healthcare Research and Quality. (2000). *Outcomes research fact sheet* (AHRQ Publication no. 00-P011). Rockville, MD: Author.

Agency for Healthcare Research and Quality. (2014). *AHRQ methods guide for effectiveness and comparative effectiveness reviews* (AHRQ Publication no. 10(14)-EHC063-EF). Rockville, MD: Author. Retrieved from http://effectivehealthcare.ahrq.gov/ehc/products/60/318/CER-Methods-Guide-140109.pdf [Chapters available at: http://www.effectivehealthcare.ahrq.gov/ehc/products/60/318/CER-Methods-Guide-140109.pdf]

Agency for Healthcare Research and Quality. (2015). *AHRQ healthcare cost and utilization project (HCUP)*. Retrieved from http://www.ahrq.gov/research/data/hcup

Benner, S. (2009). *Clinical decision support systems: State of the Art* (AHRQ Publication no. 09-0069-EF). Rockville, MD: Agency for Healthcare Research and Quality. Retrieved from http://healthit.ahrq.gov/sites/default/files/docs/page/09-0069-EF_1.pdf

Carter, H. B., Albertsen, P. C., Barry, M. J., Etzioni, R., Freedland, S. J., Greene, K. L., . . . Zietman, A. L. (2013). *Early detection of prostate cancer: AUA guideline*. Retrieved from https://www.auanet.org/common/pdf/education/clinical-guidance/Prostate-Cancer-Detection.pdf

Chao, T. E., Sharma, K., Mandigo, M., Hagander, L., Resch, S. C., Weiser, T. G., & Meara, J. G. (2014). Cost-effectiveness of surgery and its policy implications for global health: A systematic review and analysis. *Lancet Global Health*, 2(6), e334–e345. doi:10.1016/s2214-109x(14)70213-x

Clancy, C. M., & Eisenberg, J. M. (1998). Outcomes research: Measuring the end results of health care. *Science*, 282, 245–246.

Dreyer, N. A., Schneeweiss, S., McNeil, B. J., Berger, M. L., Walker, A. M., Ollendorf, D. A., & Gliklich, R. E. (2010). GRACE principles: Recognizing high-quality observational studies of comparative effectiveness. *American Journal of Managed Care*, 16(6), 467–471.

Dwan, K., Kirkham, J. J., Williamson, P. R., & Gamble, C. (2013). Evidence-based practice: Selective reporting of outcomes in randomised controlled trials in systematic reviews of cystic fibrosis. *BMJ Open, 3,* e002709. doi:10.1136/bmjopen-2013-002709

Fu, R., Gartlehnerb, G., Grant, M., Shamliyan, T., Sedrakyan, A., Wilt, T. J., . . . Trikalinosi, T. A. (2011). Conducting quantitative synthesis when comparing medical interventions: AHRQ and the Effective Health Care Program. *Journal of Clinical Epidemiology, 64*(11), 1187–1197. [Update available in Chapter 12 of AHRQ Methods Guide (2014) at: http://effectivehealthcare.ahrq.gov]

Glascow, R. E., & Steiner, J. F. (2012). Comparative effectiveness research to accelerate translation: Recommendations for an emerging field of science. In R. C. Brownson, G. A. Colditz, & E. K. Proctor (Eds.), *Dissemination and implementation research in health: Translating science to practice* (pp. 72–93). New York, NY: Oxford University Press.

Higgins, J. P. T., & Green, S. (2011). *Cochrane handbook for systematic reviews of interventions Version 5.1.0. The Cochrane Collaboration.* Retrieved from http://handbook.cochrane.org

Holve, E., & Pittman, P. (2009). *A first look at the volume and cost of comparative effectiveness research in the United States. Academy Health Publication.* Retrieved from http://www.academyhealth.org/files/publications/CERMonograph09.pdf

Levsky, J. M., Haramati, L. B., Taub, C. C., Spevack, D. M., Menegus, M. A., Travin, M. I., . . . Garcia, M. J. (2014). Rationale and design of a randomized trial comparing initial stress echocardiography versus coronary CT angiography in low-to-intermediate risk emergency department patients with chest pain. *Echocardiography, 31*(6), 744–750.

McCauley, K., Bradway, C., Hirschman, K. B., & Naylor, M. (2014). Studying nursing interventions in acutely ill, cognitively impaired older adults. *American Journal of Nursing, 114*(10), 44–52. doi:10.1097/01.NAJ.0000454851.22018.5d

Naylor, M. D., Hirschman, K. B., Hanlon, A. L., Bowles, K. H., Bradway, C., McCauley, K. M., & Pauly, M. V. (2014). Comparison of evidence-based interventions on outcomes of hospitalized, cognitively impaired older adults. *Journal of Comparative Effectiveness Research, 3*(3), 245–257.

OCEBM Levels of Evidence Working Group. (2011). *The Oxford 2011 levels of evidence table. Oxford Centre for Evidence-Based Medicine.* Retrieved from http://www.cebm.net/wp-content/uploads/2014/06/CEBM-Levels-of-Evidence-2.1.pdf

Patient Protection and Affordable Care Act. Subtitle D—Patient-Centered Outcomes Research Institute. (2010) *PUBLIC LAW 111–148—MAR. 23, 2010.* Retrieved from http://www.pcori.org/sites/default/files/PCORI_Authorizing_Legislation.pdf

Patient-Centered Outcomes Research Institute. (2012). *Patient-centered outcomes research definition revision.* Retrieved from http://www.pcori.org/research-results/patient-centered-outcomes-research

Pearson, S. D., & Bach, P. B. (2010). How Medicare could use comparative effectiveness research in deciding on new coverage and reimbursement. *Health Affairs, 29,* 1796–1804.

Relevo, R., & Balshem, H. (2011). Finding evidence for comparing medical interventions: AHRQ and the Effective Health Care Program. *Journal of Clinical Epidemiology, 64*(11), 1168–1177.

Reynolds, W. S., McPheeters, M., Blume, J., Surawicz, T., Worley, K., Wang, L., & Hartmann, K. (2015). Comparative effectiveness of anticholinergic therapy for overactive bladder in women: A systematic review and meta-analysis. *Obstetrics and Gynecology, 125*(6), 1423–1432.

Riveros, C., Perrodeau, E., Dechartres, A., Boutron, I., Haneef, R., & Ravaud, P. (2013). Timing and completeness of trial results posted at ClinicalTrials.gov and published in journals. *PLoS Medicine, 10,* e1001566. Retrieved from http://journals.plos.org/plosmedicine/article?id=10.1371/journal.pmed.1001566

Root, E. D., Thomas, D. S. K., Campagna, E. J., & Morrato, E. H. (2014). Adjusting for geographic variation in observational comparative effectiveness studies: A case study of antipsychotics using state Medicaid data. *BMC Health Services Research, 14,* 355. doi:10.1186/1472-6963-14-355

Santaguida, P. L., & Raina, P. (2008). McMaster Quality Assessment Scale of Harms (McHarm) for Primary Studies: Manual for use of the McHarm. Edited by CCOHTA Canadian Coordinating Office for Health Technology Assessment. Retrieved from http://www.citeulike.org/user/SRCMethods Library/article/13308169

Schalet, B. D., Revicki, D. A., Cook, K. F., Krishnan, E., Fries, J. F., & Cella, D. (2015). Establishing a common metric for physical function: Linking the HAQ-DI and SF-36 PF Subscale to PROMIS physical function. *Journal of General Internal Medicine*, *30*(10), 1517–1523. doi:10.1007/s11606-015-3360-0

Schneider, E. C., Timbie, J. W., Fox, D. S., Van Busum, K. R., & Caloyeras, J. P. (2013). Dissemination and adoption of comparative effectiveness research findings when findings challenge current practices, and was conducted for RAND Health, a division of the RAND Corporation. U.S. Department of Health and Human Services Publication. Retrieved from http://aspe.hhs.gov/health/reports/2013/CERDissemination/rpt_RANDFinal.pdf

Stefan, M. S., Nathanson, B. H., Higgins, T. L., Steingrub, J. S., Lagu, T., Rothberg, M. B., & Lindenauer, P. K. (2015). Comparative effectiveness of noninvasive and invasive ventilation in critically ill patients with acute exacerbation of chronic obstructive pulmonary disease. *Critical Care Medicine*, *43*(7), 1386–1394.

Stillwell, S. B., Fineout-Overholt, E., Melnyk, B. M., & Williamson, K. M. (2010). Evidence-based practice, step-by-step: Asking the clinical question: A key step in evidence-based practice. *American Journal of Nursing*, *110*(3), 58–61.

Taveras, E. M., Marshall, R., Horan, C. M., Gillman, M. W., Hacker, K., Kleinman, K. P., . . . Simon, S. R. (2013). Rationale and design of the STAR randomized controlled trial to accelerate adoption of childhood obesity comparative effectiveness research. *Contemporary Clinical Trials*, *34*(1), 101–108.

Timbie, J. W., Ringel, J. S., Fox, D. S., Waxman, D. A., Pillemer, F., Carey, C., . . . Kellermann, A. L. (2012). *Allocation of scarce resources during mass casualty events.* Evidence Report No. 207. (Prepared by the Southern California Evidence-Based Practice Center under Contract No. 290-2007-10062-I; AHRQ Publication no. 12-E006-EF). Rockville, MD: Agency for Healthcare Research and Quality. Retrieved from www.effectivehealthcare.ahrq.gov/reports/final.cfm

U.S. Federal Coordinating Council for Comparative Effectiveness Research. (2009). *Report to the President and the Congress.* Retrieved from http://www.med.upenn.edu/sleepctr/documents/FederalCoordinatingCoucilforCER_2009.pdf

Velentgas, P., Dreyer, N. A., Nourjah, P., Smith, S. R., & Torchia, M. M. (Eds.). (2013). *Developing a protocol for observational comparative effectiveness research: A user's guide* (AHRQ Publication no. 12(13)-EHC099). Rockville, MD: Agency for Healthcare Research and Quality. Retrieved from http://effectivehealthcare.ahrq.gov/ehc/products/440/1166/User-Guide-Observational-CER-130113.pdf

Walker, K. L., Kirillova, O., Gillespie, S. E., Hsiao, D., Pishchalenko, V., Pai, A. K., . . . Hazlehurst, B. L. (2014). Using the CER Hub to ensure data quality in a multi-institution smoking cessation study. *Journal of the American Medical Information Association*, *21*(6), 1129–1135.

Wang, Y., Wu, Y., Wilson, R. F., Bleich, S., Cheskin, L., Weston, C., . . . Segal, J. (2013). *Childhood obesity prevention programs: Comparative effectiveness review and meta-analysis. Comparative effectiveness review No. 115.* (Prepared by the Johns Hopkins University Evidence-Based Practice Center under Contract No. 290-2007-10061-I; AHRQ Publication no. 13-EHC081-EF). Rockville, MD: Agency for Healthcare Research and Quality. Retrieved from http://www.ncbi.nlm.nih.gov/pubmedhealth/PMH0057623/pdf/TOC.pdf

Wilke, R. J., & Mullins, C. D. (2011). "Ten commandments" for conducting comparative effectiveness research using "real-world data." *Journal of Managed Care Pharmacy*, *17*(Suppl. 9A), s10–s15.

Xian, Y., Hammill, B. G., & Curtis, L. H. (2013). Data sources for heart failure comparative effectiveness research. *Heart Failure Clinics*, *9*(1), 1–13.

APPENDIX 6.1 COMPARATIVE EFFECTIVENESS RESOURCES

Name of Resource URL of Resource Description of Resource
• Journal of Comparativeness Effectiveness Research (CER) • www.futuremedicine.com/loi/cer • An international, peer-reviewed, and open-access journal focusing on CER in health care
• Developing a Protocol for Observational Comparative Effectiveness Research: A User's Guide • http://effectivehealthcare.ahrq.gov/ehc/products/440/1166/User-Guide-Observational-CER-130113.pdf • Detailed guide for conducting observational CER
• Good ReseArch for Comparative Effectiveness (GRACE) Principles • www.graceprinciples.org • Resources with checklists and publications to improve the quality of observational CER and facilitate decision making on therapeutic alternatives
• The ISPE (International Society for Pharmacoepidemiology) Guidelines for Good Pharmacoepidemiology Practices • www.pharmacoepi.org/resources/guidelines_08027.cfm • Concise overview for developing research protocols and conducting CER research
• Strengthening the Reporting of Observational Studies in Epidemiology (STROBE) guidelines • www.strobe-statement.org • Checklists and recent publications on observational studies in epidemiology
• Methodological Standards for Patient-Centered Outcomes Research by Patient-Centered Outcomes Research Institute (PCORI) • www.pcori.org/research-results/research-methodology • Section of PCORI website that focuses on getting the "methods" right
• National Library of Medicine (NLM) Resources for Informing Comparative Effectiveness • www.nlm.nih.gov/nichsr/cer/cerqueries.html • Supports specialized searches of published research (PubMed) and research still in progress—HSRProj and ClinicalTrials.gov—to help inform investigations for CER
• Substance Abuse and Mental Health Service Administration (SAMSA) CER Resources • www.nrepp.samhsa.gov/CERResources.aspx • Links to web pages, print/media resources, CER databases, and funding/training areas
• CONSORT (CONsolidated Standards of Reporting Trials) 2010 guideline • www.consort-statement.org/consort-2010 • Provides a checklist, flow diagram, and sample studies for reports of clinical trials
• Agency for Healthcare Research and Quality (AHRQ) Practice-Based Research Networks • http://pbrn.ahrq.gov • Resources for pragmatic (practice based) research, including the PRagmatic-Explanatory Continuum Indicator Summary (PRECIS) tool
• Academy Health: Methods of CER • www.hsrmethods.org/SuggestedReadings/Journal%20Articles/Comparative%20Effectiveness.aspx • Lists recommended articles on CER methods by types of studies

APPENDIX 6.2 EXAMPLES OF CER ABSTRACTS FROM THE PUBLISHED LITERATURE

Abstract #1

Nursing interventions for the frail elderly are the subject of the first two CER abstracts related to RCTs as examples of research that is guiding policy development. A third abstract presents a CER study related to using a systematic review method to determine effectiveness of pharmacological (anticholinergic) therapy for women with overactive bladder. The fourth abstract is an example of an observational CER study designed to compare patient outcomes after treatment with non-invasive ventilation (NIV) or invasive mechanical ventilation in COPD (chronic obstructive pulmonary disease) patients in the ICU using a large multicenter database of ICU patients.

McCauley, K., Bradway, C., Hirschman, K. B., & Naylor, M. D. (2014). Studying nursing interventions in acutely ill, cognitively impaired older adults. *American Journal of Nursing, 114*(10), 44–52.

Abstract #2

Overview

Although it increases the risk of poor outcomes and raises the costs of care, cognitive impairment in hospitalized older adults is often neither accurately identified nor well managed. In conducting a two-phase, comparative-effectiveness clinical trial of the effects of three nursing interventions—augmented standard care (ASC), resource nurse care (RNC), and the transitional care model (TCM)—on hospitalized older adults with cognitive deficits, a team of researchers encountered several challenges. For example, in assessing potential subjects for the study, they found that nearly half of those assessed had cognitive impairment, yet many family caregivers either could not be identified or had no interest in participating in the study. One lesson the researchers learned was that research involving cognitively impaired older adults must actively engage clinicians, patients, and family caregivers, as well as address the complex process of managing post-discharge care.

www.ncbi.nlm.nih.gov/pubmed/25251126

Naylor, M. D., Hirschman, K. B., Hanlon, A. L., Bowles, K. H., Bradway, C., McCauley, K. M., & Pauly, M. V. (2014, May). Comparison of evidence-based interventions on outcomes of hospitalized, cognitively impaired older adults. *Journal of Comparative Effectiveness Research, 3*(3), 245–257.

Abstract #3

Aim

This article reports the effects of three evidence-based interventions of varying intensity, each of which is designed to improve outcomes of hospitalized cognitively impaired older adults.

Materials and Methods

In this comparative effectiveness study, 202 older adults with cognitive impairment (assessed within 24 hours of index hospitalization) were enrolled at one of the three hospitals within an academic health system. Each hospital was randomly assigned one of the following interventions: ASC (lower dose: $n = 65$), RNC (medium dose: $n = 71$), or the TCM (higher dose: $n = 66$). Since randomization at the patient level was not feasible due to potential contamination, generalized boosted modeling that estimated multigroup propensity score weights was used to balance baseline patient characteristics between groups. Analyses compared the three groups on time with first rehospitalization or death, the number and days of all-cause rehospitalizations per patient, and functional status through 6-month postindex hospitalization.

Results

In total, 25% of the ASC group were rehospitalized or died by day 33 compared with day 58 for the RNC group versus day 83 for the TCM group. The largest differences between the three groups on time to rehospitalization or death were observed early in the Kaplan–Meier curve (at 30 days: ASC = 22% vs. RNC = 19% vs. TCM = 9%). The TCM group also demonstrated lower mean rehospitalization rates per patient compared with the RNC ($p < .001$) and ASC groups ($p = .06$) at 30 days. At 90-day postindex hospitalization, the TCM group continued to demonstrate lower mean rehospitalization rates per patient only when compared with the ASC group ($p = .02$). No significant group differences in functional status were observed.

Conclusion

Findings suggest that the TCM intervention, compared with interventions of lower intensity, has the potential to decrease costly resource use outcomes in the immediate postindex hospitalization period among cognitively impaired older adults.

Keywords

cognitive impairment; functional status; rehospitalizations; transitional care

Free PMC Article

www.ncbi.nlm.nih.gov/pubmed/24969152

Reynolds, W. S., McPheeters, M., Blume, J., Surawicz, T., Worley, K., Wang, L., & Hartmann, K. (2015). Comparative effectiveness of anticholinergic therapy for overactive bladder in women: A systematic review and meta-analysis. *Obstetrics & Gynecology, 125*(6), 1423–1432.

Abstract #4

Objective

To summarize evidence about reduction in voiding and resolution of urine loss in overactive bladder by comparing data from the active drug arms with the placebo arms of randomized trials.

Data Sources

We searched MEDLINE, EMBASE, Cumulative Index to Nursing and Allied Health Literature, and ClinicalTrials.gov in March 2014.

Methods of Study Selection

Multiple reviewers screened original research published in English on community-dwelling women with a non-neurogenic overactive bladder undergoing pharmaco-therapy with medications that are available in the United States. Studies in which women comprised less than 75% of the population or those with a sample size less than 50 were excluded. Study designs included RCTs for meta-analysis and cohorts, case-control series, and case series for harms data. Our search identified 50 RCTs from among 144 candidate publications (one was of good quality, 38 were fair, and 11 were poor).

Tabulation, Integration, and Results

Multiple team members performed data extraction independently with a secondary review of data entry to ensure quality and validity. Studies were assessed for risk of bias. Meta-analysis was performed using fixed-effects regression models. The primary outcomes and measurements were the numbers of daily voids and urge incontinence episodes. Medications delivered as a daily dose reduced urge incontinence by 1.73 episodes per day (95% confidence interval [CI] 1.37–2.09) and voids by 2.06 per day (95% CI 1.66–2.46) from 2.79 (95% CI 0.70–4.88) to 11.28 (95% CI 7.77–14.80) at baseline, respectively. Placebo reduced urge incontinence episodes by 1.06 (95% CI 0.7–1.42) and voids by 1.2 (95% CI 0.72–1.67) per day. No individual agent demonstrated superiority over another. The majority (98%) of studies reporting funding were sponsored by the industry.

Conclusion

Evidence from more than 27,000 women participating in RCTs suggests that improvement in symptoms with anticholinergic management of an overactive bladder is modest and rarely fully resolves symptoms.

www.ncbi.nlm.nih.gov/pubmed/26000514

Stefan, M. S., Nathanson, B. H., Higgins, T. L., Steingrub, J. S., Lagu, T., Rothberg, M. B., & Lindenauer, P. K. (2015). Comparative effectiveness of noninvasive and invasive ventilation in critically ill patients with acute exacerbation of chronic obstructive pulmonary disease. *Critical Care Medicine, 43*(7), 1386–1394. doi: 10.1097/CCM.0000000000000945

Abstract #5

Objectives

To compare the characteristics and hospital outcomes of patients with an acute exacerbation of chronic obstructive pulmonary disease treated in the ICU with initial NIV or invasive mechanical ventilation.

Design

A retrospective, multicenter cohort study of prospectively collected data was used. We used propensity matching to compare the outcomes of patients treated with NIV to those treated with invasive mechanical ventilation. We also assessed predictors for NIV failure.

Setting

Thirty-eight hospitals participated in the Acute Physiology and Chronic Health Evaluation database from 2008 through 2012.

Subjects

A total of 3,520 patients with a diagnosis of chronic obstructive pulmonary disease exacerbation, including 27.7% who received NIV and 45.5% who received invasive mechanical ventilation, participated.

Interventions

None

Measurements and Main Results

NIV failure was recorded in 13.7% from patients ventilated noninvasively. Hospital mortality was 7.4% for patients treated with NIV; 16.1% for those treated with invasive mechanical ventilation; and 22.5% for those who failed NIV. In the propensity-matched analysis, patients initially treated with NIV had a 41% lower risk of death compared with those treated with invasive mechanical ventilation (relative risk, 0.59; 95% CI, 0.36–0.97). Factors that were independently associated with NIV failure were Simplified Acute Physiology Score II (relative risk = 1.04 per point increase; 95% CI, 1.03–1.04) and the presence of cancer (2.29; 95% CI, 0.96–5.45).

Conclusions

Among critically ill adults with chronic obstructive pulmonary disease exacerbation, the receipt of NIV was associated with a lower risk of in-hospital mortality compared with that of invasive mechanical ventilation; NIV failure was associated with the worst outcomes. These results support the use of NIV as a first-line therapy in appropriately selected critically ill patients with chronic obstructive pulmonary disease while also highlighting the risks associated with NIV failure and the need to be cautious in the face of severe disease.

www.ncbi.nlm.nih.gov/pubmed/25768682

CHAPTER SEVEN

DISSEMINATION RESEARCH

JANE T. GARVIN, AMBER B. McCALL, AND
DEVITA T. STALLINGS

OBJECTIVES

After reading this chapter, readers will be able to:

1. Describe dissemination research within the context of translation research
2. Discuss the importance of dissemination research
3. Differentiate dissemination research from implementation research
4. Identify key components of methods used in dissemination research
5. List key resources for learning more about this evolving translation research method

DEFINING DISSEMINATION RESEARCH

Dissemination research is the "systematic study of processes and factors that lead to widespread use of an evidence-based intervention by the target population" (Rabin, Brownson, Haire-Joshu, Kreuter, & Weaver, 2008, p. 119). Distinct from other types of research, the goal of dissemination research is to determine the best methods to achieve widespread intervention use (Rabin et al., 2008). Dissemination research does not involve modifying the intervention to fit into a particular setting; instead, it focuses on processes involved in transmitting the unedited message of a successful intervention to a target audience for widespread use.

Placing Dissemination Research in the Research Trajectory: Bench to Bedside to Practice

In order to identify where dissemination research fits in the research translation process, it is helpful to review the research trajectory, which includes both translational research and translation research. Clinicians are familiar with the term *bench to bedside*. The process of moving findings from basic science research to clinical practice involves three areas of translation (Westfall, Mold, & Fagnan, 2007). The first two areas of translation are referred to as *translational research*. The first area, *translation to humans*, begins when phase 1 and 2 basic science (bench) clinical trials are translated to human clinical trials (bedside). Next, controlled observational studies and phase 3 clinical trials take place at the bedside. Much occurs between human clinical trials (bedside) and clinical practice (practice) when the aim is to get the right treatment to the right patient at the right time. Between bedside and practice is another step (practice-based research) where phase 3 and 4 clinical trials along with observational studies and survey research are conducted. The second area of translation, *translation to patients*, involves systematic reviews, meta-analyses, and guideline development as research is translated to patients (practice-based research). The third area of translation, *translation to practice*, moves practice-based research to real-world clinical practice. In this final step, referred to as *translation research*, both dissemination research and implementation research are conducted, moving research to clinical practice.

Placing Dissemination Research in Translation Research

Dissemination research falls under the umbrella of translation research. Translation research includes three types of research: dissemination, implementation, and diffusion (Schillinger, 2010). Dissemination research and implementation research are often addressed together by authors and even by the National Institutes of Health (NIH) and are referred to as dissemination and implementation (D&I) research (Brownson, Colditz, & Proctor, 2012; NIH—Office of Behavioral and Social Sciences Research, 2015). Diffusion research involves more passive approaches, builds on earlier research, and focuses on the broadest use of evidence-based interventions (EBIs; Rabin et al., 2008; Schillinger, 2010).

Because of the relevance of these evolving, more active translation research approaches (D&I) to nurse scholars, this book includes chapters on D&I research. This chapter addresses dissemination research, and the next chapter (Chapter 8) addresses implementation research.

Clarification of Terms

Translation research is an emerging field. As such, terms were blurred in the past. In 2008, the first resource was written to clarify some of the key terms (Rabin et al., 2008). Since then, key terms have been defined with a public health focus (Schillinger, 2010), and further defined and documented in the key reference book for D&I research written by leaders in this field, Brownson et al. (2012). To further clarify the terms of D&I research, the terms are compared in Table 7.1 with emphasis placed on key concepts.

TABLE 7.1   Dissemination Research Compared With Implementation Research

Dissemination Research	Implementation Research
Dissemination research is the study of how the **targeted distribution** of information ***to a specific audience*** can lead to **widespread use** of the EBI.	*Implementation research* is the study of how to **fit or integrate** an EBI ***into a specific setting*** for use in that specific setting.

EBI, evidence-based intervention.
Source: Definitions provided here are based on definitions in text (Rabin et al., 2008; Schillinger, 2010).

Translation research characterizes the sequence of events (i.e., process) in which a proven scientific discovery (i.e., evidence-based public health intervention) is successfully institutionalized (i.e., seamlessly integrated into established practice and policy). . . . Translation research takes effectiveness studies and attempts to understand the process that moves discoveries to sustained adoption (Schillinger, 2010).

Dissemination is an active approach of spreading evidence-based interventions to the target audience via determined channels using planned strategies (Rabin et al., 2008). Dissemination is the targeted distribution of information and intervention materials to a specific public health or clinical practice audience (Schillinger, 2010).

Dissemination research is the systematic study of processes and factors that lead to widespread use of an evidence-based intervention by the target population (Rabin et al., 2008). Dissemination research is the systematic study of how the targeted distribution of information and intervention materials to a specific public health audience can be successfully executed so that increased spread of knowledge about the evidence-based public health interventions achieves greater use and impact of the intervention (Schillinger, 2010).

Implementation is the process of putting to use or integrating evidence-based interventions within a setting (Rabin et al., 2008). Implementation is the use of strategies to adopt and integrate evidence-based health interventions and to change practice patterns within specific settings (Schillinger, 2010).

Implementation research seeks to understand the processes and factors that are associated with successful integration of evidence-based interventions within a particular setting (e.g., worksite or school; Rabin et al., 2008). Implementation research is the systematic study of how a specific set of activities and designed strategies are used to successfully integrate an evidence-based public health intervention within specific settings (e.g., primary care clinic, community center, school; Schillinger, 2010).

Diffusion is the passive, untargeted, unplanned, and uncontrolled spread of new interventions (Rabin et al., 2008).

Diffusion research is the systematic study of the factors necessary for successful adoption by stakeholders and the targeted population of an evidence-based intervention which results in widespread use (e.g., state or national level) and specifically includes the uptake of new practices or the penetration of broad scale recommendations through dissemination and implementation efforts, marketing, laws and regulations, systems research, and policies (Schillinger, 2010).

IMPORTANCE OF DISSEMINATION RESEARCH

The value of scientific evidence is related to how widely it is applied. Dissemination research is critical to expand and accurately measure the reach of a specific area of research. *Reach* refers to accessibility and uptake of an intervention (Schillinger, 2010). Dissemination research is an important step toward getting the right care to the right patient at the right time. The aims of dissemination research are to identify the best methods to (a) move information about well-researched interventions to the targeted health care providers or patient groups and (b) motivate the targeted providers or patient groups to use that information. Dissemination research is vital to the mission of improving health care.

Reasons for Using Dissemination Research

There are many reasons for using dissemination research. Dissemination research provides information about effective as well as ineffective methods of (a) moving information about well-researched effective interventions to the target health care provider and patient populations and (b) moving target populations from awareness of well-researched effective interventions to adoption of those well-researched effective interventions. Researchers and clinicians use the published findings from dissemination research to guide future dissemination plans. Many interventions and health promotion strategies have been well researched and found to be effective but not readily adopted. Dissemination research provides the evidence to fill the gap between effective interventions and adoption. Researchers and clinicians use findings from dissemination research to choose effective dissemination strategies with desired outcomes and avoid wasting resources on ineffective strategies.

METHODS OF CREATING DISSEMINATION RESEARCH

Choosing the Intervention to Disseminate

Dissemination research differs from other types of research in that this research starts with a well-researched, effective intervention. The effective intervention is strong enough to warrant widespread dissemination. In addition, the effective intervention addresses an important clinical or public health problem. Research on how to disseminate EBIs is clear that dissemination does not occur spontaneously (Brownson et al., 2012).

Clinical practice guidelines offer a starting point when choosing an intervention to disseminate. Ideally, clinical practice guidelines are based on well-researched effective interventions. However, there are a number of reasons that clinical practice guidelines might not be based on well-researched effective interventions. In particular, clinicians often seek guidance on important issues when the research on the topic has not been fully developed; therefore, the related guidelines may be based on weak evidence or solely expert opinion. It is vital to choose well-researched interventions as the basis for dissemination research regardless of inclusion in a clinical practice guideline.

Choosing a Population to Target

Dissemination research may target a variety of groups. Primary targets include *health care providers, patients,* or *the public in general.* The target population will depend on the EBI chosen; thus, it is important to understand for whom the intervention was designed as well as to choose a strategy to move the intervention forward toward widespread use.

Choosing the Dissemination Strategy

Dissemination research aims to have a wide or broad reach. Strategies should be designed to achieve adoption by a large portion of the target population, for example, television, electronic methods such as e-mail, social media, and health care applications for mobile devices. The strategy should employ a creative and/or novel approach to move information and gain adoption by the target population. If the strategy employs familiar resources, the resources should be engaged in an innovative manner that differs from the status quo. The strategy could employ a specific product or involve developing a new product for the purpose of disseminating the intervention and gaining intervention adoption. Strategies should be designed to enhance motivation such as engaging key leaders, social networks, rewards, and ideal timing of the dissemination intervention and to make the disseminated materials easy to use, such as specific resources (e.g., laptop computer) or training to use the dissemination method (e.g., computer skills, application skills on handheld devices; Agency for Healthcare Research and Quality [AHRQ], 2012). Consider strategies that intervene on multiple levels (individuals, groups, and larger groups—similar to the socioecological model; AHRQ, 2012). In addition, strategies might be designed to target high-risk groups.

Choosing a Comparison Strategy

Ideally, a dissemination research study with a strong design would include a comparison strategy and randomization. Options for comparison may include current strategies that are commonly used, low-cost strategies, or dissemination strategies with the best outcomes known to date.

Choosing an Outcome

Although there is not much in the literature on dissemination outcomes, several constructs that can serve as measurable outcomes have emerged (Proctor & Brownson, 2012). Dissemination is a two-step process. The first step is to reach the target population with the message. This generates the opportunity for an outcome related to awareness of the intervention. The second step focuses on adoption or use of the intervention. As a result, it is necessary to determine whether the information about the intervention is being used, by whom, and to what degree (Proctor & Brownson, 2012). Therefore, a variety of outcomes could be measured (e.g., adoption or not, description of users, frequency of use, or participation rates).

Choosing Variables That Influence the Outcome

A number of variables may influence the process of dissemination (awareness and adoption). Variables that influence information movement, uptake, and regular use are worthy of study and may be included in quantitative analyses or qualitative inquiry. Influential variables for consideration may include ease of use (i.e., How easy is it to use the information delivery system?), realistic implementation (i.e., How easy is it to perform the intervention?), cost (i.e., Does it fit within the target audience's budget?), barriers, accelerants/motivators (e.g., additional supporting influences such as health care coverage or reimbursement), subsample characteristics (i.e., Does the intervention work better or worse for specific groups?), and any number of other influencing variables.

Choosing the Time or Interval for Follow-Up

Although every study should have a baseline assessment, a number of factors may dictate the time or interval for appropriate follow-up. Health care priorities, available resources, and seasons are just a few of the factors that may influence one's choice of time for follow-up. An appropriate interval for follow-up would allow the target population sufficient opportunity to receive the message and to use the information about the well-researched intervention. However, any time is better than not having a follow-up time.

Examples of Aims Related to Dissemination Research

Several broad examples of aims are provided. Details of one's research can be used to modify these broad examples to develop specific aims.

- Describe the experience of a person in the target group who adopted the intervention being disseminated.
  - Describe the factors (facilitators and barriers) involved in initial adoption
  - Describe the process of adoption.
  - Describe the factors involved in continued use of the intervention.
- Describe the factors that influence the creation, packaging, transmission, and receipt of valid health research knowledge. Some of the variables may include funding, culture, format (electronic or paper), cost, or readiness. Influential variables may also be discovered through qualitative inquiry.
- Determine effectiveness of individual and systemic strategies to acquire, maintain, and use knowledge in decision making and practice. Effectiveness can be measured in terms of awareness, adoption, or degree of use. Reviews of health records can be conducted to determine who used the intervention and to what degree when examining, for example, point-of-decision resources as a dissemination strategy.
- Determine effectiveness of alternative strategies targeting rural, minority, and other underserved populations. Without modifying the intervention, determine the effectiveness of a given method of moving information to a target population. The method to deliver the message may differ based on the target population but the message (EBI) itself remains unchanged.
- Determine awareness of a specific clinical practice guideline by a target audience (e.g., specialty nurses).
- Determine whether a target audience (e.g., specialty nurses) uses a specific clinical practice guideline.

- Describe factors that influence a target audience (e.g., specialty nurses) to use a specific evidence-based clinical practice guideline following a targeted dissemination intervention (e.g., distributing information via guideline publication, adding information to electronic guideline database, tweeting, electronic device application).

Choosing the Design of Dissemination Research

Dissemination research is suited to research designs involving qualitative, quantitative, and mixed methods (Gaglio & Glasgow, 2012; Proctor & Brownson, 2012). The study aims drive the methodological approach and analysis. Therefore, a methodologist should be consulted early in the planning process regardless of the approach (qualitative or quantitative). The methodologist or statistician plays a vital role in framing the question and clarifying the analysis required to address the aims and answer the research questions.

Dissemination research often requires initial qualitative inquiry to determine which variables influence the process. In addition, observational studies and surveys are well suited to dissemination research. Studies employing randomization are desirable, as it is difficult to control for outside influences. Studies that measure moderators (variables associated with the degree of adoption and the time to adoption) and mediators (process variables) are particularly well suited to dissemination research, because they identify factors and processes associated with adoption or rejection of an intervention.

ANALYSIS OF DATA RELATED TO DISSEMINATION RESEARCH

Analysis varies widely between qualitative and quantitative studies. The aims of the study determine the analytical approach. Some examples follow.

- Qualitative studies
  - Interviews and focus groups can be conducted for deeper understandings of the processes of obtaining and using the specific intervention. Data are coded and examined for themes.
- Quantitative studies
  - Descriptive data
    - Who uses the information and intervention materials?
  - Chi-square (comparisons of the percentage of adoption from one dissemination method with another or for one group with another)
    - Is there a difference between one dissemination method and another?
    - Is there a difference between one group's adoption of the intervention and another group's adoption of it?
  - Logistic regression (where the dependent variable [DV] is adoption/use of the intervention [yes/no] and the independent variables [IVs] are the personal/agency characteristic along with other variables related to the method of dissemination)
    - What influences use of the information?

- Linear regression (where the DV is the number of times information was used over some period and the IVs are the personal/agency characteristic and other variables related to the method of dissemination)
  - What influences the frequency of using the information and intervention material?
- Structural equation modeling (to describe the process of adoption of the intervention)
  - What is the relationship between variables of interest and the outcome, use of information, or intervention material?

INTERPRETATION AND PRESENTATION OF DISSEMINATION RESEARCH

Dissemination research yields information about who uses the intervention, what information or components of an intervention are used, which variables influence the process of dissemination, where and when the information is accessed and used, why the information is accessed and used (or not), and how the information is accessed and used. Dissemination research is challenged by many potential confounding variables—factors outside of the study design that may influence the outcome. Therefore, it is important to acknowledge these limitations when interpreting the findings.

What the findings are and how they are reported depend on the type of inquiry used to address the aim or research question. For example, qualitative studies present the findings as themes or processes involved in adoption in a narrative format and may not use a table to describe characteristics of the target group involved in the study. Quantitative studies most often use tables to describe the target group and to present findings. Tables are descriptive enough to stand alone, whereas texts are used to interpret key findings for the reader. Guidelines with checklists are available to ensure that key information is included when reporting findings of the study. The guidelines and checklists vary based on the type of study conducted. An extensive list of the guidelines has been compiled (Simera, Moher, Hoey, Schulz, & Altman, 2010). Some of the more commonly used guidelines for nursing are provided next.

- Qualitative
  - Consolidated Criteria for Reporting Qualitative Research (COREQ) for interviews and focus groups (Tong, Sainsbury, & Craig, 2007)
- Quantitative
  - STrengthening the Reporting of OBservational Studies in Epidemiology (STROBE) for observational studies (von Elm et al., 2008)
  - Transparent Reporting of Evaluations With Nonrandomized Designs (TREND) for nonrandomized intervention studies (Des Jarlais, Lyles, Crepaz, & The Trend Group, 2004)
  - CONsolidated Standards of Reporting Trials (CONSORT) for randomized, controlled intervention studies (Schulz, Altman, & Moher, 2010)

Dissemination research is similar to other types of research in terms of presenting research findings. Regardless of the type of study or the guideline used, the report should include the following: a description of the sample, details about the intervention and any comparison intervention, and results of the study. Aspects of each element are highlighted next along with general comments and comments specific to dissemination research.

- Population (Sample)
  - Describe the sample/target population.
  - Use tables with frequencies, percentages, means, and standard deviations, as they are ideal.
  - Report sample (participant/subject/patient/clinician) characteristics.
    - Age, gender, race, socioeconomic status, region or geographic area, and other variables of interest that describe the sample are used.
    - Other personal or agency variables that influence obtaining or using information and intervention material (e.g., access to a computer with Internet service) are included.
    - If a comparison intervention is used, the sample may be described as one group, and as two separate groups (treatment and comparison) to demonstrate similarities and differences among the treatment and comparison groups.
- Intervention: Dissemination strategies
  - Identify the EBI, but the focus of this section is the strategy to move information and gain adoption of the EBI.
  - Provide details of the strategy.
    - Details may be presented in the text, text box, or table.
    - Include the following.
      - Communication techniques
      - Combinations of techniques used to move the information to the target population
      - Presentation format (e.g., reading level, photos, diagrams, hypothetical cases, photos reflecting different groups—age, gender, race)
      - Strategies to enhance motivation
      - Strategies to enhance ability to use the dissemination materials
  - Describe in detail the use of the strategy or participation in the text or a table.
    - Report in a separate table the participation or use of the dissemination strategy (e.g., accessed the online intervention application on average X times in the first month [or other observed study period], percentage of those who accessed the application at least five times per week).
- Comparison
  - If a comparison dissemination strategy is used, describe it in detail and in the same format as the previously mentioned primary intervention.
- Outcome
  - Describe outcomes in detail in the text or tables; the outcome, or DV, may be depicted in equations, graphs, diagrams, or tables.
  - Include the following.
    - Awareness of the information and/or intervention materials
    - Knowledge about the information and/or intervention materials
    - Discussions about the information and/or intervention materials
    - Self-efficacy to use the information and/or intervention materials

          – Intentions to use or apply the information and/or intervention materials
          – Behavior demonstrating use or application of the information and/or intervention materials
          – Clinical outcomes for patients or recipients of health care

- Time
  - Specify the time of follow-up after delivery of the information and/or intervention material.
  - Describe time in the text; in addition, time may be presented in graphs or figures with other results.
  - If time to adoption is a variable in a regression analysis, present it in a table with other variables.

EXAMPLES OF PUBLISHED DISSEMINATION RESEARCH

Two examples of completed dissemination research are highlighted here. Topics include adoption of feeding tube placement verification recommendation and adoption of a guideline related to type 2 diabetes (T2D) management using metformin mono-therapy (Bourgault et al., 2014; Huang, Zdon, Moore, Jane Moran, & Quick, 2010). Other examples of likely dissemination research topics that come to mind may not be found in the literature, as dissemination research may fall into the category of marketing research. For example, dissemination research related to vaccines and other medications is often conducted by pharmaceutical companies and that information may be considered proprietary; therefore, it would not be found in the literature.

Feeding Tube Placement Verification

Bourgault et al. (2014) studied factors that influence critical care nurses' adoption of the American Association of Critical-Care Nurses (AACN) evidence-based clinical guideline, the practice alert to verify correct placement of feeding tubes. The target population or *specific group* was critical care nurses across the United States (Bourgault et al., 2014). The dissemination intervention aimed to move information to the critical care nurses. The study was guided by Rogers's diffusion of innovations theory, which influenced the selection of study variables. The DV was the adoption of this specific evidence-based clinical practice guideline. An elegant analytical model depicting the theoretical and empirical structure of this dissemination study was published in this article.

Through an electronic AACN newsletter, all AACN members were invited to participate in the online survey. Although the survey's response rate was low (0.6%, $n = 619$), and about 40% of the surveys were excluded from the analysis, resulting in a final sample of 370 critical care nurses, the findings were interesting. Fifty-five percent of respondents were aware of the practice alert, and 45% reported they had adopted it into their practice. However, less than a third of the adopters reported adopting all four of the clinical practices.

Data were analyzed using logistic regression to examine factors influencing critical care nurses' adoption of the specialty organization's recommended four clinical practices, which constituted the key study outcome. Controlling for other variables, only the perceived presence of a policy prevailed as a significant predictor of adoption of all four practices (odds ratio, 6.77; 95% confidence interval [CI], 3.12–14.72). It is worth noting that this research was conducted by a nurse scholar as part of a doctoral program and is an example of how a dissertation can be converted into a continuing education manuscript (Bourgault et al., 2014).

Diabetes Management

Huang et al. (2010) studied the impact of the national and international clinical guidelines published by the American Diabetes Association (ADA) and the European Association for the Study of Diabetes (EASD) of their consensus algorithm for the initiation and adjustment of T2D therapy. The target population or specific group was health care providers in the United States. The dissemination intervention aimed to move information to health care providers by these two specialty guidelines recommending early metformin monotherapy for newly diagnosed diabetics.

The study outcome was the guideline adoption. Data on patients newly diagnosed with T2D and their treatment 30 days post-diagnosis were retrieved from an integrated database of medical claims, pharmaceutical claims, and laboratory results from a diverse group of health insurance plans. The trend in the incidence of guideline adoption, early metformin monotherapy, was analyzed using joinpoint regression modeling (Joinpoint regression modeling is a complex statistical modeling technique that assesses for statistically significant changes in incidence trends over time). The analysis showed that the publication of the guidelines by ADA and EASD was associated with a significant acceleration in the incidence of early metformin monotherapy (Huang et al., 2010).

Other Resources

Resources for more information are listed here. D&I science and research often lump together both dissemination research and implementation research (see Chapter 8 for implementation research).

D&I news can be found at the following website maintained by the NIH: http://obssr.od.nih.gov/scientific_areas/translation/dissemination_and_implementation

Example of one dissemination research framework:
https://depts.washington.edu/hprc/docs/dissemination-research.pdf

Moving health services research into policy and practice:
www.academyhealth.org/lessons

SUMMARY

Factors influencing adoption of clinical practice guidelines among nurses are surprisingly understudied (Bourgault et al., 2014), and they are an important area for future nursing research. As such, the interdisciplinary field of dissemination research continues to grow. Nurse scholars can have a significant role in advancing knowledge of salient dissemination processes and factors that successfully result in widespread adoption of clinical and public health evidence-based practice (EBP) interventions.

REFERENCES

Agency for Healthcare Research and Quality. (2012). *Evidence-based practice center systematic review protocol: Communication and dissemination strategies to facilitate the use of health and health care evidence.* Retrieved from http://www.effectivehealthcare.ahrq.gov

Bourgault, A. M., Heath, J., Hooper, V., Sole, M. L., Waller, J. L., & NeSmith, E. G. (2014). Factors influencing critical care nurses' adoption of the AACN practice alert on verification of feeding tube placement. *American Journal of Critical Care, 23*(2), 134–144. doi:10.4037/ajcc2014558

Brownson, R., Colditz, G., & Proctor, E. (Eds.). (2012). *Dissemination and implementation research in health: Translating science to practice.* New York, NY: Oxford University Press.

Des Jarlais, D. C., Lyles, C., Crepaz, N., & The Trend Group. (2004). Improving the reporting quality of nonrandomized evaluations of behavioral and public health interventions: The TREND statement. *American Journal of Public Health, 94*(3), 361–366.

Gaglio, B., & Glasgow, R. E. (2012). Evaluation approaches for dissemination and implementation research. In R. C. Brownson, G. Colditz, & E. Proctor, E. (Eds.). *Dissemination and implementation research in health: Translating science to practice* (pp. 327–356). New York, NY: Oxford University Press.

Huang, E. A., Zdon, G. S., Moore, R. J., Jane Moran, H., & Quick, W. W. (2010). The impact of publishing medical specialty society guidelines on subsequent adoption of best practices: A case study with type 2 diabetes. *International Journal of Clinical Practice, 64*(5), 558–561. doi:10.1111/j.1742-1241.2009.02319.x

National Institutes of Health—Office of Behavioral and Social Sciences Research. (2015). *Dissemination and implementation.* Retrieved from http://obssr.od.nih.gov/scientific_areas/translation/dissemination_and_implementation

Proctor, E., & Brownson, R. C. (2012). Measurement issues in dissemination and implementation research. In R. C. Brownson, G. Colditz, & E. Proctor (Eds.). *Dissemination and implementation research in health: Translating science to practice* (pp. 261–280). New York, NY: Oxford University Press.

Rabin, B. A., Brownson, R. C., Haire-Joshu, D., Kreuter, M. W., & Weaver, N. L. (2008). A glossary for dissemination and implementation research in health. *Journal of Public Health Management and Practice, 14*(2), 117–123. doi:10.1097/01.PHH.0000311888.06252.bb

Schillinger, D. (2010). *An introduction to effectiveness, dissemination and implementation research. From the series: UCSF Clinical and Translational Science Institute (CTSI) resource manuals and guides to community engaged research.* San Francisco, CA: Clinical Translational Science Institute Community Engagement Program, University of California San Francisco.

Schulz, K. F., Altman, D. G., & Moher, D. (2010). CONSORT 2010 statement: Updated guidelines for reporting parallel group randomized trials. *Annals of Internal Medicine, 152*(11), 726–732. doi:10.7326/0003-4819-152-11-201006010-00232

Simera, I., Moher, D., Hoey, J., Schulz, K. F., & Altman, D. G. (2010). A catalogue of reporting guidelines for health research. *European Journal of Clinical Investigation, 40*(1), 35–53. doi:10.1111/j.1365-2362.2009.02234.x

Tong, A., Sainsbury, P., & Craig, J. (2007). Consolidated criteria for reporting qualitative research (COREQ): A 32-item checklist for interviews and focus groups. *International Journal for Quality in Health Care, 19*(6), 349–357. doi:10.1093/intqhc/mzm042

von Elm, E., Altman, D. G., Egger, M., Pocock, S. J., Gøtzsche, P. C., & Vandenbroucke, J. P. (2008). The Strengthening the Reporting of Observational Studies in Epidemiology (STROBE) statement: Guidelines for reporting observational studies. *Journal of Clinical Epidemiology, 61*(4), 344–349. doi:10.1016/j.jclinepi.2007.11.008

Westfall, J. M., Mold, J., & Fagnan, L. (2007). Practice-based research—"blue highways" on the NIH roadmap. *Journal of the American Medical Association, 297*(4), 403–406. doi:10.1001/jama.297.4.403

CHAPTER EIGHT

IMPLEMENTATION RESEARCH

JOAN R. BLOCH, MYRA L. CLARK, AND JUDY FAUST

OBJECTIVES

After reading this chapter, readers will be able to:

1. Describe implementation research
2. Discuss terminology used in implementation science research
3. Identify and define discrete implementation strategies
4. Design an implementation research or practice project
5. Interpret results from published implementation research

Evidence-based practice (EBP) has been described as the "gold standard" for clinical practice; however, the challenge comes in translating that evidence from research into actual day-to-day clinical practice. Discrepancies exist within health care organizations and systems regarding whether or not the evidence is applicable to that individual organization. How will incorporating the evidence progress the outcomes of the organization? The question also arises as to whether or not the evidence truly provides the best practice or is easily adapted to improve patient outcomes. To that extent, implementation research provides some answers.

Implementation research is important for practice-based clinical inquiry. It is relatively new and an emerging interdisciplinary field with multiple definitions (Powell et al., 2015; Proctor et al., 2009). Research on implementation aims to improve the knowledge base to guide efforts to fit health interventions within real-world clinical and public health systems. The definition of *implementation research* has changed over time; for purposes of this chapter, implementation research is defined as:

> the study of methods, interventions, and variables that promote the uptake and use of research findings and other EBP's by individuals and organizations to improve clinical and operational decision-making in health care with the goal of improving health care quality. (Newhouse et al., 2013)

Within this definition is the process to achieve translation of research into practice. Thus, implementation research is categorized as a translation research method (discussed in Chapter 7). Dissemination research is related to implementation research, but it differs in definition and scope in that dissemination research involves the distribution of findings to a specific population whereas implementation research is the use of the research findings for change within a population or institution (Proctor et al., 2009). Chapter 7 focuses on dissemination research. This chapter focuses on implementation research.

The purpose of implementation research is to address health care gaps by strategically developing questions that will advance knowledge about implementing evidence-based interventions (EBIs) that are generalizable beyond an individual practice setting (Proctor, Powell, Baumann, Hamilton, & Santens, 2012). EBI implementation can be accomplished through a systems approach, thereby incorporating the best evidence into policy and practice to improve the health of populations (Lobb & Colditz, 2013). It is estimated that translation of research results into practice and health systems arenas would decrease greater than 50% of the health care burden that exists today (Lobb & Colditz, 2013). Although research tells us what we *should* do, the knowledge gap that actually exists is how to *really* do it so that it sticks in the real world of health care systems.

Designing an implementation research project, a complicated iterative process, can be simplified and described as having four basic phases (Damschroder et al., 2009):

- Plan
- Engage
- Execute
- Reflect and Evaluate (see Figure 8.1)

The planning phase describes the focused activities for advance preparation for the project (Damschroder et al., 2009). It is during the planning that determination is made for the framework or theory to guide the project. Questions to be asked during this phase include: (a) Who are the stakeholders? (b) What are the cultural, demographic, and organizational identities of the stakeholders? (c) What is the preferred means of communication? (d) What type of monitoring and analysis is needed? Advanced planning with inclusion of all stakeholders must be thorough and may require modification until agreed upon as acceptable to all parties.

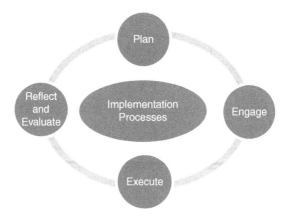

Figure 8.1 Key implementation processes.

Engaging includes identification and collaboration with appropriate individuals within the community and health care organization. This includes finding champions who are early adapters within the intended organization. Questions to be asked include: (a) How does one identify potential champions for this project? (b) What is the role of the champion in the organization? (c) Does the champion reflect the demographics of the organization? (d) What type of influence does the champion have within the organization (formal or informal)? (e) What is the role of the champion in the project? Engaging appropriate key team members prior to execution of the implementation project will aid in adoption of the intervention (Damschroder et al., 2009).

Executing is the actual performance of the implementation project. Detailed planning and engaging will provide availability of quality data for analysis. Key factors to be considered during the execution phase are: (a) fidelity, (b) intensity, (c) timeliness, and (d) stakeholder engagement (Damschroder et al., 2009).

Reflecting and evaluating "relates to implementation efforts" and not to project goals (Damschroder et al., 2009). Regular team meetings to solicit reflection and feedback allow for project improvement and learning opportunities. It is important to recognize that this process is not linear but involves multiple points of reflection throughout the project implementation (Damschroder et al., 2009).

Development of Implementation Science and Research

Knowledge of the historical development of implementation research assists with providing a foundation for both past and future studies. Early stages of implementation science were present during the 1960s to 1970s. The question arose during this period as to why it was difficult to implement practice-based initiatives on a national basis, especially since the Centers for Disease Control and Prevention (CDC) closely monitored progress in reaching national health goals and objectives through its Healthy People initiatives. The Healthy People benchmarks with measurable objectives continued the development of implementation research. Toolkits and implementation strategies were developed and distributed to state and local health departments to strive toward attainment of established Healthy People benchmarks (Lobb & Colditz, 2013). However, even with the establishment of evaluation measures and toolkits to ensure progress toward the benchmarks, there still existed a gap between research, policy, and practice, specifically in mental health research. In efforts to understand how to close these gaps, the term *implementation science* evolved. In this chapter, implementation science is used broadly and refers to the interdisciplinary discipline dedicated to using scientific methods to advance knowledge of implementation phenomena.

Implementation research focuses on advancing knowledge about processes used during implementation phases that are required for successful translation of research evidence into policy and practice. Increased investment and activity in implementation and implementation research are critical to achieve these goals. Stimulus for this paradigm shift was found in *Crossing the Quality Chasm: A New System for the 21st Century,* published by the Institute of Medicine (IOM, 2001), and in increased funding from the National Institutes of Health (NIH; Lobb & Colditz, 2013). The NIH encouraged translation of research findings from bench to bedside— to the community—with initiation of the Roadmap Initiative in 2007 (Lobb & Colditz, 2013). Implementation research seeks to evaluate the real-world use of

EBIs and implementation strategies by organizations and individuals. From here, stakeholder involvement to improve population health has emerged. Collaborative efforts between academic researchers, practitioners, and key stakeholders to identify and implement sustainable solutions that work in the real world are needed. Implementation processes must be better understood if science-based interventions are to be used and improvements in health outcomes and health care practices are to be realized (Proctor & Rosen, 2008).

Implementation science continues to evolve with a focus on developing theoretical frameworks, methods, and related terminology (Damschroder et al., 2009; Glasgow, Brownson, & Kessler, 2013; Proctor, Powell, & McMillen, 2013; Rabin, Brownson, Haire-Joshu, Kreuter, & Weaver, 2008). Table 8.1 provides a brief list of commonly used terms in this growing field of implementation science. Some terms will be familiar, as they are also used in other chapters in this book. Dissemination and implementation (D&I) science builds on many of the translation research methods that have been gaining attention since *Crossing the Quality Chasm* (IOM, 2001) was first published.

TABLE 8.1 Defining Key Implementation Science Terms

Term	Definition
Adoption	Decision to commit and initiate an EBP (Rabin & Brownson, 2012)
Diffusion	The passive, untargeted, unplanned, and uncontrolled spread of new interventions (Rabin & Brownson, 2012)
EBI	Intervention with demonstrated efficacy and effectiveness (Rabin et al., 2008)
Efficacy research	The initial impact of an intervention with a focus on internal validity or establishment of a causal relationship (Rabin et al., 2008)
Fidelity	The degree that the actual implementation project matches the planned EBI, as designed from the planning phase (Damschroder et al., 2009)
Implementation	Deliberate use of iterative processes and strategies to integrate evidence and EBI into health care policy and practice (Schillinger, 2010)
Implementation research	Systematic study of how a specific set of processes and methods leading to activities and designed strategies are used to successfully integrate EBI (Schillinger, 2010)
Implementation science	Interdisciplinary discipline dedicated to pursuing knowledge about implementation phenomena
Implementation strategy	The processes, activities, and resources used to integrate interventions into real-world settings (Rabin & Brownson, 2012)
Intensity	The quality and depth of the implementation project (Pearson et al., 2005)
Scalability	Describes the adoption of an intervention in a wider usage with sustainability (Schillinger, 2010)
Scaling up	Expanding the coverage of successful interventions to additional settings (Rabin & Brownson, 2012)

(continued)

TABLE 8.1	Defining Key Implementation Science Terms (*continued*)
Term	**Definition**
Stakeholder	Individuals or organizations that will be affected by the intervention (Damschroder et al., 2009)
Stakeholder engagement	Level of participation, commitment, and accountability (Proctor et al., 2012)
Stakeholder participation	The role of the stakeholder during the intervention (Damschroder et al., 2009)
Sustainability	Achieving long-term adoption of EBI (Schillinger, 2010)
Translation	The process of applying basic research findings into interventions that improve the health of individuals and populations (National Center for Advancing Translational Sciences, 2015)

EBI, evidence-based intervention; EBP, evidence-based practice.

Scientific Attention to External Validity

In essence, implementation research methods emphasize external validity in contrast to traditional research methods that emphasize internal validity (Green & Nasser, 2012). There is a lack of data on the external validity of many EBIs when they are implemented in real-world practice settings, despite the elegant design of randomized controlled trials (RCTs) to prove their causality of treatment. This concern has garnered interdisciplinary interest to think of new ways to generate broader and innovative EBPs for advancing knowledge of the best implementation strategies to improve health and health care systems (Ammerman, Smith, & Calancie, 2014; Brownson, Diez Roux, & Swartz, 2014).

WHY NURSE SCHOLARS SHOULD USE IMPLEMENTATION SCIENCE IN RESEARCH AND PRACTICE

Implementation science is conceptually congruent to nursing science and the nursing process, which constitute the organizing framework for professional nurses worldwide. Implementation, one of the five constructs of the nursing process, guides clinical and population-health nursing practice. Figure 8.2 shows the steps of the nursing process: (a) assess, (b) diagnose, (c) plan, (d) implement, and (e) evaluate. Nurses are taught from their entry-level education to use this dynamic nursing process to do what needs to be done to optimize health outcomes for individuals, families, and communities.

The nursing profession has been at the forefront of bringing knowledge to action. Using nursing science, nurses apply knowledge in practice to improve the health of their patients and health care delivery systems. Nursing practice includes implementation of treatment plans to patients and their families based on clinical phenomena and related patient needs. Implementation of system- and community-wide health programs and policies is associated with the roles and responsibilities

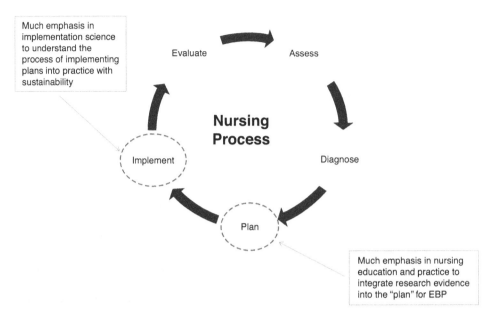

Figure 8.2 The nursing process: translating research into practice through planning and implementation processes.
EBP, evidence-based practice.

inherent in nursing practice. Thus, the discipline of nursing has much to contribute to advance broader and deeper understandings of implementation science. However, nursing scholars must conceptualize and articulate their knowledge and professional efforts within this transdisciplinary context of implementation science. Figure 8.2 shows the overall nursing process and places where growing implementation science falls in contrast to the planning phase, which is the current emphasis of much attention in nursing science and EBP.

The procedure to actually implement EBP using similar language and frameworks as funded implementation scientists has lagged behind in the profession of nursing. Implementation scientists are more concerned with advancing knowledge about how to implement plans into practice. Perhaps this is where applied nursing knowledge excels; as a profession, we have not recognized the importance of unraveling the complex processes within the black boxes of what nurses do so well in the context of implementation science. Explicating how plans are moved into action in successful ways is the crux of implementation science. So as we continue forth in furthering health care science, nursing has a critical role in advancing implementation science by elucidating the salient processes of what works in successful implementation of health care plans, programs, and policies.

Furthermore, implementation science, by design, lends itself to exemplar collaborations between PhD and Doctor of Nursing Practice (DNP) nurses. Fundamentally different scientific approaches that have been traditionally taught to advance nursing and medical science are needed to accelerate integration of EBI into practice. Nurses, as exemplar implementers, have an important role to play in advancing knowledge in implementation science.

HOW TO USE IMPLEMENTATION SCIENCE

Theories and Models to Guide Implementation Research

There is no one underlying theory or conceptual model that is driving this field, but a variety of theories and models (Brownson, Colditz, & Proctor, 2012). The most common theories and models are those related to change (e.g., Diffusion of Innovations, persuasive communication, and social marketing) and implementation evaluation (e.g., reach, effectiveness, adoption, implementation, and maintenance [RE-AIM], consolidated framework for implementation research [CFIR]; Brownson, Dreisinger, Colditz, & Proctor, 2012; Damschroder et al., 2009). Key characteristics of implementation science are that it is contextual, complex, multicomponent, nonlinear, transdisciplinary, multilevel, and multi-method (Glasgow & Chambers, 2012). Thus, relevant systems and complexity theories are also applied. Specific frameworks guiding implementation planning and evaluation research have surfaced in the published literature within recent years. Table 8.2 provides a list, but it is not meant to be exhaustive. Brownson et al. (2012) note that the most commonly used frameworks have been PRECEDE–PROCEED and RE-AIM (Brownson, Dreisinger, et al., 2012). The most important is that the theoretical model and design fit the questions asked. Ample models are being used to push forward a body of knowledge of how to successfully adopt, implement, and sustain EBIs.

TABLE 8.2   Frameworks for Implementation Planning and Evaluation

Framework's Acronym	Full Name of Implementation Framework	Published Reference for More Information
CFIR	Consolidated framework for implementation research	Damschroder et al. (2009)
GTO	Getting to outcomes	Chinman et al. (2008)
KTO	Knowledge to action	Field, Booth, Ilott, and Gerrish (2014)
PARiHS	Promoting action on research implementation in health services	Kitson et al. (2008)
PRISM	Practical robust implementation and sustainability model	Feldstein and Glasgow (2008)
PRECEDE–PROCEED	Predisposing, reinforcing, and enabling constructs in educational/environmental diagnosis and evaluation–policy, regulatory, and organizational constructs in educational/environmental development	Green and Kreuter (1999)
RE-AIM	Reach, effectiveness, adoption, implementation, and maintenance	Glasgow, Vogt, and Boles (1999)

Implementation Strategies

Implementation strategies are the "how to" component of changing health care practice (Proctor et al., 2013). These include all the specific processes that are involved in introducing, gaining support, and then implementing changes or improvements in practice. The science of implementation seeks to advance knowledge about these processes. What is problematic is that the knowledge of methods used to enhance the adoption, implementation, and sustainability of translating EBIs into clinical and population health practices have been hampered by a lack of conceptual clarity (Powell et al., 2015; Proctor et al., 2013). Additionally, implementation strategies (a) are often inconsistently labeled and poorly described; (b) lack operational definitions or manuals to guide their use; and (c) are a part of "packaged" approaches whose specific elements are poorly understood (Proctor et al., 2013). For instance, the same term is used but has different meanings or just the opposite happens, that is, different terms are used but have the same meaning. In response to these shortcomings, implementation scientists collaborated together through the Expert Recommendations for Implementing Change (ERIC) project to reach consensus on a comprehensive compilation of implementation strategies. Using a modified Delphi process to generate consensus, they compiled a comprehensive list of discrete strategies with conceptual definitions that serve as guidelines when naming, defining, and operationalizing implementation strategies (Powell et al., 2015). Table 8.3 provides this list compiled from the ERIC study. The list is intentionally comprehensive enough to include multistage implementation strategies that are relevant to a wide range of stakeholders with respect to the actors, actions, targets, and the temporality and dose of implementation (Proctor et al., 2013).

Table 8.3 is important for PhD–DNP nurse scholars, as it provides implementation science nomenclature for those who actively engage in various phases of translating research to improve nursing and health care practices. Until now, the discipline of nursing has focused more on the language of evidence-based nursing practice (Craig & Smyth, 2012; Melnyk & Fineout-Overholt, 2015) without much integration of the language put forth by D&I scientists. Consequently, the discipline of nursing is surprisingly minimally represented in this interdisciplinary scientific endeavor. However, nurses have been, and will continue to be, actively

TABLE 8.3 Results From the ERIC Study: Compilation of Discrete Implementation Strategies

Strategy	Definition
Access new funding	Access new or existing money to facilitate the implementation.
Alter incentive/ allowance structures	Work to incentivize the adoption and implementation of the clinical innovation.
Alter patient/ consumer fees	Create fee structures where patients/consumers pay less for preferred treatments (the clinical innovation) and more for less preferred treatments.

(continued)

TABLE 8.3   Results From the ERIC Study: Compilation of Discrete Implementation Strategies (*continued*)

Strategy	Definition
Assess for readiness and identify barriers and facilitators	Assess various aspects of an organization to determine its degree of readiness to implementations, barriers that may impede implementation, and strengths that can be used in the implementation effort.
Audit and provide feedback	Collect and summarize clinical performance data over a specified period and give them to clinicians and administrators to monitor, evaluate, and modify provider behavior.
Build a coalition	Recruit and cultivate relationships with partners in the implementation effort.
Capture and share local knowledge	Capture local knowledge from implementation sites on how implementers and clinicians made something work in their setting and then share it with other states.
Centralize technical assistance	Develop and use a centralized system to deliver technical assistance focused on implementation issues.
Centralize accreditation or membership requirements	Strive to alter accreditation standards so that they require or encourage use of the clinical innovation. Work to alter membership organization requirements so that those who want to affiliate with the organization are encouraged or required to use the clinical innovation.
Change liability laws	Participate in liability reform efforts that make clinicians more willing to deliver the clinical innovation.
Change physical structure and equipment	Evaluate current configurations and adapt, as needed, the physical structure and/or equipment (e.g., changing the layout of a room, adding equipment) to best accommodate the targeted innovation.
Change record systems	Charge records systems to allow better assessment of implementation or clinical outcomes.
Change service sites	Change the location of clinical service sites to increase access.
Conduct cyclical, small tests of change	Implement changes in a cyclical fashion using small tests of change before making system-wide changes. Tests of change benefit from systematic measurement, and results of the tests of change are studied for insights on how to do better. This process continues serially over time, and refinement is added with each cycle.
Conduct educational meetings	Hold meetings targeted toward different stakeholder groups (e.g., providers, administrators, other organizational stakeholders, and community, patient/consumer, and family stakeholders) to teach them about the clinical innovation.
Conduct educational outreach visits	Have a trained person meet with providers in their practice settings to educate providers about the clinical innovation with the intent of changing the provider's practice.

(continued)

TABLE 8.3   Results From the ERIC Study: Compilation of Discrete Implementation Strategies (*continued*)

Strategy	Definition
Conduct local consensus discussions	Include local providers and other stakeholders in discussions that address whether the chosen problem is important and whether the clinical innovation that addresses it is appropriate.
Conduct local needs assessment	Collect and analyze data related to the need for the innovation.
Conduct ongoing training	Plan for and conduct training in the clinical innovation in an ongoing way.
Create a learning collaborative	Facilitate the formation of groups of providers or provider organizations and foster a collaborative learning environment to improve implementation of the clinical innovation.
Create new clinical teams	Change who serves on the clinical team, adding different disciplines and different skills to make it more likely that the clinical innovation is delivered (or is more successfully delivered).
Create or change credentialing and/or licensure standards	Create an organization that certifies clinicians in the innovation or encourage an existing organization to do so. Change governmental professional certification or licensure requirements to include delivering the innovation. Work to alter continuing education requirements to shape professionals toward the innovation.
Develop a formal implementation blueprint	Develop a formal implementation blueprint that includes all goals and strategies. The blueprint should include the following: (a) aim/purpose of the implementation; (b) scope of the change [e.g., what organization units are affected]; (c) time frame and milestones; and (d) appropriate performance/progress measures. Use and update this plan to guide the implementation effort over time.
Develop academic partnerships	Partner with a university or an academic unit for the purposes of shared training and bringing research skills to implementation projects.
Develop an implementation glossary	Develop and distribute a list of terms describing the innovation, implementation, and stakeholders in the organizational change.
Develop and implement tools for quality monitoring	Develop, test, and introduce the right input into quality monitoring systems—the appropriate language, protocols, algorithms, standards, and measures (of processes, patient/consumer outcomes, and implementation outcomes) that are often specific to the innovation being implemented.
Develop and organize quality monitoring systems	Develop and organize systems and procedures that monitor clinical processes and/or outcomes for the purpose of quality assurance and improvement.

(*continued*)

TABLE 8.3 Results From the ERIC Study: Compilation of Discrete Implementation Strategies (*continued*)

Strategy	Definition
Develop disincentives	Provide financial disincentives for failure to implement or use the clinical innovation.
Develop educational materials	Develop and form manuals, toolkits, and other supporting materials in ways that make it easier for stakeholders to learn about the innovation and for clinicians to learn how to deliver the clinical innovation.
Develop resource-sharing agreements	Develop partnerships with organizations that have resources needed to implement the innovation.
Distribute educational materials	Distribute educational materials (including guidelines, manuals, and toolkits) in person, by mail, and/or electronically.
Facilitate relay of clinical data to providers	Provide as close to real-time data as possible about key measures of process/outcomes using integrated modes/channels of communication in a way that promotes use of the targeted innovation.
Facilitation	A process of interactive problem solving and support that occurs in a context of recognized need for improvement and a supportive interpersonal relationship.
Fund and contract for the clinical innovation	Governments and other payers of services issue requests for proposals to deliver the innovation, use contracting processes to motivate providers to deliver the clinical innovation, and develop new funding formulas that make it more likely that providers will deliver the innovation.
Identify and prepare champions	Identify and prepare individuals who dedicate themselves to supporting, marketing, and driving through an implementation, overcoming indifference or resistance that the intervention may provoke in an organization.
Identify early adopters	Identify early adopters at the local site who learn from their experiences with the practice innovation.
Increase demand	Attempt to influence the market for the clinical innovation to increase competition intensity and to increase the maturity of the market for the clinical innovation.
Inform local opinion leaders	Inform providers identified by colleagues as opinion leaders or "educationally influential" about the clinical innovation in the hopes that they will influence colleagues to adopt it.
Intervene with patients/ consumers to enhance uptake and adherence	Develop strategies with patients to encourage and problem solve around adherence.
Involve executive boards	Involve existing governing structures (e.g., boards of directors, medical staff boards of governance) in the implementation effort, including the review data on the implementation process.

(*continued*)

TABLE 8.3 Results From the ERIC Study: Compilation of Discrete Implementation Strategies (continued)

Strategy	Definition
Involve patients/ consumers and family members	Engage or include patients/consumers and families in the implementation effort.
Make billing easier	Make it easier to bill for the clinical innovation.
Make training dynamic	Vary the information delivery methods to cater to different learning styles and work contexts, and shape the training in the innovation to be interactive.
Mandate change	Have leadership declare the priority of the innovation and their determination to have it implemented.
Model and simulate change	Model or simulate the change that will be implemented prior to implementation.
Obtain and use patients/ consumers and family feedback	Develop strategies to increase patient/consumer family feedback on the implementation effort.
Obtain formal commitments	Obtain written commitments from key partners that state what they will do to implement the innovation.
Organize clinician implementation team meetings	Develop and support teams of clinicians who are implementing the innovation and give them protected time to reflect on the implementation effort, share lessons learned, and support one another's learning.
Place innovation on fee-for-service lists/formularies	Work to place the clinical innovation on lists of actions for which providers can be reimbursed (e.g., a drug is placed on a formulary, a procedure is now reimbursable).
Prepare patients/ consumers to be active participants	Prepare patients/consumers to be active in their care, ask questions, and, specifically, inquire about care guidelines, the evidence behind clinical decisions, or about available evidence-supported treatments.
Promote adaptability	Identify the ways in which clinical innovation can be tailored to meet local needs and clarify which elements of the innovation must be maintained to preserve fidelity.
Promote network weaving	Identify and build on existing high-quality working relationships and networks both within and outside the organization, organizational units, teams, and so on, to promote information sharing, collaborative problem solving, and a shared vision/goal related to implementing the innovation.
Provide clinical supervision	Provide clinicians with ongoing supervision focusing on the innovation. Provide training for clinical supervisors who will supervise clinicians who provide the innovation.

(continued)

TABLE 8.3   Results From the ERIC Study: Compilation of Discrete Implementation Strategies (*continued*)

Strategy	Definition
Provide local technical assistance	Develop and use a system to deliver technical assistance focused on implementation issues using local personnel.
Provide ongoing consultation	Provide ongoing consultation with one or more experts in the strategies used to support implementing the innovation.
Purposely reexamine the implementation	Monitor progress and adjust clinical practices and implementation strategies to continuously improve the quality of care.
Recruit, designate, and train for leadership	Recruit, designate, and train leaders for the change of effort.
Remind clinicians	Develop reminder systems designed to help clinicians recall information and/or to prompt them to use the clinical innovation.
Revise professional roles	Shift and revise roles among professionals who provide care, and redesign job characteristics.
Shadow other experts	Provide ways for key individuals to directly observe experienced people and engage with or use the targeted practice change/innovation.
Stage implementation scale-up	Phase implementation efforts by starting with small pilot or demonstration projects and gradually move on to a system-wide rollout.
Start a dissemination organization	Identify or start a separate organization that is responsible for disseminating the clinical innovation. It could be a for-profit or nonprofit organization.
Tailor strategies	Tailor the implementation strategies to address barriers and leverage facilitators that were identified through earlier data collection.
Use advisory boards and work groups	Create and engage a formal group of multiple kinds of stakeholders to provide input and advice on implementation efforts and to elicit recommendations for improvements.
Use an implementation advisor	Seek guidance from experts in implementation.
Use capitated payments	Pay providers or care systems a set amount per patient/consumer for delivering clinical care.
Use data experts	Involve, hire, and/or consult experts to inform managements on the use of data generated by implementation efforts.
Use data warehousing techniques	Integrate clinical records across facilities and organizations to facilitate implementation across systems.

(continued)

TABLE 8.3 Results From the ERIC Study: Compilation of Discrete Implementation Strategies (*continued*)

Strategy	Definition
Use mass media	Use media to reach large numbers of people to spread the word about the clinical innovation.
Use other payment schemes	Introduce payment approaches (in a catch-all category).
Use train-the-trainer strategies	Train designated clinicians or organizations to train others in clinical innovations.
Visit other sites	Visit sites where a similar implementation has been considered successful.
Work with educational institutions	Encourage educational institutions to train clinicians in the innovation.

ERIC, Expert Recommendations for Implementing Change.

Source: Powell et al. (2015). This table was reprinted with permission.

involved in the operations of moving EBIs into the real world of health care practice. Thus, for recognition of nursing efforts in pushing forward this domain of science, PhD–DNP nurse scholars should use the interdisciplinary terminology in Table 8.2 when appropriate. The following case example illustrates this in a real-world application of implementing and scaling up an EBI.

Discrete Implementation Strategies in Action: Case Example of Implementing Centering Pregnancy®

Background of the Clinical Problem
Infant mortality in the United States averages just more than six per 1,000 live births, which is embarrassingly higher than all other countries of comparable wealth (IOM, 2013; Mathews & MacDorman, 2013). Among socioeconomically disadvantaged urban neighborhoods, infant mortality rates are twice as high. There is research evidence that a nontraditional group visit prenatal care model, Centering Pregnancy, improves perinatal outcomes in communities burdened with adverse social determinants of health (Baldwin, 2006; Ickovics et al., 2011). Centering Pregnancy was developed in 1994 as a new model of care to "provide high quality service within a system that is mandating more economy and efficiency" (Rising, 1998, p. 46). This EBP model of prenatal care has been implemented worldwide; however, the uptake in changing, or transforming, from the traditional model of prenatal care in the United States to this newer EBP model has been minimal.

Charged with implementing this EBP Centering Pregnancy model of care, strategic actions were carefully planned for implementation success within this particular health system that serves women living in an underserved urban area. The health system's nurse executive, a coauthor of this chapter (J.F.), was the operations manager responsible for implementation. In this case example, organizational values driven by the philosophy of nursing practice were integrated with implementation science to improve health care and health outcomes through implementing Centering Pregnancy.

Jean Watson's Theory of Human Caring provides the theoretical underpinnings of nursing practice in this urban health system (Watson, 2008). As such, this group model of care is theoretically congruent. Guided by implementation science, the plan, do, study, act (PDSA) model serves as the framework guiding implementation of Centering Pregnancy (Langley, Moen, Nolan, Norman, & Provost, 2009). Using the language of implementation strategies compiled from the ERIC study, Table 8.4 describes the discrete strategies used that led to the successful implementation of this EBP model of prenatal care. It is noteworthy that key to achieving successful funding for this implementation was the championship and collaboration received from senior leadership in this health care system.

TABLE 8.4 Description of ERIC's Discrete Implementation Strategies Used to Implement EBP Model of Centering Pregnancy in an Urban Area With High Infant Mortality Rates

ERIC's Discrete Implementation Strategies	Description of These Strategies in Implementing Centering Pregnancy
Access new funding	In 2012, the OB/GYN department of the hospital received funding from the State of Pennsylvania to pilot a Centering Pregnancy prenatal care model at a faith-based site (church) located in the zip code with the second highest infant mortality rate in Philadelphia.
Alter incentive/allowance structures	Incentive was the ability to bill for OB care under insurance/Medicaid. Under the current financial model, there would be no negative impact to other providers who would refer patients to the Centering Pregnancy program.
Alter patient/consumer fees	There was no need to alter billing or costs to patients. Billing was done as usual. Patients were assisted with enrollment in Medicaid.
Assess for readiness and identify barriers and facilitators	Barriers: (a) Lack of knowledge about the model; (b) Challenge of getting women to the faith-based site. Facilitators: (a) hired midwife experienced in Centering Pregnancy model; (b) hired facilitator for group sessions, and to assist with program; and (c) program staff sent for Centering Pregnancy training.
Audit and provide feedback	Limited initial success: Enrollment was challenging, because women did not know about the Centering Pregnancy model; getting women to go to a church for prenatal care was a challenge; and two buses were required to get to church from the hospital clinic.
Build a coalition	Gained support from some providers and staff. Support was received from the March of Dimes—they coordinated a State Centering Pregnancy seminar for providers who were able to learn and share successes and challenges. A PhD/NP local university faculty member supportive of the Centering Pregnancy model agreed to attend the training session and provide a Grand Rounds presentation for the OB/GYN department on Centering Pregnancy.

(continued)

TABLE 8.4　Description of ERIC's Discrete Implementation Strategies Used to Implement EBP Model of Centering Pregnancy in an Urban Area With High Infant Mortality Rates (*continued*)

ERIC's Discrete Implementation Strategies	Description of These Strategies in Implementing Centering Pregnancy
Capture and share knowledge	Held discussions with other Centering Pregnancy sites across states and with the National Centering Healthcare Institute.
Change liability laws	Not needed for the Centering Pregnancy program.
Change physical structure and equipment	Utilized existing PCP site in church, but slightly adapted.
Change record systems	Used web-based OB electronic medical record utilized by the hospital OB site. Created a list of data elements that should be captured based on the data that the March of Dimes requested.
Change service sites	Set up a PCP site for OB care and education. Use group room near office space at church for Centering Pregnancy group sessions.
Conduct cyclical, small tests of change	Regular review of data, pilot various changes using PDSA model to encourage patients to attend Centering Pregnancy prenatal care at the church. Offered tokens if transportation was a challenge for patients.
Conduct educational meetings	Provided Grand Rounds on Centering Pregnancy model for OB providers and nursing staff. Conducted dissemination with academic public health forums.
Conduct educational outreach visits	Attended state-wide Centering Pregnancy provider meeting sponsored by March of Dimes.
Conduct needs assessment	High infant mortality in city and specific zip code, high level of Medicaid-enrolled or eligible patients.
Conduct ongoing training	Updates provided for staff at location used to recruit patients.
Create a learning collaborative	Participated in bimonthly Centering Pregnancy sites all across the state, sponsored by March of Dimes.
Create new clinical teams	Hired health educator as a facilitator and to assist with recruitment. Also hired a medical assistant for group sessions and to assist with recruitment at OB site.
Create or change credentialing and/or licensure standards	Not needed for the Centering Pregnancy program.
Develop a formal implementation blueprint	The initial implementation program outlined by the hospital's OB/GYN department was provided to and approved by the state Department of Health.
Develop academic partnerships	NP/PhD faculty member at local university provided input related to the program.

(continued)

TABLE 8.4   Description of ERIC's Discrete Implementation Strategies Used to
Implement EBP Model of Centering Pregnancy in an Urban Area With High Infant
Mortality Rates (*continued*)

ERIC's Discrete Implementation Strategies	Description of These Strategies in Implementing Centering Pregnancy
Develop an implementation glossary	Not done, resulting in some challenges because of clients and providers not understanding the model and/or not supporting it.
Develop and implement tools for quality monitoring	Database developed to track data for the state and March of Dimes.
Develop and organize quality monitoring systems	OB quality nurse provided input and chart reviews.
Develop incentives	Provided enrollees with Centering Pregnancy book, snacks, and small incentives (hand lotion, baby wipes, small gift bag at postpartum reunion visit).
Develop educational materials	Purchased materials from the Centering Healthcare Institute, and other pregnancy education materials.
Facilitate relay of clinical data to providers	Providers have access to their own data. Provided updates to all department members at monthly business meetings regarding enrollment and outcomes.
Fund and contract for the clinical innovation	Funding obtained from the state Department of Health, obtained 10% additional funding needed from the hospital.
Identify and prepare champions	Key OB medical and nursing administrators. Conducted Grand Rounds; administrator for service line trained in the model and educated clinic staff.
Identify early adopters	Program staff hired for program; also, sister site at our other suburban hospital had been providing Centering Pregnancy on a small scale.
Increase demand	Advertised program in the community, through newspapers, billboards, and handouts at community sites.
Inform opinion leaders	Educated Women, Infants, and Children staff and other community agencies regarding the program.
Intervene with patients/ consumers to enhance uptake and adherence	Ongoing challenges educating patients/consumers regarding the group model of prenatal care; once patients understood the model, they would usually attend most prenatal sessions.
Involve executive boards	Senior leadership meetings on a monthly and then a quarterly basis to evaluate the program and make suggestions on how to enhance it.
Involve patients/ consumers and family members	Patients encouraged their friends to seek prenatal care via the Centering Pregnancy model. Women were offered the option to bring a person with them to the Centering Pregnancy sessions.

(*continued*)

TABLE 8.4   Description of ERIC's Discrete Implementation Strategies Used to Implement EBP Model of Centering Pregnancy in an Urban Area With High Infant Mortality Rates (*continued*)

ERIC's Discrete Implementation Strategies	Description of These Strategies in Implementing Centering Pregnancy
Make billing easier	Billing completed based on standard electronic billing process.
Make training dynamic	Ongoing training provided for program staff, including level II Centering Pregnancy training.
Mandate change	In 2013, received federal funds from CMS Innovations Center for second Centering Pregnancy program under the Strong Start funding, which focused on women with high-risk conditions. The site started a process to transition to opt out of the Centering Pregnancy model. With two programs (high-risk care and normal prenatal care), all patients had the Centering Pregnancy option. Because of challenges with recruitment to an off-campus faith-based site, the state allowed us to move the program to the main campus.
Model and simulate change	Hired and trained additional staff for a new program. Three internal employees were transferred to the Strong Start model.
Obtain and use patients/ consumers and family feedback	Patients' and support persons' feedback obtained regarding the Centering Pregnancy model.
Obtain formal commitments	Formal commitment from health care network for space for Centering Pregnancy model at main campus.
Organize clinician implementation team meetings	Leadership team formed to support, monitor, and evaluate both programs.
Place innovation on fee-for-service lists/ formularies	Adapted appointment system to allow for group Centering Pregnancy appointments.
Prepare patients/ consumers to be active participants	Created a short video that included patients and providers who participated in the Centering Pregnancy prenatal care model; video shown in the prenatal clinic and on other TVs within the network.
Promote adaptability	Other providers interested in participating in the model as guest speakers when the second program started on the main campus; adapted Centering Pregnancy sessions to allow for guest speakers (interpersonal violence, dental care, mental health, postpartum depression, newborn care).
Promote networking	Continued to promote the model at local meetings within the city as well as provided a presentation to the health care network board of directors.

(continued)

TABLE 8.4   Description of ERIC's Discrete Implementation Strategies Used to Implement EBP Model of Centering Pregnancy in an Urban Area With High Infant Mortality Rates (*continued*)

ERIC's Discrete Implementation Strategies	Description of These Strategies in Implementing Centering Pregnancy
Provide clinical supervision	Maternal fetal medicine physicians provided clinical supervision for the providers; administrator/clinical director provided supervision for other staff.
Provide local technical assistance	Health care network IT staff provided support for the program, including data collection. (Funders require evaluation data.)
Provide ongoing consultations	Providers would reach out to other sites, providing care via Centering Pregnancy model, as well as reach out to the Centering Healthcare Institute for suggestions. Annual review completed by state Department of Health funder. Bi-weekly calls and then monthly calls with CMS staff. Onsite evaluation after first year of grant program was completed.
Purposely reexamine the implementation	Ongoing discussion with key stakeholders. Continued challenges, increasing enrollment, patients "show" rate for the first appointment and lack of understanding that Centering Pregnancy sessions are prenatal care and not education sessions.
Recruit, designate, and train for leadership	In 2014, the hospital received a second federal grant from HRSA under the Healthy Start Program. This program provides enhanced services for Centering Pregnancy prenatal patients and allows for the funding of a Centering Parenting® program. HRSA funding allowed for a program manager position.
Remind clinicians	Ongoing education provided at departmental meetings.
Revise professional roles	Added physicians and pediatric residents to the Centering Parenting program.
Shadow other experts	Two pediatricians traveled to another site to observe Centering Parenting sessions, and learned from the providers who had been using this model for several years.
Stage implementation scale-up	Opt-out model only, resulting in 37% of eligible patients being enrolled in Centering Pregnancy care. Met with clinic staff and developed a new process for "new OB day" to allow for a quick introduction to Centering Parenting with snacks provided. Women learn to take their BP. Instead of waiting in the waiting room for their appointment, women are actively involved in their care, education is provided, and the women enjoy snacks and the chance to speak with other new moms instead of sitting alone in the waiting room. At the time for the exam, a member of the staff escorts the patients upstairs to the OB office. Three pilot sessions of the new model are completed, and 100% of the women are introduced to Centering Parenting via the new model enrolled in the program. Will monitor show rate for first Centering Parenting session to see whether this new model increases first visit show rate.

(*continued*)

TABLE 8.4 Description of ERIC's Discrete Implementation Strategies Used to Implement EBP Model of Centering Pregnancy in an Urban Area With High Infant Mortality Rates (*continued*)

ERIC's Discrete Implementation Strategies	Description of These Strategies in Implementing Centering Pregnancy
Start a dissemination organization	Educated pediatric providers on D&I as part of the design and implementation of the Centering Parenting program, as well as education for the Centering Pregnancy team members.
Tailor strategies	Continue to adapt the models to attract patients to the program, but maintain the fidelity of the key elements of the Centering model.
Use advisory boards and workgroups	HRSA grant also funded two other Healthy Start programs in the city. Citywide action group to be formed.
Use an implementation advisor	PhD academic faculty and hospital administrator attended the 2014 national conference on D&I. HRSA grant provides education sessions on implementation strategies for the HRSA program, including the concept of collective impact.
Use capitated payments	Services billed via traditional billing models.
Use data experts	Increase the amount of support provided from IT department. New program manager has a background in quality and data analysis.
Use data warehousing techniques	Developed a web-based tool to track data to replace the current data tracking tools.
Use mass media	Started marketing program again; press releases on the Centering Parenting program.
Use other payment schemes	Obtained internal funding for construction of Centering Parenting space, as well as for snacks and small incentives for participants.
Use train-the-trainer strategies	After site receives accreditation from Centering Healthcare Institute two staff members will be trained by Centering Healthcare Institute as trainers, in order for us to provide internal training.
Visit other sites	Attended statewide meeting of Centering Pregnancy providers in Winter 2015. Shared successes with other sites providing Centering Parenting care.
Work with educational institutions	Continue work with university faculty members to enhance team members' understanding of D&I science.

BP, blood pressure; CMS, Centers for Medicare and Medicaid Services; D&I, dissemination and implementation; EBP, evidence-based practice; ERIC, Expert Recommendations for Implementing Change; GYN, gynecology; HRSA, Health Resources and Services Administration; IT, information technology; NP, nurse practitioner; OB, obstetrics; PCP, primary care practice; PDSA, plan, do, study, act.

Source: Implementation of Centering Pregnancy was funded, in part, by grants from the Pennsylvania Department of Health and the U.S. Department of Health and Human Services (HHS), Health Resources and Services Administration, Maternal and Child Health Bureau, Division of Healthy Start and Perinatal Services. The project described is also supported by Funding Opportunity Number CMS-1D1-12-001 from the Centers for Medicare & Medicaid Services, Center for Medicare & Medicaid Innovation. The contents of this document do not necessarily represent the official views of HHS or any of its agencies. This project does not limit a fee-for-service Medicare, Medicaid, or CHIP patient's freedom to choose a particular health care provider.

Role of Leadership to Develop Strategic Climate for EBP Implementation

In the case example described earlier, championship from leadership was paramount for success. Senior leadership must be engaged in the process of implementing EBP programs into health care systems through an understanding that EBP can improve both administrative and clinical outcomes. Engagement of senior leaders will set the stage, and be important champions, for implementing changes instead of status quo organizational operations. Adoption of a framework at the organizational level, such as the Evidence-Based System of Innovation Support (EBSIS) health care providers' ability to implement the EBP, should be considered (Leeman, et al., 2015).

Support from senior leaders to create an EBP environment for the health system is necessary. Nurses need access to research databases, educational time to search the literature for EBPs, training on how to identify high-quality research, and formal education on implementation science. Additionally, financial support from the organization for the activities described earlier is critical for the success of creating an EBP environment (Ellen et al., 2014).

Communication plays a key role in the process of EBP implementation in order to ensure organizational uptake. During this stage, leaders need to ensure that communication occurs in a transformational manner rather than in a transactional manner (Manojjlovich, Squires, Davies, & Graham, 2015). Once EBP is adopted, leadership must assure sustainability. If EBP implementation is grant supported, both staff and leadership must identify beneficial outcomes on clinical care and/or administrative processes to ensure continued use of the EBP in the organization even after the grant funding has ended (Proctor et al., 2015).

THE INTERPRETATION AND PRESENTATION OF IMPLEMENTATION RESEARCH

In this section of the chapter, examples of actual funded implementation studies are provided so readers can see what is actually considered implementation research by reviewers of research grant applications. By showing examples of the most highly regarded research in this field, readers can learn exactly what is considered implementation research. Because the NIH recognizes that closing the gap between research discovery and program delivery is a complex challenge but an absolute necessity, if all populations are to benefit from scientific discoveries, the NIH funds D&I research (NIH, 2015). The NIH's priorities for advancing the interdisciplinary field of implementation are listed in Table 8.5.

Next, Table 8.6 provides a list of NIH-funded implementation studies and some of the publications that resulted from them. The list is organized alphabetically by the name of the principal investigator (PI) with the exact title of the funded implementation study. The NIH reference number is given so readers, if interested, can go to the NIH's website RePORTER (https://projectreporter.nih.gov/reporter.cfm; retrieved June 1, 2015) to learn more details about the study. In Table 8.6, two publications from each study are provided so readers have research articles to read from these NIH-funded implementation studies. Additional resources to read are the following two journals, *Worldviews of EBP* and *Implementation Science*.

Figure 8.3 shows a screenshot from this website where the PI went to learn more.

TABLE 8.5 Examples of NIH Priority Implementation Research Topics Supported by the NIH Program Announcement, PAR-13-055

- Studies of efforts to scaffold multiple EBPs within care settings, to meet the needs of complex patients, systems of care, and service integration.

- Longitudinal and follow-up studies on the factors that contribute to the sustainability of research-based improvements in public health and clinical practice.

- Studies testing the effectiveness and cost-effectiveness of dissemination or implementation strategies to reduce health disparities and improve quality of care among rural, minority, low literacy and numeracy, and other underserved populations.

- Studies that address context in descriptive and innovative ways and investigate the relationship between context and adoption, implementation, and maintenance.

- Comparative effectiveness research that addresses D&I issues and approaches, and that evaluates the cost, resource requirements, and other economic and policy outcomes.

- Studies of the adoption, implementation, and sustainability of health policies and their interaction with programs and contextual factors.

- Studies of complex health problems, comorbid patients, and complex interventions using innovative methods, models, and analyses that fit these needs.

- Studies on the fidelity/adaptation of implementation efforts, including the identification of components of implementation that will enable fidelity to be assessed meaningfully.

- Studies of systems interventions that impact organizational structure, climate, culture, and processes to enable D&I of clinical/public health information and effective clinical/public health interventions.

- Studies of efforts to implement health promotion, prevention, early detection, and diagnostic interventions, as well as effective treatments, clinical procedures, or guidelines into existing care systems across the life span to measure the extent to which such procedures are utilized, adhered to, and sustained, by patients, providers, and consumers.

- Studies of the capacity of specific care delivery settings (primary care, schools, worksites, community health settings, health departments, etc.) to incorporate D&I efforts within current organizational forms.

- Studies that focus on the development and testing of theoretical and evaluation models for D&I processes, or use such models to conduct reviews of the D&I literature.

- Development of D&I relevant outcome and process measures and suitable methodologies for D&I approaches that accurately assess the success of an approach to move evidence into practice (i.e., not just clinical outcomes). Applicants are encouraged to review available resources, where possible, and to use more harmonized and standard measures, rather than developing their own measures for each study.

- Studies testing D&I strategies of symptom management interventions that reduce the symptom burden in patients with chronic conditions, including multiple chronic conditions.

- Studies of how approaches to shared decision making may be implemented and sustained among practitioners.

(continued)

TABLE 8.5 Examples of NIH Priority Implementation Research Topics Supported by the NIH Program Announcement, PAR-13-055 (*continued*)

- Studies of how successful screening promotion approaches and policies are implemented in health care and community practice, and especially in international or low-resource settings.

- Studies of the adoption, implementation, and sustainability of data and surveillance reporting tools and techniques.

- Studies of the D&I of effective and cost-effective strategies for incorporating genomic medicine, sequence-based diagnostics, and therapeutics in clinical care.

- Studies testing the incorporation and use of genomic information, family history risk information, and/or pharmacogenetic information for improved diagnosis and treatment.

D&I, dissemination and implementation; EBPs, evidence-based practices; NIH, National Institutes of Health.

Source: The table was created from the information that appeared in the NIH's website explaining the grant program announcement (PAR-13-055). This program announcement was posted January 2013 and expires January 2016 (http://grants.nih.gov/grants/guide/pa-files/PAR-13-055.html, retrieved June 1, 2015).

TABLE 8.6 List of NIH-Funded Implementation Studies and Some of Their Publications

Principal Investigator and Grant Number	Title	Overall Aim of Funded Project	Publications**
Aarons, Gregory (R01MH092950)	Interagency collaborative teams to scale up EBP	Examine whether or not the interagency collaborative team can develop system-wide safe care expertise and maintain fidelity.	Aarons et al. (2014); Yeh et al. (2014)
Bogner, Hillary (R21MH094940)	Implementing care for depression and diabetes	Assess how implementation core components are adopted and by whom and how to develop interventions that are adapted to the practice environment and that are sustainable.	de Vries McClintock, Morales, Small, and Bogner (2015); de Vries McClintock, Wiebe, et al. (2015)
Dolcini, Margaret (R01MH085502)	Influences on the translation of an evidence-based HIV/STI intervention into practice	Use diffusion theory and RE-AIM to guide assessment of adoption and implementation of RESPECT in 30 participating agencies.	Catania, Dolcini, Gandelman, Narayanan, and McKay, (2014); Dolcini et al. (2010)

(continued)

TABLE 8.6 List of NIH-Funded Implementation Studies and Some of Their Publications (*continued*)

Principal Investigator and Grant Number	Title	Overall Aim of Funded Project	Publications**
Kegeles, Susan (R01MH065196)	Moving a research-based intervention into practice	Guided by a conceptual model of implementation effectiveness, study the implementation of an EBP, the Mpowerment project, across 80 community-based organizations.	Kegeles et al. (2012); Rebchook, Kegeles, and Huebner (2006)
Novins, Douglas (R01DA022239)	EBPs and substance abuse treatment for Native Americans	Describe EBPs in substance abuse treatment programs serving AI/AN communities and what factors are associated with the decision to implement EBP programs. Treatment programs serve AI/AN communities.	Legha, Raleigh-Cohn, Fickenscher, and Novins (2014); Moore, Aarons, Davis, and Novins (2015)
Ouslander, Joseph (R01NR012936)*	Implementing interventions to reduce hospitalizations of nursing home residents	Use RCT to test the implementation of a quality improvement program, INTERACT, on hospitalization rates among nursing home residents.	Ouslander (2013); Ouslander, Bonner, Herndon, and Shutes (2014)
Reid, Manney Carrington (R03NR010093)*	Implementing a cognitive/exercise therapy for back pain in the community setting	Use a CBPR approach to refine our intervention prior to implementation.	Beissner et al. (2013); Townley et al. (2010)
Saint, Sanjay (R01NR010700)*	Implementing evidence to prevent urinary infection and enhance patient safety	Describe the adoption and implementation of a Catheter-Associated Urinary Tract Infection Prevention Bundle (Bladder Bundle)	Fakih et al. (2012); Saint, Gaies, Fowler, Harrod, and Krein (2014)
Solberg, Lief (R01MH080692)	Evaluation of a natural experiment to improve statewide depression care in Minnesota	Evaluate the effects of an impending statewide change in reimbursement combined with facilitated implementation of that best-practice model.	Solberg et al. (2013); Whitebird et al. (2014)

(continued)

TABLE 8.6 List of NIH-Funded Implementation Studies and Some of Their Publications (*continued*)

Principal Investigator and Grant Number	Title	Overall Aim of Funded Project	Publications**
Weiner, Bryan (R01CA124402)	Implementing systemic interventions to close the discovery–delivery gap	Examine the implementation and sustainability of a federally funded national PBRN, the community clinical oncology program, as a model for PBRNs in other disease areas.	Jacobs, Weiner, and Bunger (2014); Penn et al. (2015)

*These studies were funded by the National Institute of Nursing Research.

**For the sake of this table, there was a limit of only two publications per funded study. Thus, this is not intended to be an exhaustive list of publications from the cited NIH-funded projects.

AI/AN, American Indian/Alaska Native; CBPR, community-based participatory research; EBPs, evidence-based practices; NIH, National Institutes of Health; PBRN, practice-based research network; RCT, randomized controlled trial; RE-AIM, reach, effectiveness, adoption, implementation, and maintenance; STI, sexually transmitted infection.

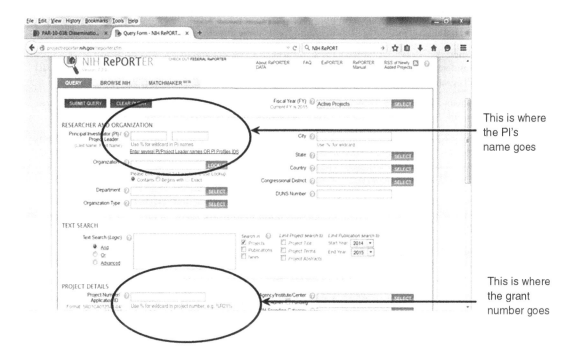

Figure 8.3. NIH's RePORTER website to find more information about funded implementation studies.

PI, principal investigator.

SUMMARY

Implementation research is important for practice-based clinical inquiry. Implementation science is an evolving and growing interdisciplinary science forging forward with theories and language to fill in important knowledge gaps of how to translate research into real-world health care practice. This chapter provides a brief history of the evolution of implementation science along with research approaches that are evolving. Nurses, as change agents, are often charged to forward implementation of scientific evidence into practice at clinical and population levels of health care systems. Thus, nurse scholars have much to offer by conducting implementation research to elucidate successful implementation processes and strategies. Resources for nurse scholars to contribute to and learn from are presented in this chapter, thereby providing the means to move implementation and nursing science forward and to ensure that the health of the people improves.

REFERENCES

Aarons, G. A., Green, A. E., Willging, C. E., Ehrhart, M. G., Roesch, S. C., Hecht, D. B., & Chaffin, M. J. (2014). Mixed-method study of a conceptual model of evidence-based intervention sustainment across multiple public-sector service settings. *Implementation Science, 9*, 183–195. doi:10.1186/s13012-014-0183-z

Ammerman, A., Smith, T. W., & Calancie, L. (2014). Practice-based evidence in public health: Improving reach, relevance, and results. *Annual Review of Public Health, 35*, 47–63.

Baldwin, K. (2006). Comparison of selected outcomes of Centering Pregnancy versus traditional prenatal care. *Journal of Midwifery and Women's Health, 51*, 266–272.

Beissner, K., Bach, E., Murtaugh, C., Parker, S. J., Trachtenberg, M., & Reid, M. C. (2013). Implementing a cognitive-behavioral pain self-management program in home health care, part 1: Program adaptation. *Journal of Geriatric Physical Therapy, 36*(3), 123–129.

Brownson, R., Colditz, G. A., & Proctor, E. K. (2012). *Dissemination and implementation research in health: Translating science to practice.* New York, NY: Oxford University Press.

Brownson, R., Dreisinger, M., Colditz, G. A., & Proctor, E. K. (2012). The path forward in dissemination and implementation research. In R. Brownson, G. Colditz, & E. K. Proctor (Eds.), *Dissemination and implementation research in health: Translating science to practice* (pp. 498–508). New York, NY: Oxford Press University.

Brownson, R. C., Diez Roux, A. V., & Swartz, K. (2014). Commentary: Generating rigorous evidence for public health: The need for new thinking to improve research and practice. *Annual Review Public Health, 35*, 1–7.

Catania, J. A., Dolcini, M. M., Gandelman, A. A., Narayanan, V., & McKay, V. R. (2014). Fiscal loss and program fidelity: Impact of the economic downturn on HIV/STI prevention program fidelity. *Translational Behavioral Medicine, 4*(1), 34–45.

Chinman, M., Hunter, S. B., Ebener, P., Paddock, S. M., Stillman, L., Imm, P., & Wandersman, A. (2008). The getting to outcomes demonstration and evaluation: An illustration of the prevention support system. *American Journal of Community Psychology, 41*(3–4), 206–224.

Craig, J., & Smyth, R. (2012). *The evidence-based practice manual for nurses* (3rd ed.). London, UK: Churchill Livingstone Elsevier.

Damschroder, L. J., Aron, D. C., Keith, R. E., Kirsh, S. R., Alexander, J. A., & Lowery, J. C. (2009). Fostering implementation of health services research findings into practice: A consolidated framework for advancing implementation science. *Implementation Science, 4*, 50. doi:10.1186/1748-5908-4-50 de Vries McClintock, H. F., Morales, K. H., Small, D. S., & Bogner, H. R. (2015). A brief adherence intervention that improved glycemic control: Mediation by patterns of adherence. *Journal of Behavioral Medicine*, *38*(1), 39–47.

de Vries McClintock, H. F., Wiebe, D. J., O'Donnell, A. J., Morales, K. H., Small, D. S., & Bogner, H. R. (2015). Neighborhood social environment and patterns of adherence to oral hypoglycemic agents among patients with type 2 diabetes mellitus. *Family and Community Health*, *38*(2), 169–179.

Dolcini, M., Gandelman, A. A., Vogan, S. A., Kong, C., Leak, T. N., King, A. J., . . . O'Leary, A. (2010). Translating HIV interventions into practice: Community-based organizations' experiences with the diffusion of effective behavioral interventions (DEBIs). *Social Science and Medicine*, *71*(10), 1839–1846.

Ellen, M. E., Leon, G., Bouchard, G., Ouiment, M., Grimshaw, J. M., & Lavis, J. N. (2014). Barriers, facilitators and views about next steps to implementing supports for evidence-informed decision-making in health systems—a qualitative study. *Implementation Science*, *9*(179), 1–12.

Fakih, M. G., Watson, S. R., Greene, M. T., Kennedy, E. H., Olmsted, R. N., Krein, S. L., & Saint, S. (2012). Reducing inappropriate urinary catheter use: A statewide effort. *Archives of Internal Medicine*, *172*(3), 255–260.

Feldstein, A. C., & Glasgow, R. E. (2008). A practical, robust implementation and sustainability model (PRISM) for integrating research findings into practice. *Joint Commission Journal on Quality and Patient Safety*, *34*(4), 228–243.

Field, B., Booth, A., Ilott, I., & Gerrish, K. (2014). Using the knowledge to action framework in practice: A citation analysis and systematic review. *Implementation Science*, *9*, 172.

Glasgow, R. E., Brownson, R. C., & Kessler, R. S. (2013). Thinking about health-related outcomes: What do we need evidence about? *Clinical Translation Science*, *6*(4), 286–291.

Glasgow, R. E., & Chambers, D. (2012). Developing robust, sustainable, implementation systems using rigorous, rapid and relevant science. *Clinical Translation Science*, *5*(1), 48–55.

Glasgow, R. E., Vogt, T. M., & Boles, S. M. (1999). Evaluating the public health impact of health promotion interventions: The RE-AIM framework. *American Journal of Public Health*, *89*(9), 1322–1327.

Green, L., & Kreuter, M. (1999). *Health promotion planning: An educational and environmental approach*. Mountain View, CA: Mayfield.

Green, L., & Nasser, M. (Eds.). (2012). *Furthering dissemination and implementation research: The need for more attention to external validity*. New York, NY: Oxford University Press.

Ickovics, J. R., Reed, E., Magriples, U., Westdahl, C., Rising, S. S., & Kershaw, T. S. (2011). Effects of group prenatal care on psychosocial risk in pregnancy: Results form a randomized controlled trial. *Psychology and Health*, *26*(2), 235–250.

Institute of Medicine (IOM). (2001). Crossing the quality chasm: A new health care system for the 21st century. *National Academy of Sciences*. Retrieved from http://iom.nationalacademies.org/Reports/2001/Crossing-the-Quality-Chasm-A-New-Health-System-for-the-21st-Century.aspx

Institute of Medicine. (2013). Health in international perspective: Shorter lives, poorer health. *National Academy of Sciences*. Retrieved from http://iom.nationalacademies.org/Reports/2013/US-Health-in-International-Perspective-Shorter-Lives-Poorer-Health/Report-Brief010913.aspx

Jacobs, S. R., Weiner, B. J., & Bunger, A. C. (2014). Context matters: Measuring implementation climate among individuals and groups. *Implementation Science*, *9*, 46. doi:10.1186/1748-5908-9-46

Kegeles, S. M., Rebchook, G., Pollack, L., Huebner, D., Tebbetts, S., Hamiga, J., . . . Zovod, B. (2012). An intervention to help community-based organizations implement an evidence-based HIV prevention intervention: The Mpowerment project technology exchange system. *American Journal of Community Psychology*, *49*(1–2), 182–198.

Kitson, A. L., Rycroft-Malone, J., Harvey, G., McCormack, B., Seers, K., & Titchen, A. (2008). Evaluating the successful implementation of evidence into practice using the PARiHS framework: Theoretical and practical challenges. *Implementation Science*, *3*, 1. doi:10.1186/1748-5908-3-1

Langley, G. J., Moen, R. D., Nolan, K. M., Norman, C. L., & Provost, L. P. (2009). *The improvement guide*. San Francisco: Jossey-Bass.

Leeman, J., Calancie, L., Hartman, M. A., Escoffery, C. T., Herrmann, A. K., & Tague, L (2015). What strategies are used to build practitioners' capacity to implement community-based interventions and are they effective?: A systematic review. *Implementation Science, 10*, 80.

Legha, R., Raleigh-Cohn, A., Fickenscher, A., & Novins, D. (2014). Challenges to providing quality substance abuse treatment services for American Indian and Alaska Native communities: Perspectives of staff from 18 treatment centers. *BioMed Central Psychiatry, 14*, 181–191. doi:10.1186/1471-244x-14-181

Lobb, R., & Colditz, G. A. (2013). Implementation science and its application to population health. *Annual Review of Public Health, 34*, 235–251.

Manojjlovich, M., Squires, J. E., Davies, B., & Graham, I. D. (2015). Hiding in plain sight: Communication theory in implementation science. *Implementation Science, 10*, 58., doi:10.1186/s13012-015-0244-y

Matthews, T. J., & MacDorman, M. F. (2013). Infant mortality statistics from the 2009 period linked birth/infant death data set. *National Vital Statistics Report, 61*(8), 1–27.

Melnyk, B., & Fineout-Overholt, E. (2015). *Evidence-based practice in nursing and healthcare: A guide to best practice* (3rd ed.). Philadelphia, PA: Wolters Kluver.

Moore, L. A., Aarons, G. A., Davis, J. H., & Novins, D. K. (2015). How do providers serving American Indians and Alaska Natives with substance abuse problems define evidence-based treatment? *Psychological Services, 12*(2), 92–100.

National Center for Advancing Translational Sciences. (2015). *Translational science spectrum*. Retrieved from http://www.ncats.nih.gov/translation

National Institutes of the U.S. Department of Health and Human Services. (2015). *Dissemination and implementation research in health (R01)*. Retrieved from grants.nih.gov/grants/guide/pa-files/PAR-13-055.html

Newhouse, R., Bobay, K., Dykes, P. C., Stevens, K. R., & Titler, M. (2013). Methodology issues in implementation science. *Medical Care, 51*(4:2), S32–S40.

Ouslander, J. G. (2013). The triple aim: A golden opportunity for geriatrics. *Journal of American Geriatric Society, 61*(10), 1808–1809.

Ouslander, J. G., Bonner, A., Herndon, L., & Shutes, J. (2014). The interventions to reduce acute care transfers (INTERACT) quality improvement program: An overview for medical directors and primary care clinicians in long term care. *Journal of the American Medical Directors Association, 15*(3), 162–170.

Pearson, M. L., Wu, S., Schaefer, J., Bonomi, A. E., Shortell, S. M., . . . Keeler, E. B. (2005). Assessing the implementation of the chronic care model in quality improvement collaboratives. *Health Services Research, 40*(4), 978–996.

Penn, D. C., Chang, Y., Meyer, A. M., DeFilippo Mack, C., Sanoff, H. K., Stitzenberg, K. B., & Carpenter, W. R. (2015). Provider-based research networks may improve early access to innovative colon cancer treatment for African Americans treated in the community. *Cancer, 121*(1), 93–101.

Powell, B. J., Waltz, T. J., Chinman, M. J., Damschroder, L. J., Smith, J. L., Matthieu, M. M., . . . Kirchner, J. E. (2015). A refined compilation of implementation strategies: Results from the Expert Recommendations for Implementing Change (ERIC) project. *Implementation Science, 10*(1), 21. doi:10.1186/s13012-015-0209-1

Proctor, E., Luke, D., Calhoun, A., McMillen, C., Brownson, R., McCrary, S., & Padek, M. (2015). Sustainability of evidence-based healthcare: Research agenda, methodological advances, and infrastructure support. *Implementation Science, 10*, 88.

Proctor, E. K., Landsverk, J., Aarons, G., Chambers, D., Glisson, C., & Mittman, B. (2009). Implementation research in mental health services: An emerging science with conceptual, methodological, and training challenges. *Administration and Policy in Mental Health, 36*(1), 24–34.

Proctor, E. K., Powell, B. J., Baumann, A. A., Hamilton, A. M., & Santens, S. L. (2012). Writing implementation research grant proposals: Ten key ingredients. *Implementation Science, 7,* 96. doi:10.1186/1748-5908-7-96

Proctor, E. K., Powell, B. J., & McMillen, J. C. (2013). Implementation strategies: Recommendations for specifying and reporting. *Implementation Science, 8,* 139. doi:10.1186/1748-5908-8-139

Proctor, E. K., & Rosen, A. (2008). From knowledge production to implementation: Research challenges and imperatives. *Research on Social Work Practice, 18*(4), 285–291.

Rabin, B., & Brownson, R. (2012). Developing the terminology for dissemination and implementation research. In R. Brownson, G. Colditz, & E. K. Proctor (Eds.), *Dissemination and implementation research in health* (pp. 23–51). New York, NY: Oxford University Press.

Rabin, B. A., Brownson, R. C., Haire-Joshu, D., Kreuter, M. W., & Weaver, N. L. (2008). A glossary for dissemination and implementation research in health. *Journal of Public Health Management and Practice, 14*(2), 117–123.

Rebchook, G. M., Kegeles, S. M., & Huebner, D. (2006). Translating research into practice: The dissemination and initial implementation of an evidence-based HIV prevention program. *AIDS Education Prevention, 18*(4 Suppl. A), 119–136.

Rising, S. S. (1998). Centering Pregnancy: An interdisciplinary model of empowerment. *Journal of Nurse-Midwifery and Women's Health, 43,* 46–54.

Saint, S., Gaies, E., Fowler, K. E., Harrod, M., & Krein, S. L. (2014). Introducing a catheter-associated urinary tract infection (CAUTI) prevention guide to patient safety (GPS). *American Journal of Infection Control, 42*(5), 548–550.

Schillinger, D. (2010). An introduction to effectiveness, dissemination and implementation research. In P. Goldstein & E. Fleisher (Eds.), *UCSF Clinical and Translation Science Institute (CTSI) resource manuals and guides to community-engaged research.* San Francisco, CA: Clinical Translational Science Institute Community Engagement Program, University of California San Francisco.

Solberg, L. I., Crain, A. L., Jaeckels, N., Ohnsorg, K. A., Margolis, K. L., Beck, A., . . . Van de Ven, A. H. (2013). The DIAMOND initiative: Implementing collaborative care for depression in 75 primary care clinics. *Implementation Science, 8,* 135.

Townley, S., Papaleontiou, M., Amanfo, L., Henderson, C. R., Jr., Pillemer, K., Beissner, K., & Reid, M. C. (2010). Preparing to implement a self-management program for back pain in New York City senior centers: What do prospective consumers think? *Pain Medicine, 11*(3), 405–415.

Watson, J. (2008). *Nursing: The philosophy and science of caring.* Boulder, CO: University Press.

Whitebird, R. R., Solberg, L. I., Jaeckels, N. A., Pietruszewski, P. B., Hadzic, S., Unutzer, J., . . . Rubenstein, L. V. (2014). Effective implementation of collaborative care for depression: What is needed? *American Journal of Managed Care, 20*(9), 699–707.

Yeh, M., Aarons, G. A., Ho, J., Leslie, L. K., McCabe, K., Tsai, K., & Hough, R. (2014). Parental etiological explanations and longitudinal medication use for youths with attention deficit hyperactivity disorder. *Administration and Policy in Mental Health, 41*(3), 401–409.

PART III

A TOOLBOX FOR GREATER IMPACT AND SUCCESS

CHAPTER NINE

USING GEOGRAPHIC INFORMATION SYSTEMS IN CLINICAL AND POPULATION HEALTH RESEARCH

JOAN R. BLOCH AND SARAH CORDIVANO

OBJECTIVES

After reading this chapter, readers will be able to:

1. Describe geographic information systems (GIS)
2. Become familiar with basic GIS terminology and tools
3. Identify important reasons to use GIS for generating and disseminating data-driven knowledge about clinical and population health
4. Explain steps to incorporate GIS into scholarly PhD-DNP clinical inquiry research
5. Provide examples of research that used GIS from the published peer-review literature

Geographic locations and environments in which individuals and their families live, work, and play are important to their health and overall well-being. Promotion of optimal population health and disease prevention require knowledge of geographical patterns of health and illness and environmental factors that impact populations. In the 21st century, having access to excessive amounts of data combined with innovative computer engineering provides tremendous opportunities to connect large amounts of data about people and their local, regional, national, and global environments. One can generate knowledge from the plethora of geographic data to promote human health and wellness by integrating geographic computer database software with health science research. This geographic database software is referred to as *geographic information systems* and is most commonly referred to by its acronym, GIS. GIS also refers to the academic discipline of working with geographic information systems within the discipline of geoinformatics (Blaschke et al., 2014; Kounadi & Leitner, 2014; Moss & Schell, 2004).

The purpose of this chapter is to provide an overview of GIS and to introduce PhD and Doctor of Nursing Practice (DNP) scholars to the potential contributions of GIS to their scholarship. The key objectives of this chapter are to describe GIS; explain how it has been used in health science research and practice; and propose how scholars can use it as a tool to advance knowledge that, ultimately, will be translated into practice to positively impact the health and well-being of individuals, families, and communities. This chapter also provides a brief overview of the language, tools, and uses of GIS to enhance collaboration between clinical scholars and geographers or spatial scientists that could lead to funded research or health program projects.

GEOGRAPHIC INFORMATION SYSTEMS

GIS software provides a database for storing, interactively querying, and editing data in maps; analyzing geographic data; and presenting the results in a variety of figures, tables, and powerful visual maps (Mitchell, 2009). Through GIS, data are assigned spatially to where they belong geographically. Geographic units of analysis can be small, such as an actual street address based on the longitudinal (X) and latitudinal (Y) coordinates, or aggregated to larger geographic units to reflect local, regional, or national areas. These data can be aggregated to represent characteristics of neighborhoods, cities, counties, states, and countries. A wide variety of data can be entered into GIS to display and explore spatial data, which may or may not lead to more rigorous, complex analysis. Descriptive and hypothesis-testing spatial analyses are possible with GIS, depending on the research purpose and specific research questions.

Health and Health Care Data Can Be Geographically Assigned

GIS is an important tool to better understand the spatial relationships between health and illness. Obtaining answers to clinical research questions through GIS analyses provides insight so that intelligent decisions are made about the macro-level contextual factors and relationships that would not be possible without the GIS data (Mitchell, 2009). GIS tools and methods can create new data that can be displayed visually on a map for further analyses and interpretations.

Unlike other disciplines that are concerned primarily with the environment, the health care sciences, including nursing, public health, and medicine, have been slow to adopt GIS tools in research and practice. Since the 1970s, GIS tools have been adopted by environmental management and the biological sciences (Taylor, Yeager, Ouimet, & Menachemi, 2012). Only recently has GIS gained momentum in the health sciences, particularly in public health research (Auchincloss, Gebreab, Mair, & Diez Roux, 2012; Kurland & Gorr, 2009). Recognizing the geographic patterns of health and illness has important implications for developing and evaluating targeted and tailored interventions to promote health and prevent illness.

GIS Mapping: A Powerful Tool

GIS mapping is a valuable tool in helping bridge the gap between data producers, users, and decision makers (Detres, Lucio, & Vitucci, 2014). Maps can be powerful tools to illustrate the environment in which people live, work, and play. Providing striking visual patterns of salient factors that influence the health and well-being of communities is often much more effective than just reporting tables of statistics. GIS results are visually displayed through maps. Depending on the desired purpose, a great variety of GIS maps can be produced.

Any element of data related to the attainment of health services occurs within a geographic context: patient location, service provider location, pharmacy location, and environmental factors affecting health, such as neighborhood safety, location of pollutants or contaminates, and air quality. Beyond being explored in a traditional database or spreadsheet, these elements can be visualized on a map within a GIS database, which greatly increases the likelihood of recognizing important spatial patterns within the data. The power of GIS lies in its ability to present problems in multiple ways, including any geographic relationships that exist (Cromley & McLafferty, 2012). Consider, for example, community-focused safe-sex interventions through condom distribution sites that are aimed at preventing sexually transmitted infections and unplanned pregnancies. This chapter's coauthor (S. C.) created Figures 9.1 and 9.2 to illustrate how GIS can be used for exploratory spatial descriptive analysis. These GIS maps were created from a descriptive analysis (a) to explore the geographic distribution of the areas in which most of the young urban population resides in Philadelphia and (b) to determine whether sites for condom distribution were located appropriately, that is, where most of the high-risk populations live. Notice how clear and powerful these GIS-created maps are in showing this relationship. Figure 9.1 is called a chloropleth map, or a thematic map, because it uses graded differences in shading of predetermined geographic areas to reflect differences in proportions of the characteristic displayed. In this map, the predetermined area is a census tract, the most widely used proxy for neighborhood research (Krieger et al., 2003). A census tract represents a geographic unit of about 4,000 to 8,000 households (Kawachi & Berkman, 2003). Data are aggregated to the geographic unit and then represented on the map with a color or shaded gradient that represents a proportion. In contrast to Figure 9.1, Figure 9.2 is considered a density map. The dots represent population density of the characteristic under examination. Each dot represents an actual point of a specific location, such as the exact street address. With density maps, privacy issues are of concern if one is mapping sensitive data that are not highly prevalent among the population. The data are not aggregated to a preselected geographic area, so a breach of confidentially of the data may occur because displaying the location of a particular characteristic may reveal the identity of the person with the characteristic (Kounadi & Leitner, 2014). An extreme example of this phenomenon is creating a density map of Ebola contractions for a city with only two residents who contracted Ebola.

There are multiple unique ways to analyze geographic data through using GIS. GIS can be used to simply explore data in a geographic context. This approach requires first identifying the geographic location of data on a map (commonly known as *geocoding*). Inspection of geographic data is often powerful, as shown earlier, in gaining a snapshot of the geographic distribution of data. This first step is analogous to the important step of in-depth exploratory descriptive analyses in quantitative research. This allows the researchers to assess how the data are distributed spatially and what further analyses may be possible on the basis of spatial patterns. To determine what further robust spatial analyses may be possible, one needs a trained spatial analyst to test for possible statistically significant spatial relationships between multiple variables. Connecting data from various sources is a tremendous strength of GIS software. Multiple data sets can be linked as long as geographic locations are assigned to the data, and those locations can function as the common identifiable linking variables.

Assessing geographic patterns of health is not really new to health research. What is new is GIS computer software. More than 150 years ago, a non-computer-based GIS was used by physician John Snow to investigate the source of a cholera outbreak.

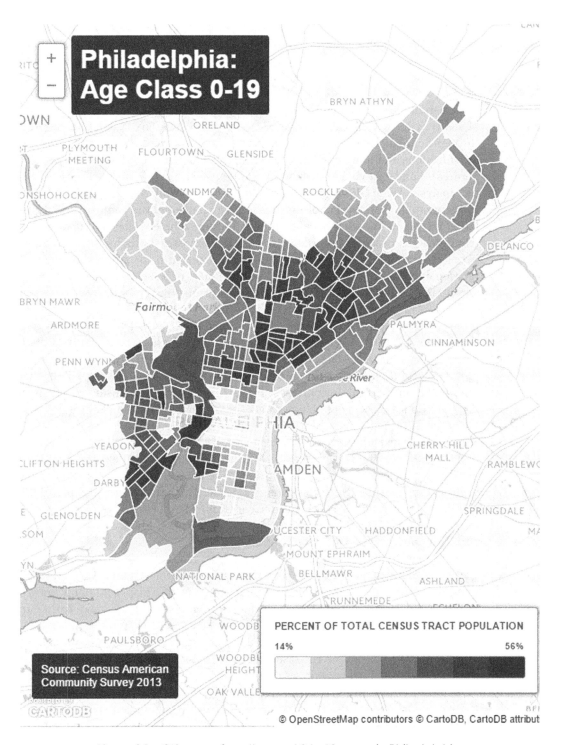

Figure 9.1 GIS map of youth, aged 0 to 19 years, in Philadelphia.
GIS, geographic information systems.
Source: Census American Community Survey (2013).

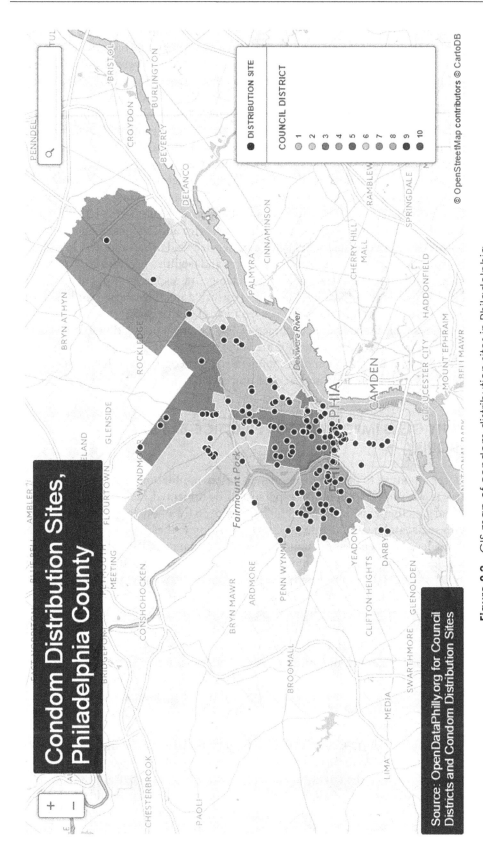

Figure 9.2 GIS map of condom distribution sites in Philadelphia.

GIS, geographic information systems.

Source: OpenDataPhilly.org for Council Districts and Condom Distribution Sites.

By mapping the locations of the cases of cholera deaths in 1849, he was able to identify the contaminated water pump in London, England (Friis & Sellers, 2009; Johnson, 2007). The geographic patterns of cholera deaths were elemental in establishing the vector (water pump), which was the source of the outbreak. John Snow, who is now recognized as the father of epidemiology, used mapping to determine the etiology and specific vector (the water pumps) of the cholera outbreak (Friis & Sellers, 2009). Thus, it is no surprise that, in the 21st century, GIS software has become a powerful tool for public health research, especially in the specialized areas of environmental health and social epidemiology.

Another key application of GIS is in health services research. Ensuring equitable access and utilization of needed health care is an important goal of a health care delivery system (Aday, 2001; Aday, Begley, Lairson, & Slater, 1998). GIS is a valuable tool for planning and evaluating health care service allocations. Being able to identify the geographic element of health care service void or saturation is key in planning locations for future health care services and facilities (Cordivano, 2011), which is especially important when geographic changes in resources or populations occur and services must adjust accordingly to ensure equitable access. Understanding population demographics and utilization rates of health care services is important, because not all services are consumed evenly among a population in a given area. Income, culture, race, sex, and age are some of the many demographic factors that affect access and utilization of recommended and required health care services for optimal health promotion and disease prevention.

REASONS WHY GIS IS IMPORTANT FOR PRACTICE-BASED CLINCAL INQUIRY

Closer attention to developing evidence-based, population-focused nursing activities is warranted in lieu of the persistent documented racial and ethnic health disparities that exist locally and globally, especially among populations burdened with social and health inequities. Closer attention to these issues will help advance a broader and deeper understanding about the characteristics of the places where people lead their lives. The built environment matters, because the physical and social attributes of environments vary considerably. Simply understood, generating and sustaining optimal well-being and functioning for individuals and their families are easier in healthy environments than in unhealthy environments. In unhealthy environments, physical, chemical, and psychosocial stressors can cause health to deteriorate. Individuals and entire communities burdened with chronic and cumulative environmental exposures such as poverty and violence are documented to be at risk for life course trajectories of adverse health outcomes (Kawachi & Berkman, 2003; Love, David, Rankin, & Collins, 2010). How nursing activities could be most efficiently and effectively targeted in relation to the environment is largely unexplored.

GIS is an important tool for clinical inquiry aimed at improving health and well-being. Applying GIS to this burgeoning field of geography and health illustrates relationships between the environment and health. Exploring critical health problems (e.g., disease outbreak and spread, medical resource allocation, health outcome disparity) with geospatial methods allows for a much more comprehensive analysis. Considering geography when addressing these issues provides a greater context and allows for more comprehensive and informed solutions. For example, disease outbreak and spread rely heavily on geographic factors such as navigability of terrain and the built environment; resource allocation is directly concerned with location and saturation of existing medical resources; and health outcome disparity correlates to the demographic distribution of wealth of a region. All of these important health issues require the inclusion of key geographic data in addressing and developing solutions. Omitting this important aspect of analysis is akin to leaving the research question half written or arbitrarily throwing out a subset of data.

Studying interactions between health and the environment is not new for the discipline of nursing. What is new is the ability to capture, analyze, and visually illustrate attributes of the environment using sophisticated computer software programs that can spatially appoint huge amounts of data to provide deeper and broader understandings of the places in which people live, work, and play. GIS software transforms large amounts of data into relevant nursing knowledge in ways never before possible.

GIS: A Data-Driven Method to Study the Nursing Metaparadigm Concept of the Environment

Contemporary nurse theorists postulate that the scientific basis of nursing knowledge comprises four key metaparadigm concepts: the environment, human beings, health, and nursing. Leading nursing theorist Fawcett (2005, p. 6) defines the metaparadigm concept of the environment as the physical surroundings in which human beings and their families are situated and in which the provision of nursing care occurs. She then expands the definition to include "the local, regional, national, and global cultural, social, political, and economic conditions that are associated a human being's health."

Attention to the interplay between health, the environment, human beings, and nursing care has been documented since the days of Florence Nightingale. The science of nursing generates and translates knowledge to promote health and prevent illness among individuals, families, and communities, especially among vulnerable populations burdened with life course trajectories of health and health care disadvantages. As mentioned earlier, unhealthy environments underlie health disadvantage. Being able to locate these environments and delve deeper to identify ways to help improve health and health care is a paramount concern for nurses. GIS software applications allow the capture, description, and analysis of data about the environment in ways never before possible.

Integrating GIS Into Clinical Inquiry Scholarship: Understanding Populations

Identifying Patterns of Hot Spots or Clusters

GIS can answer all the following questions: How are the characteristics of interest distributed in the geographic area? What is the pattern of these characteristics in the geographic area? Are there *hot spots* or *clusters* of certain characteristics in the geographic area?

The ability of GIS to efficiently identify hot spots of whatever phenomenon nurse scholars are concerned about is unmatched. Visualization of the geographic patterns points nurse scholars to where they need to go to study the phenomenon of concern. It is well documented that patterns of transmission of infectious disease follow geographic patterns (Goswami et al., 2012); it is also true that adverse health outcomes are more prevalent in areas with a larger burden of adverse social determinants of health, such as preterm birth (Bloch, 2011; O'Campo et al., 2008) and breast cancer (Highfield, 2013).

Visualizing Social Determinants of Health

An incredible strength of GIS is its ability to illustrate spatial relationships between social science and health variables. Visualizing social determinants of health by mapping social constructs such as poverty, violence, and racial segregation with documented health disparities is powerful. Figures 9.3 and 9.4 contain GIS maps of Philadelphia produced during a study that investigated whether neighborhood exposures to the stressors of poverty and violence may, in part, explain the observed health advantage of foreign-born Blacks compared with native U.S.-born Blacks based on residential addresses (Bloch, 2011).

The aforementioned study of preterm births in Philadelphia concluded that neighborhood trumped nativity. From the GIS analysis, it appeared that the foreign-born advantage did not hold up among the foreign-born Black mothers who lived in the neighborhoods with the highest exposures to the stressors of poverty and violence (Bloch, 2011). There was no statistically significant difference in preterm birth rates on the basis of nativity among all the Black mothers living in these neighborhoods. These findings were instrumental in redirecting this researcher's program of perinatal health disparities research.

The previous research example may be categorized as social epidemiology research. However, GIS is also a robust tool to use in health services research. Using the same geographic location of Philadelphia and its neighborhoods, Cordivano (2011) studied the impact of closing 13 maternity units from 1996 to 2008 in Philadelphia. Use of GIS demonstrated the value of spatial analytical methods in assessing the impact of changes in closures of health care facilities. More importantly, GIS proved to be an important data-driven tool to use when proposing equitable locations for health care delivery services.

Ground Truthing GIS Results to the Population of Concern

Using results of GIS analyses by creating maps can facilitate bringing together key interdisciplinary stakeholders within academia, clinical practice, and the community to accelerate health care action and innovation (Detres et al., 2014). As underscored throughout this chapter, GIS-informed research reveals powerful spatial relationships between the built environment and health. The term *ground truth* basically refers to any verification of mapped data against true ground conditions. *Ground truth* is not a common term in health care research, but we have introduced it because it is an important construct that can be used to compare maps generated from GIS-aggregated data with information obtained from the stakeholders, including health care professionals, in the communities themselves. The illuminating information thus obtained can be used to make point-of-care changes as needed.

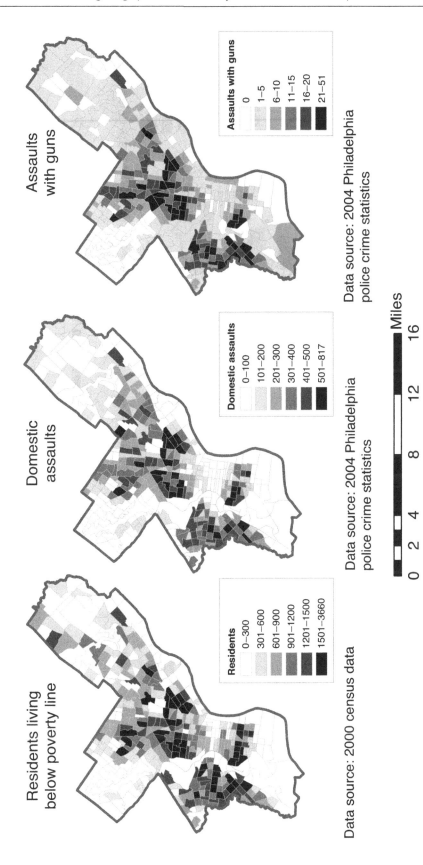

Figure 9.3 Neighborhood stressors.
Reproduced with permission from JOGNN (Bloch, 2011).

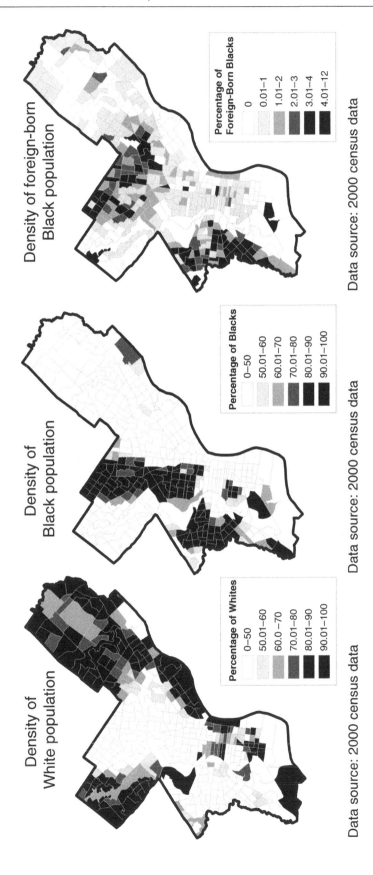

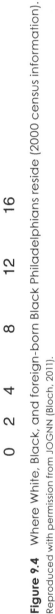

Figure 9.4 Where White, Black, and foreign-born Black Philadelphians reside (2000 census information).

Reproduced with permission from JOGNN (Bloch, 2011).

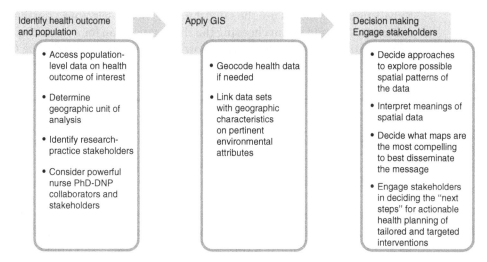

Figure 9.5   Ground truthing GIS aggregated population-level data to the people for full and complete meanings.

DNP, Doctor of Nursing Practice.

Asking for input about GIS-generated maps from the people at the ground level, the people affected the most within the geographic areas, can include performing a critical step in developing feasible, implementable programs designed to improve health. Using GIS data is an important area for future PhD-DNP scholarship and collaborations, especially for those seeking to mitigate harm from adverse social determinants and built environments. Salient questions need to be elicited from GIS findings among all stakeholders to obtain sufficient understanding to help clarify what actions may be taken.

The steps to be taken when using GIS for stakeholder-engaged decision making are described in Figure 9.5. GIS is an excellent tool to use in community-based participatory research (CBPR; Detres et al., 2014; Hites et al., 2013; Smith & Miller, 2013). Community members can be invited to participate during the initial phases of exploratory spatial data analysis before GIS maps are even created. Prudence is especially warranted when mapping sensitive information about populations. One demonstrates respect for the community by engaging with them in deciding which GIS maps are the best for dissemination.

HOW TO USE GIS IN NURSING CLINICAL INQUIRY RESEARCH

Choosing a GIS Analyst as a Collaborator Is Important

Integral to using GIS in nursing research is having access to someone who is trained in using GIS software and spatial analysis. The field of GIS software and spatial analysis is fast growing and constantly evolving. The application of GIS in health care has grown with the exponentially growing field of social epidemiology. Nurse scholars who are beginning to use GIS may want to consider collaborating with a nurse or public health scientist who has advanced training in social epidemiology and special training in using GIS. Choosing a well-trained professional GIS spatial analyst for the project is crucial. Keeping up with the advancements in GIS is a challenge. One should use the same due diligence in selecting a qualified GIS analyst that one would use in choosing the right statistician for a research project. (See Chapter 10 for more information on how to choose a statistician.) The GIS consultant should know what GIS application, specific tools, and appropriate accessible data sources are best suited to one's specific projects. Integrating GIS into one's program of clinical inquiry also necessitates familiarity with basic GIS terminology.

GIS Terminology

GIS has a unique vocabulary. Embarking on a project that incorporates GIS requires knowledge of some of the terms that collaborators trained in GIS may use. Table 9.1 provides a brief list of common geospatial terms. For a complete list of GIS, see the excellent interdisciplinary resource published by Wade (2006), *A to Z GIS: An Illustrated Dictionary of Geographic Information Systems*. This book includes more than 1,800 defined terms in alphabetical order and about 400 full-color

TABLE 9.1   GIS Terminology

Term	Definition
Attribute table*	A tabular file containing information about the GIS map layer often displayed with rows and columns. (Data with some GIS applications can be shared back and forth fairly easily with Microsoft Excel.)
Basemap	A map including streets, water, or place-name features that can be used beneath symbolized data to provide additional context.
Cartography**	The study and practice of map visualization and design. This discipline specializes in legibility and effective communication of mapped data.
Choropleth map	A thematic map for visualizing data in which areas are shaded using color gradients in proportion to the measurement of a variable per geographic area. Each color or shade represents a different measurement interval for the attribute.
Geographic data*	Information describing the location and attributes of things, including their shapes and representation. Geographic data are the composite of both spatial and attribute data.
Geographic data types: Vector	Representation of geographic data as points, lines, or polygons with tabular attributes associated with each feature.
Geographic data types: Raster	Geographic data in a grid format with each grid cell having associated size, value, and location coordinates.
Geocoding	The process of identifying the geographic location (coordinates) of an address or a spreadsheet of addresses using comprehensive street reference data.
Geographic data formats	There are numerous geographic data formats. Some have a closed format, meaning they can only be opened with proprietary software, whereas others have an open format and can be opened with numerous programs.

(continued)

TABLE 9.1 GIS Terminology (*continued*)

Term	Definition
Geoprocessing*	A GIS operation used to manipulate GIS data. A typical geoprocessing operation takes an input data set, performs an operation on that data set, and returns the result of the operation as an output data set. Common geoprocessing operations include overlay, clip, buffer, and spatial join.
GIS*	Acronym for geographic information systems. An integrated collection of computer software and data used to view and manage information about geographic places, analyze spatial relationships, and model spatial processes.
Joining*	Appending the fields of one table to those of another through the variable common to both tables. A join is usually used to attach additional attributes to the attribute table of a geographic layer.
Legend*	The map legend is usually displayed in the map layout to briefly indicate what each symbol or graphic on the map represents.
Map elements	These elements provide additional context to a map and include title, scale bar, north arrow, and source information.
Print map	A static map produced by GIS that can be included in a print publication or distributed via PDF or any other static file format.
Raster map**	Map created from images created with software that are stored in digital image files as a rectangular array, or raster, of tiny square pixels.
Shapefile**	Shapefiles are the most common digital storage format for vector spatial data. They are used for storing the location, shape, and attributes of geographic features. A shapefile is stored in a set of related files and contains one feature class.
Spatial analysis*	The process of examining the locations, attributes, and relationships of features in spatial data through overlay and other analytical techniques in order to address a question or gain useful knowledge.
Spatial analyst	A practitioner of spatial analysis. Analysts might have a formal background in geography, statistics, urban planning, computer science, or any other applicable area of study.
Spatial data**	Data about the locations and shapes of geographic features, in the form of either vector or raster data.
Vector maps**	Maps that are created from layers that consist of geographic points, lines, and polygons. A polygon is a closed area with a distinct boundary.
Web map	An interactive map that can have multiple layers, with zoom control or pan control enabled for the user. These allow for interactivity and exploration by the user.

*Kurland and Gorr (2009).

**GIS Dictionary (2014).

GIS, geographic information systems.

illustrations. It is considered one of the best resources in the field, even 9 years after it was first published.

GIS Applications and Tools

Several GIS applications are available. It can be confusing, because there are different GIS computer software applications with many optional add-on tools available for spatial exploration and analysis of geographically appointed data. GIS software tools, available in both desktop and web format, fulfill a wide variety of purposes with specialties in different disciplinary fields (e.g., environmental biology, criminology, public health) and types of spatial analysis. The sets of tools available, their costs, and the accompanying resources (training and support) are evolving as the market changes and geographic awareness becomes more ubiquitous. Traditionally, the software company Esri® was almost the exclusive provider of a desktop GIS solution, a comprehensive suite of desktop geoprocessing tools for data analysis.

Open source tools, built by a community of GIS experts who contribute their code to the public, have recently gained prominence. Online tools with analytical and visualization features are also more readily available. The newer online tools have simplified sharing capabilities, offering a practical option for those not seeking to use an entire desktop processing suite, which is sometimes quite expensive.

Some of the key elements of GIS software applications to be considered are the computer platform (desktop, web), cost and licensing (proprietary, open source), and functionality (comprehensive, limited). Table 9.2 lists some of the leading GIS tools and their characteristics. Because GIS software tools constantly evolve, be sure to investigate new options when determining what is the most appropriate option for a project.

Spatial Measurements and Statistics

Using data that are spatially assigned to describe geographic patterns and relationships is referred to as *spatial measurements* and *spatial statistics* (Mitchell, 2009). Spatial statistics is an advanced specialty within the disciplines of geography and statistics and is mathematically complicated. Computational analysis of geographic patterns to find optimum routes, site selection, and advanced predictive spatial modeling is at the very heart of GIS technology. Spatial measurements are collected and entered into the GIS database. GIS analysis uses specialized spatial statistics to identify patterns and relationships in the data that are contained within the map layers (Mitchell, 2009). Specialized descriptive and analytic spatial statistics can be categorized into the following four functional categories: (a) measuring geographic sizes, shapes, and distributions; (b) determining how places are related; (c) finding the best locations and paths; and (d) detecting and quantifying geographic patterns. Many specialized spatial statistical packages are available for performing these functions. GIS add-ons are available for specialized spatial statistics. Table 9.2 contains a list of GIS software tools and add-ons, together with pricing information, to be used in preparation of grant applications to potential funders (e.g., National Institutes of Health [NIH], Health Resources and Services Administration [HRSA]).

TABLE 9.2 GIS Software Applications With Associated Characteristics

GIS Application	Advantages	Weaknesses	Computer Platform
ArcGIS® Desktop	Comprehensive suite of geoprocessing computer software tools. Most prevalent software application used for GIS applications across multiple disciplines. Upgraded spatial analyst and geostatistical analyst extensions available for additional licensing fees. Excellent technical support and services for academia. Active R&D division.	Proprietary software Prohibitive cost Steep learning curve Short-term academic license that prevents utilization of software beyond expiration	Desktop (Windows only) application with some web interactivity GIS maps created are saved easily as pdf files or other image formats
QGIS®	Comprehensive suite of geoprocessing tools. Open source with significant documentation and support by community of users. Free software.	Slow industry adoption due to open-source software	Desktop (Windows, Mac, and Linux) application with some web interactivity
GeoDa®	Desktop GIS application intended specifically for statistical spatial analysis. Tools include advanced statistical geoprocessing tools. Free software.	Limited cartographic capability. Primary function on spatial statistical analysis	Desktop (Windows and Mac)
ArcGIS® Online	Online platform for sharing and analyzing mapped data.	Free personal tier or $2,500 annual organizational fee	Web
CartoDB*	Online platform for sharing and analyzing mapped data.	Free tier or paid tiers based on usage of $29 to $299 per month	Web

*CartoDB (cartodb.com).

GIS, geographic information systems; R&D, research and development.

One cannot perform the necessary analyses without the appropriate software tools, which must be budgeted when planning the project.

Although training programs and college-level courses teach GIS for interdisciplinary applications, expertise in spatial statistics requires more advanced education. Testing hypotheses about population health with spatial analytical statistics warrants caution, because epidemiologists are not routinely taught methods to test spatial hypotheses (Auchincloss et al., 2012). Spatial analytic methods can be categorized into three key categories: (a) cluster detection; (b) spatial interpolation and smoothing, and (c) multivariable spatial regression methods that account for the spatial dependencies of the data (Auchincloss et al., 2012). Therefore, it is best to collaborate with an appropriately trained GIS spatial analyst to avoid obtaining biased results when testing spatial hypotheses. Dissemination of incorrect conclusions could be harmful to the entire population.

Software Applications for Spatial Measurement and Statistics

As the geographic context becomes more commonplace in statistical analysis and research, statistical tools often have spatial libraries or plug-ins available to assess geographic location in addition to traditional statistical methods. Tools, plug-ins, and libraries are constantly developed and retired. Table 9.3 contains an incomplete list of commonly used statistical applications with their accompanying spatial tools, plug-ins, or libraries. The application of spatial statistics to social epidemiology is growing and is also an important focus area for developing innovative methods of spatial biostatistics (Auchincloss et al., 2012). Spatial measurement and analytical statistical tools are undergoing tremendous growth. The most up-to-date information on the functionality of spatial tools for analyzing geographic data can be found by reading the documentation and user guides for these resources.

TABLE 9.3 Statistical Software With Specialized Spatial Measurement and Analysis Applications

Statistical Application	Spatial Application Plug-ins or Libraries
R	Base R automatically supports many spatial functions, but additional packages such as maps, raster, spatial are available, which add additional spatial functionality to R.
Microsoft Excel	MapPoint is a product that can be used to visualize data stored in Excel. Advanced geospatial processing is impossible with MapPoint. Another product, Power Map, will let you visualize data on a three-dimensional glove.
Matlab	The Mapping and Image Processing toolboxes are used for geospatial image and data analysis within Matlab.
SPSS	The SPSS Statistics Package allows for the visualization of geographic data and comes with geographic boundary files along with the software.
SAS	SAS/GIS provides GIS functionality, including tools, features, and capabilities for visualizing and manipulating geographic data within the SAS system. Geocoding and thematic mapping are also possible with this product.
STATA	Modules spmap and shp2dta, among others, provide spatial interoperability and functionality to the Stata package.
JMP	Beginning with JMP 9, graphic visualization of geographic data is now supported. Built-in basemap data are also included.

GIS, geographic information systems.

TABLE 9.4   Additional Resources for GIS and Health

Type of Resource	Name of Resource
Practical GIS for health	Blatt (2012, 2014); Gatrell and Elliott (2014); Johnson (2007); Koch (2005, 2011)
Technical cartographic and GIS tips	Brewer (2008); Mitchell (2009); Peterson (2012); Wade (2006)

GIS, geographic information systems.

Interpretation and Presentation of GIS in Health Research

When interpreting geographic data, one must address many important issues. For example, it is important to determine the distribution of a disease in the population by calculating the prevalence of the disease per 1,000 population in a given geographic area. This approach will help identify an unexpectedly high incidence of disease in a given population. It is important to present legible, clearly mapped data. The following are some simple guidelines to ensure that the mapped data are clear:

1. Provide enough map detail (street and place names) to give sufficient context but not too much detail to cause clutter or confusion.
2. Use small multiples, that is, a series of small maps with minimal detail showing a variety of variables, spanning years, or categories of data for one geographic area. These facilitate easy comparisons.
3. If your map is to be printed in a black-and-white journal, be sure to use a color palette that converts clearly to grayscale, or better still, design your map in grayscale to ensure it is discernible when printed.
4. If your map is to be printed in color, be sure to use a color-blind-safe palette so individuals with impaired vision will have no issue with interpretation.

An excellent resource that has numerous tips for accurately analyzing and representing visualized data, including mapped data, is Yau's (2013) *Data Points: Visualization That Means Something*. Additional resources such as *Designing Better Maps: A Guide for GIS Users* (Brewer, 2005) and *Designed Maps: A Sourcebook for GIS Users* (Brewer, 2008) provide ample guidance for creating clear maps that communicate effectively. Table 9.4 contains a list of other resources that also serve as good references. This list is a guide and not meant to be exhaustive.

EXAMPLES OF PUBLISHED LITERATURE

Table 9.5 lists examples of research articles published in scholarly journals. This list of publications was formulated to provide a variety of examples of GIS applications that would be relevant to readers. The articles span the range of research

TABLE 9.5 Examples of Published Research Reports That Used GIS

Author	Study Purpose	GIS Applications	Sample and Setting	Key Results
Angier et al. (2014)	Assess feasibility of using GIS to visualize patient's insurance coverage status and as tool to engage stakeholders.	Geocoded EHR *Health care access; health disparities research*	Oregon used EHR data from 52 clinics that are within a practice-based research network	GIS maps illustrated areas with higher densities of uninsured residents. This was used to target outreach interventions.
Bloch (2011)	Determine whether the places in which mothers live explain disparities in preterm birth rates between U.S.-born and foreign-born Black mothers.	GIS used to study spatial patterns of preterm births among Black mothers by nativity, racial segregation, crime, and poverty. *Health Disparities Research (nursing journal)*	Philadelphia, Pennsylvania, used census tracts as a unit of analysis (neighborhood level)	Clear spatial neighborhood patterns existed. Stressful neighborhood exposures trumped protective effect of being foreign born.
Cordivano (2011)	Determine impact of closing 13 maternity units from 1996 to 2008 in a city burdened with documented racial/ethnic perinatal health disparities.	Used GIS methods innovatively to assess spatial implications of the closure of 13 maternity units in Philadelphia. *Health care access; health service research*	Philadelphia, Pennsylvania, used census tracts as the unit of analysis (neighborhood level)	Demonstrated value of GIS spatial analytical methods to assess impact of changes and closures of health care facilities. GIS can be used to propose equitable locations for health care delivery services.
Detres et al. (2014)	Describe use of GIS in CBPR research in developing implementation strategies to improve birth outcomes.	Used GIS to map infant deaths and preterm births. Used maps to engage community stakeholders. *CBPR research*	Pinellas County, Florida Infant deaths and preterm births from 2007 to 2009. Unit of analysis was zip code	Community engagement and feedback were fostered by using GIS maps. GIS maps revealed some surprises with areas not known to be at risk.
Faruque, Lofton, Doddato, and Mangum (2003)	Assess feasibility of using GIS for community health assessments.	Used GIS to locate target population to acquire a representative sample for subsequent field data collection. *Community Health Planning (nursing journal)*	Nursing students of the University of Mississippi geocoded locations of all potential survey centers in low-income, densely populated areas	GIS technology is an important tool for systematic approaches to acquire representative samples of targeted populations.

Source	Purpose	Methods	Data/Sample	Findings
Ghosh, Sterns, Drew, and Hamera (2011)	Identify geographic regions with shortages of PMH-APNs.	GIS hot spot analysis tool used to identify geographical shortages of hot spots. *Health Care Access Research (nursing journal)*	Obtained national sample through the ANCC. Geocoded employment zip codes of certified PMH-APNs	GIS is an efficient tool to identify geographic areas with PMH-APN shortages. Findings have implications for nursing education, practice, and policy.
Goswami et al. (2012)	Determine spatial variation efficient screening for TB, HIV, and syphilis.	GIS density maps identified hot spots. *Health care access; health disparities research*	Wake County, North Carolina HIV, syphilis, and TB cases, 2005 to 2007	GIS-based screening can effectively penetrate populations with high disease burden and poor access to care.
Highfield (2013)	Assess spatial correlation between breast cancer incidence and prevalence of uninsured women aged 40 to 64 years.	GIS special autocorrelation analyses applied to the data (Moran's I statistic). *Breast Health Disparities Research* *Health care access; health disparities research*	Harris County, Texas. Used breast cancer incidence data from 1995 to 2004. Unit of analysis was census tract	GIS analyses revealed negative spatial correlation between breast cancer incidence and areas with a high prevalence of uninsured women.
Hillier et al. (2015)	Investigate the relationship between tobacco advertising, tobacco retailers, and places that accept WIC and SNAP vouchers.	GIS spatial statistics (Ripley's K-function) used to test for significant spatial clustering. *Built environment*	Philadelphia, Pennsylvania. Geocoded results from field work that identified existing licensed tobacco retailers and advertising	GIS results showed that there were more tobacco advertising and retailers in low-income, racial/ethnic, segregated, and minority neighborhoods.
Hites et al. (2013)	Determine whether there are spatial patterns of unsafe conditions on a specific college campus.	Mixed-method approach using GIS. GIS quantitative and qualitative data triangulated, followed by focus groups. *Community assessment*	One large research—an intensive university with more than 17,000 students; students ($n = 61$) participated in focus groups. Geospatial analysis of crime data identified hot spots	Mixed methods using GIS geocoded crime data facilitated engaged discussions, leading to a more complete understanding of multifaceted issues related to campus safety.

(continued)

TABLE 9.5 Examples of Published Research Reports That Used GIS (continued)

Author	Study Purpose	GIS Applications	Sample and Setting	Key Results
Kramer, Cooper, Drews-Botsch, Waller, and Hogue (2010)	Assess misclassification and measurement bias between two different GIS methods to measure residential racial segregation.	Focused on GIS approach to measure residential segregation, an important variable when measuring social determinants of health. *Health disparities research*	Used 231 metropolitan areas in the United States representing the northeast, south, midwest, and west.	Misclassification and measurement bias needs to be considered by researchers when using GIS to measure neighborhood residential segregation. The first step in analysis is exploring place–health variations on the spatial scale analyzed. Because of variations of spatial scales, careful attention must be given to the role and variation in spatial scales across geographic regions with regard to the study of place and health outcomes.
Madigan, Wiencek, and Vander Schrier (2009)	Assess community-based providers for end-of-life care to the elderly in rural geographical areas.	Used GIS to locate hot spots that were underserved. *Health Care Access Research (nursing journal)*	Eight states: Used county level as unit of analysis to study rural areas.	GIS maps showed where underserved areas were located for end-of-life hospice providers. More than 85% of the rural counties in Arkansas and Louisiana were underserved.

Oreskovic et al. (2014)	Study children's physical activity by measuring the built environment's influence on method of commuting to school.	Collected geospatial data to determine whether the built environment predicted walking to school. *Built environment*	Houston, Texas Fourth-grade low-income students ($n = 149$) who participated in parent RCT study.	GIS is an important tool to contextualize built environments of students' walkability to school.
Smith and Miller (2013)	Describe the use of GIS in ecocity mapping to assess vitality of neighborhoods for health planning and intervention.	Walkability of neighborhoods. Urban Health planning *Built environment*	Pilot program engaging community in housing development in Oakland, California, 2007 to 2009.	GIS mapping is a successful tool for community organization and engagement to improve the built environment.
Taylor et al. (2012)	Use of GIS in decision making of primary care locations.	GIS network analysis tool was used as an innovative and important analytical tool. *Community Health Planning (nursing journal)*	Jefferson County, Alabama	GIS is a valuable tool for decision making to determine locations that efficiently assure access to patient care.
Topmiller, Vissman, and Miller-Francis (2015)	Describe the use of GIS in CBPR research to study physical activity in youth and their neighborhoods.	Mix-methods use of GIS to study the built environment. *Built environment*	Five neighborhoods in Covington, Kentucky. Focus groups with 15 youth (aged 11–17 years).	Engaging youth to participate in generating knowledge about their neighborhoods was productive and empowering.

ANCC, American Nurses Credentialing Center; CBPR, community-based participatory approach; EHRs, electronic health records; PMH-APNs, psychiatric mental health advanced practice nurses; RCT, randomized controlled trial; SNAP, Supplemental Nutrition Assistance Program; TB, tuberculosis; WIC, Women, Infants, and Children.

that is concerned with health disparities, community assessment, and access to health care.

SUMMARY

In the previous decade, GIS tools became much more commonplace in health research than they had been earlier. This is, in part, due to the increased availability of quality and community-supported, open-source applications; a lower technical barrier to use tools; and the ubiquity of mapping technology and geographic awareness that grew with the availability of smartphones. These assets make it easier for researchers to incorporate geographic context into their research. Therefore, to ensure that the mapped data are represented correctly and that any conclusions involving geographic data are neither distorted nor manipulated, either purposefully or accidentally, we recommend that health researchers consult with a statistician or spatial analyst with expertise in analyzing and visualizing geographic data. Monmonier (1996) describes the pitfalls of misrepresenting geographic information in his book *How to Lie With Maps*. Maintaining the integrity of the data should be the prime focus in analyzing and visualizing geographic data.

A key contribution of nursing scholarship is the generation, translation, and application of knowledge to improving health and the quality of people's lives. Using broad, holistic perspectives that capture data about the environments in which people live, work, and play, GIS is a valuable tool for nursing research and practice. Nurse scholars can further the development of GIS applications by translating geospatial data to improve health and health care systems in the clinical specialties and among the populations that they know well from their clinical practices.

REFERENCES

Aday, L. (2001). Establishment of a conceptual base for health services research. *Journal of Health Services Research*, 6(3), 183–185.

Aday, L., Begley, C. E., Lairson, D. R., & Slater, C. H. (1998). *Evaluating the healthcare system: Effectiveness, efficiency, and equity*. Chicago, IL: Health Administration Press.

Angier, H., Likumahuwa, S., Finnegan, S., Vakarcs, T., Nelson, C., Bazemore, A., . . . DeVoe, J. E. (2014). Using geographic information systems (GIS) to identify communities in need of health insurance outreach: An OCHIN practice-based research network (PBRN) report. *Journal of the American Board of Family Medicine*, 27(6), 804–810.

Auchincloss, A. H., Gebreab, S. Y., Mair, C., & Diez Roux, A. V. (2012). A review of spatial methods in epidemiology, 2000–2010. *Annual Review of Public Health*, 33, 107–122.

Blaschke, T., Hay, G. J., Kelly, M., Lang, S., Hofmann, P., Addink, E., . . . Tiede, D. (2014). Geographic object-based image analysis—towards a new paradigm. *ISPRS Journal of Photogrammetry and Remote Sensing*, 87(100), 180–191.

Blatt, A. (2012). *Perspectives in medical geography: Theory and applications for librarians*. London, UK: Routledge.

Blatt, A. (2014). *Health, science, and place: A new model (geotechnologies and the environment)*. New York, NY: Springer.

Bloch, J. R. (2011). Using geographical information systems to explore disparities in preterm birth rates among foreign-born and U.S.-born Black mothers. *Journal of Obstetric, Gynecologic, and Neonatal Nursing, 40*(5), 544–554.

Brewer, C. (2005). *Designing better maps: A guide for GIS users*. Redlands, CA: Esri Press.

Brewer, C. (2008). *Designed maps: A sourcebook for GIS users*. Redlands, CA: Esri Press.

Census American Community Survey. (2013). Retrieved from http://www.census.gov/acs/www/data/data-tables-and-tools/american-factfinder

Cordivano, S. (2011). Maternity ward closures in Philadelphia: Using GIS to measure disruptions in essential health services. *Journal of Map and Geography Libraries, 7*(2), 282–303.

Cromley, E. K., & McLafferty, S. (2012). *GIS and public health*. New York, NY: Guilford Press.

Detres, M., Lucio, R., & Vitucci, J. (2014). GIS as a community engagement tool: Developing a plan to reduce infant mortality risk factors. *Maternal and Child Health Journal, 18*(5), 1049–1055.

Faruque, F. S., Lofton, S. P., Doddato, T. M., & Mangum, C. (2003). Utilizing geographic information systems in community assessment and nursing research. *Journal of Community Health Nursing, 20*(3), 179–191.

Fawcett, J. (2005). *Contemporary nursing knowledge: Analysis and evaluation of nursing models and theories* (2nd ed.). Philadelphia, PA: F. A. Davis Company.

Friis, R. H., & Sellers, T. A. (2009). *Epidemiology for public health practice* (4th ed.). Sudbury, MA: Jones and Bartlett.

Gatrell, A., & Elliott, S. (2014). *Geographies of health: An introduction*. Hoboken, NJ: Wiley-Blackwell.

Ghosh, D., Sterns, A. A., Drew, B. L., & Hamera, E. (2011). Geospatial study of psychiatric mental health-advanced practice registered nurses (PMH-APRNs) in the United States. *Psychiatric Services, 62*(12), 1506–1509. doi:10.1176/appi.ps.000532011

GIS Dictionary. (2014). *Esri*. Retrieved from http://support.esri.com/en/knowledgebase/GISDictionary/term/spatial%20analysis

Goswami, N. D., Hecker, E. J., Vickery, C., Ahearn, M. A., Cox, G. M., Holland, D. P., . . . Stout, J. E. (2012). Geographic information system-based screening for TB, HIV, and syphilis (GIS-THIS): A cross-sectional study. *PLoS One, 7*(10), e46029. doi:10.1371/journal.pone.0046029

Highfield, L. (2013). Spatial patterns of breast cancer incidence and uninsured women of mammography screening age. *Breast Journal, 19*(3), 293–301. doi:10.1111/tbj.12100

Hillier, A., Chilton, M., Zhao, Q. W., Szymkowiak, D., Coffman, R., & Mallya, G. (2015). Concentration of tobacco advertisements at SNAP and WIC stores, Philadelphia, Pennsylvania, 2012. *Preventing Chronic Diseases, 12*, E15. doi:10.5888/pcd12.140133

Hites, L. S., Fifolt, M., Beck, H., Su, W., Kerbawy, S., Wakelee, J., & Nassel, A. (2013). A geospatial mixed methods approach to assessing campus safety. *Evaluation Review, 37*(5), 347–369.

Johnson, S. (2007). *The ghost map: The story of London's most terrifying epidemic—and how it changed science, cities, and the modern world*. New York, NY: Riverhead Trade.

Kawachi, I., & Berkman, L. F. (2003). *Neighborhoods and health*. New York, NY: Oxford University Press.

Koch, T. (2005). *Cartographies of disease: Maps, mapping, and medicine*. Redlands, CA: Esri Press.

Koch, T. (2011). *Disease maps: Epidemics on the ground*. Chicago, IL: The University of Chicago Press Books.

Kounadi, O., & Leitner, M. (2014). Why does geoprivacy matter? The scientific publication of confidential data presented on maps. *Journal of Empirical Research on Human Research Ethics, 9*(4), 34–45. doi:10.1177/1556264614544103

Kramer, M. R., Cooper, H. L., Drews-Botsch, C. D., Waller, L. A., & Hogue, C. R. (2010). Do measures matter? Comparing surface-density-derived and census-tract-derived measures of racial residential segregation. *International Journal of Health Geographics, 9*, 29. doi:10.1186/1476-072x-9-29

Krieger, N., Zierler, S., Hogan, J. W., Waterman, P. D., Chen, J., Lemieux, K., & Gjelsvik, A. (2003). Geocoding and measurement of neighborhood socioeconomic position: A U.S. perspective. In I. Kawachi & Lisa F. Berkman (Eds.), *Neighborhoods and health* (pp. 147–178). New York, NY: Oxford University Press.

Kurland, K. S., & Gorr, W. L. (2009). *GIS tutorial for health* (Vol. 3). Redlands, CA: ESRI Press.

Love, C., David, R. J., Rankin, K. M., & Collins, J. W., Jr. (2010). Exploring weathering: Effects of life-long economic environment and maternal age on low birth weight, small for gestational age, and preterm birth in African-American and White women. *American Journal of Epidemiology, 172*(2), 127–134.

Madigan, E. A., Wiencek, C. A., & Vander Schrier, A. L. (2009). Patterns of community-based end-of-life care in rural geographical areas of the United States. *Policy, Politics, & Nursing Practice, 10*(1), 71–81.

Mitchell, A. (2009). *The ESRI guide to GIS analysis: Spatial measurement and statistics* (Vol. 2). Redlands, CA: ESRI Press.

Monmonier, M. (1996). *How to lie with maps.* Chicago, IL: University of Chicago Press.

Moss, M. P., & Schell, M. C. (2004). GIS(c): A scientific framework and methodological tool for nursing research. *Advances in Nursing Science, 27*(2), 150–159.

O'Campo, P., Burke, J. G., Culhane, J., Elo, I. T., Eyster, J., Holzman, C., . . . Laraia, B. A. (2008). Neighborhood deprivation and preterm birth among non-Hispanic Black and White women in eight geographic areas in the United States. *American Journal of Epidemiology, 167*(2), 155–163.

Oreskovic, N. M., Blossom, J., Robinson, A. I., Chen, M. L., Uscanga, D. K., & Mendoza, J. A. (2014). The influence of the built environment on outcomes from a "walking school bus study": A cross-sectional analysis using geographical information systems. *Geospatial Health, 9*(1), 37–44.

Peterson, G. N. (2012). *Cartographer's toolkit: Colors, typography, patterns.* Fort Collins: PetersonGIS.

Smith, R., & Miller, K. (2013). Ecocity mapping using GIS: Introducing a planning method for assessing and improving neighborhood vitality. *Progress in Community Health Partnerships, 7*(1), 95–106. doi:10.1353/cpr.2013.0000

Taylor, D. M., Yeager, V., Ouimet, C., & Menachemi, N. (2012). Using GIS for administrative decision-making in a local public health setting. *Public Health Reports, 127*(3), 47–53.

Topmiller, M., Jacquez, F., Vissman, A. T., Raleigh, K., & Miller-Francis, J. (2015). Partnering with youth to map their neighborhood environments: A multilayered GIS approach. *Family and Community Health, 38*(1), 66–76.

Wade, T. (2006). *A to Z GIS: An illustrated dictionary of geographic information systems.* Redlands, CA: Esri Press.

Yau, N. (2013). *Data points: Visualization that means something.* Hoboken, NJ: Wiley.

CHAPTER TEN

A STATISTICAL TOOLBOX: TIPS FOR ENGAGING IN CLINICAL INQUIRY TO IMPROVE HEALTH AND HEALTH CARE

LOUIS FOGG, BETH A. STAFFILENO, AND MARCIA MURPHY

OBJECTIVES

After reading this chapter, readers will be able to:

1. Identify statistical tools to address practice-based clinical problems and inquiry
2. Explain how the statistical tools can be implemented
3. Discuss why, when, and how to work with statisticians

Respect for rigor and integrity of data in clinical inquiry is paramount. Robust meaningful clinical inquiry necessitates a working knowledge of statistics and practical knowledge of the ins and outs of working with statisticians. Thus, the purpose of this chapter is to provide useful tips when using statistics and working with statisticians, as nurse scholars use data to generate and translate knowledge that aims at positively impacting patient care outcomes. Written by three faculty members, two nurse faculty members (M.M. & B.S.), and a statistician (L.F.), this chapter is divided into two key sections. In the first section, a statistical toolbox is presented to serve as a practical guide. In the second section, the statistician (L.F.) provides his unique perspective and advice on working with statisticians. As a faculty member in the Rush University College of Nursing spanning two decades, he has collaborated with many PhD and DNP nursing faculty and students and served as the statistician on more than 25 funded National Institutes of Health (NIH) grants.

This chapter is included in this book to serve as a reminder of the critically important role that data have in the field of clinical inquiry. Integrated into this chapter is somewhat of a storytelling approach. Discussing statistics can be quite a dry topic, but understanding the use of statistics in the context of clinical inquiry is much more interesting. Through the stories and examples of several clinical inquiry projects, the reader is provided with a toolbox for tackling his or her clinical inquiry data and working with statisticians.

THE STATISTICAL TOOLBOX

There are three tools in the statistical toolbox of this chapter. The first is conventional hypothesis testing, which is the "meat and potatoes" of most statistics courses. The second is the use of effect sizes and simple descriptive statistics to explain one's findings. And finally, the third tool is the use of graphic representations to help learn about the relationships that exist in the data. With these three tools, it is possible to do two things: (a) learn how to make more useful clinical decisions; and (b) communicate findings more effectively to other clinical decision makers.

It is also important to keep in mind that the research conducted is not a "one size fits all" sort of enterprise. Nurse scholars use research to generate, disseminate, and translate new knowledge that is relevant to clinical inquiry. A statistical toolbox is needed because of the need for different tools for conducting and disseminating different types of nursing research and evidence-based practice.

The Counting Marbles Story

We begin with a background story that the statistician author (L.F.) of this chapter narrates about counting marbles. When a graduate student at the University of Chicago in the 1980s, he took several statistics courses and a recurring analogy that these courses used to analyze *sampling* and *probability* was the urns of marbles situation. The idea behind the urns of marbles is that you have two stone urns on a table, and you know that there are 70 red marbles and 30 green marbles in one urn, and 70 green marbles and 30 red marbles in the other urn. The problem is to draw samples of marbles from each of the two urns, and from these drawn samples of marbles, to determine the probability that urn one has the 70 reds or 70 greens. The idea behind the exercise is that if one is drawing a sample of marbles from the 70 red urn, one is more likely to have more red marbles in one's sample. And the primary characteristic that these urns have is that marbles are independently distributed (the choice of one marble at random does not influence the selection of the next) and identically distributed (each marble has an equal chance of being selected). Or as statisticians like to call it, i. i. d. (independently and identically distributed). When these assumptions are met, conclusions about the marbles in the urn would apply equally well to the entire universe of marble-filled urns.

He soon discovered, however, that one cannot be a graduate student forever, and he was forced to go out and obtain gainful employment while conducting statistical analyses for a psychiatric research project. The project examined psychiatric patients in various and sundry stages of recovery from their illnesses. These were very ill patients who had been unresponsive to more conventional treatment settings, and so they were sent to this research laboratory in the hopes that they could find a more effective experimental treatment for themselves.

So, on his first day of work, he sat down to look at the data that needed to be analyzed. But, to his great surprise, there were no marbles. How could this be? He had just obtained an excellent education on the analysis of urns of marbles, only to find out that he was not studying marbles at all! He was forced to actually analyze data about people. But people are nothing like marbles.

To make matters worse, the data were not i.i.d.! The observations were not independent. In fact, the subjects all had to have a mental illness, live in Illinois, and be treatment resistant. It was a big, complex mess. Not knowing how he was supposed to analyze data such as these is essentially one of the reasons he suggested writing this chapter for this book. Conducting nursing research is not only more complicated but also, in some ways, simpler than trying to characterize the number of different-colored marbles that are stored in an urn. Through evidence-based practice, nurses are trying to make clinical decisions for patients to maximize their well-being. Florence Nightingale, the first nurse researcher and statistician, made observations of soldiers returning from the Crimean War and reduced mortality rates from 43% (urn 1) to 2% (urn 2) by improving hygiene and environmental conditions (Palmer, 1977). This is, essentially, assuming that people are pretty much like marbles.

First Statistical Tool: Hypothesis Testing

The hypothetico-deductive model (Neyman & Pearson, 1992) underlies much of statistics in order to try to deduce what is true and what is not. The manner in which this is applied is that an assumption, called the *null hypothesis*, is made. The null hypothesis is the hypothesis that two populations of interest are not different from each other. So, for the urn example given earlier, the null hypothesis might be that there is the same proportion of red marbles in each of the two urns. It should be noted here that no statements are made to hypothesize how many red marbles are in each urn, but only that the proportion of red marbles (in our two-color marble universe—red/green) is the same.

To test this hypothesis, marbles are taken out of each urn. The drawn marbles are the *sample*. If the urns contain a very large number of marbles, a large sample can be drawn to get a better estimate of the proportion of red marbles in the urn. A parallel sample can be drawn from the other urn as well. Then, the magic of hypothesis testing is testing the null hypothesis that the two urns have the same proportion of red marbles. This is done by estimating the probability that the first sample (let us say there were 80 reds and 20 greens) is taken from an identically distributed urn as the second one (let us say there were 20 reds and 80 greens). This example represents a 2×2 contingency table that looks something like this (Table 10.1).

A chi-square test can be conducted to estimate the probability that the null hypothesis is true (proportion of red marbles in urn 1 equals the proportion of red marbles in urn 2). In this case, this probability is quite small ($p < .001$), and it uses a criterion probability of .05 to reject the null hypothesis that the two urns have equal proportions of red marbles. Furthermore, assuming red marbles are valued over green, urn 1 is preferred. If the marbles are relabeled as patients who recover (red marbles) and those who do not (green marbles) and the urns are relabeled as possible treatments for these patients, this pretty much describes how the hypothetico-deductive model is used in health care research.

There are a number of excellent books written about statistical analyses using the hypothetico-deductive theory. Fisher (1935/1971) wrote an excellent book on

TABLE 10.1 A 2×2 Contingency Table		
Urns	1	2
Red marbles	80	20
Green marbles	20	80

all of this, and more recently, Snedecor and Cochrane (1989) also wrote an excellent textbook in this area. Finally, if you want to combine an education on the hypothetico-deductive theory with training on how to conduct statistical analysis in Excel, Schmuller (2013) wrote an excellent text called *Statistical Analysis With Excel for Dummies*.

So, how do the urns and marbles work in the real world of nursing practice? One way to illustrate this is by providing examples of clinical inquiry. So, essentially, instead of just talking about statistics, they are described in the larger context of studies that evolved from clinical practice and clinical inquiry. Each of the following four examples highlight how nurse scholars identified a problem, developed a project, and applied methodology and statistical tools to change practice and improve patient outcomes. Elements of these processes are outlined in Table 10.2.

Example 1: Clinical Inquiry About Taking Care of Older Adults

Identifying the Problem
The proportion of adults 65 years or older in the United States is rapidly growing and expected to reach 72 million during the next two decades (Centers for Disease Control and Prevention [CDC], 2013). As many as a third of these older adults experience hospitalizations that can pose consequences to functional well-being (Stranges & Friedman, 2009). Nurses are in a key position to evaluate system processes to improve patient outcomes. For example, it has been found that nursing staff are not always educated in geriatric patient needs and care, especially certified nursing assistants who have minimal training in special populations (Gilje, Lacey, & Moore, 2007). Therefore, this study was designed to examine the effects of a geriatric education for staff nurses and certified nursing assistants in conjunction with changes in daily staff practices to increase older patient mobility (Lee, Staffileno, & Fogg, 2013).

Methods to Address the Problem
A pre/post single-group study design was selected to address the research question and measure outcomes. Although a comparison or control group would have strengthened the design of the study, the nurse scholar determined that no other unit served a similar geriatric population; therefore, it was not feasible to employ a control group (unit within the hospital) for comparison. Instead, the single-group approach was possible by comparing discharge rate and hospital complications from the previous year to evaluate the effectiveness of the intervention. The intervention included staff education on geriatric care and infrastructural change to encourage patient mobility and function. Standard measures were used for evaluating outcomes of the intervention. For example, discharge destination and length of stay (LOS) were measured using the hospital's clinical data system for patient information. Prevalence of nosocomial pressure ulcer and fall rates were obtained from the unit's existing quality outcome measures. These outcome measures were compared from data with the same period in the previous year. Functional status was measured using the Katz activities of daily living (ADL) Index, which has established reliability and validity (Katz, Down, Cash, & Grotz, 1970). Upon hospital admissions, patients were queried about their ADL over the 2-week period just prior to admission, thus serving as a baseline assessment. Patients were again queried about ADL at the time of discharge to assess for functional status change during hospitalization.

TABLE 10.2 Developing a Practice-Based Clinical Inquiry Project

What	How	Why
Identify a problem	• Clinical experience • The literature • Previous research • National initiatives • Organizational priorities • Quality and safety data	• Have a strong interest in the problem • What is already known about this problem? • Will the outcome improve quality of patient care and outcomes? • Will the findings be applicable in clinical practice?
Identify a project team	• Establish what expertise is needed to develop and execute the project • Network with key stakeholders • Determine who is the most impacted by the problem	• Who will best serve as the leader of the project? • How many people will be involved in developing and managing the project?
Develop a project question	• Review the literature • Review pertinent data • Assess clinical relevance	• Compose an argument—what is the problem? • Who is the population of interest? • Why is the problem important? (Who are the key stakeholders?) • What will happen if you fix the problem? • What will happen if the problem is not fixed?

Develop a methodology to address the problem	• Establish how to implement the project
	  ■ Identify the population
	  ■ Identify a site/location
	  ■ Develop a protocol and procedures
	  ■ Identify instruments for data collection
	  ■ Identify necessary tools, instruments, and measures
	• Establish how to evaluate the project
	  ■ Create a plan for data management and analysis
		• Having a clear method to address the problem is needed to determine a change
		• Having a mechanism for project evaluation is needed to establish sustainability

Use the statistical toolbox	• Look at your data • Describe your data using simple descriptive statistics • Test statistical hypotheses	• To examine the nature of relationships and determine if your intervention works at all • To convince your reader that your treatment or intervention actually works • To convince your reader that your results are not due to random fluctuations
Discuss and disseminate findings	• Compose a description of project findings • Present findings to key stakeholders and relevant venues • Identify next steps • Publish findings	• How does the project impact patient outcomes and extend existing knowledge? • Identify lessons learned

Consultation with a statistician was done to determine a sample size with adequate power to detect an increase in the percentage of patients returning home from hospitalization. Determination of sample size is typically a point that most clinicians will want to consult a statistician or an experienced researcher about. Another troublesome area for many is determining which statistics should be used given the type of data collected. In this case, demographic characteristics (age, gender, race, marital) were tabulated using descriptive statistics (means and standard deviations) or frequency distributions (percentages). With respect to data analysis, changes in outcomes with normally distributed mean scores, such as LOS, were compared using a paired t-test. Other outcomes involving changes using percentages or categorical data required the use of nonparametric testing. Therefore, change in ADL, rate of patients returning home, and the number of nosocomial pressure ulcers and fall rates were tested using chi-square analysis.

Pearls From the Toolbox
This is a wonderful example of how practicing nurse scholars can use nursing research to develop a new program to improve the health of patients. In addition, the hypothesis-testing tool was critical to demonstrate that the effect was robust, and it allows dissemination of this through a scholarly publication. In this case, a chi-square test demonstrated that the decrease in pressure ulcers (from 10.7% to 5.9%) was a statistically significant improvement, just as our two urns differed in the proportion of red marbles. (Yes—back to the counting marbles story!)

Lessons Learned From This Project
This study served as pilot work for subsequent inquiry that would involve implementing a research design with a control (or comparison) unit and randomization of patients. This preliminary work demonstrated that providing staff education and altering infrastructure support the transfer of knowledge to practice. Hence, promoting mobility and function improves outcomes for hospitalized older adults.

Second Statistical Tool: Effect Sizes and Simple Descriptive Statistics

The importance of finding an effect with a simple chi-square analysis is underscored here. Many statisticians will say that if you cannot find an effect with a chi-square test, it probably is not there. If the effect is that hard to find, it may not be worth much in the first place because the amount of benefit that a person will receive from the intervention is so negligible that it does not merit much time and energy. This point of view has led some researchers to begin reporting effect sizes, rather than probability statements. But what are effect sizes? One should read the Florence Nightingale story to fully understand how effect sizes matter when practice changes are needed (Box 10.1).

Example 2: Safe Patient Handling

Identifying the Problem
An advanced practice nurse (APN) determined that assessing staff perceptions of barriers and attitudes toward safe patient handling was paramount prior to introducing new lift equipment (Krill, Staffileno, & Raven, 2012). The APN wanted staff

---

BOX 10.1   The Florence Nightingale Example of How Effect Sizes Matter
Effect sizes are the simplest sorts of statistical estimates. A fine example of how effect sizes are used is found in the work of Florence Nightingale (Palmer, 1977) that was discussed earlier. Nightingale was serving with the British military in the Crimea in the mid-1800s. During this stay, she saw that the hospitals where the soldiers were treated were not very clean. The water the patients drank was not pure, and the staff did not always keep themselves and their patients clean. Nightingale instituted a program for more hygienic conditions in these hospitals, but just as importantly, she recorded the mortality rates in the hospitals both before and after she implemented her changes. The mortality rate dropped from 43% to 2% after the hygienic practices were introduced. She did not calculate a probability value or use any other statistics other than the ones just cited. And still, her findings were so striking that her practices were followed from that time on in British military hospitals. The difference between the two mortality rates was so large that the effect was convincing without having to conduct any other statistical analyses. The same thing is happening currently with nursing research. The hallmark of nursing research and nursing practice, in statistical terms, is that nursing research fosters interventions that have very large effect sizes. This is because nursing research begins at the point-of-patient care, and it is always primarily concerned with patient welfare. "Research is asking the right question—a question in clinical practice that will improve the care of patients" (Christman, 1965). The interventions that are geared to improve the care of patients are the ones that have the largest effect sizes. So, there are times when the numbers speak for themselves and are convincing without having to tie a probability value or a confidence interval to themselves. For a more technical and detailed look at various effect sizes, the reader is encouraged to look at Cohen's (1988) excellent book on the subject, *Statistical Power Analysis for the Behavioral Sciences*.

to determine what handling equipment and education was needed to successfully develop a safe patient handling program.

Methods to Address the Problem

The APN proposed a descriptive study to assess staff perceptions, identify staff needs, and involve staff in selecting equipment for safe patient handling. The APN identified two widely used national survey instruments that would assess the following: (a) staff's perceived barriers and attitudes regarding safe patient handling (Silverstein & Howard, 2006); and (b) staff's needs for equipment and education (Safe Patient Handling Risk Assessment Tool Swedish Medical Center, 2007). To reach as many as possible, it was decided to administer the surveys by using an online platform. The two surveys combined consisted of 31 questions, used a Likert scale and open-ended questions, took about 15 minutes to complete, and were available for a 1-month period to accommodate staff who were taking summer vacation. Staff also participated in a 1-hour focus group. A focus group is a form of qualitative research that encourages people to express their perceptions, opinions, beliefs, and attitudes toward a particular topic. Finally, a 1-day fair was held to evaluate a variety of lift equipment from five vendors. After an equipment trial, staff were queried as to the comfort, ease of use, versatility, stability, ease of cleaning, and willingness to use the product. Descriptive statistics were used to describe sample characteristics, the narrative themes that the participants discussed in the focus groups, and the survey data from testing the equipment. In this manner, the optimal equipment was selected.

Pearls From the Toolbox
This is a marvelous use of descriptive statistics and how they can be utilized to facilitate effective nursing practice and contribute to the efficient use of resources.

Lessons Learned From the Project
This study illustrates the use of both survey data and focus group data to tap into the professional expertise of the entire staff of the institution.

Third Statistical Tool: Graphic Representations of Data

Looking at your data through graphic representations of the data can be powerful. Often, there are certain types of relationships that are easier to see as pictures than they are to estimate as statistics (Tukey, 1977). Pictures of the data can be very helpful in answering important questions in nursing research and clinical practice. Reviewing all the possible graphic ways to illustrate data is beyond the scope of this chapter, but an example using a dose–response curve will be given (DeLean et al., 1978).

The dose–response curve is explained here through an example of showing the dose of a medication that is optimal for a patient to receive. The curve is formed by two competing mechanisms: The effectiveness of the medication in reducing symptoms or treating an illness and the toxicity of the medication when given in doses that are too high. So, as the dose of the medication is increased from zero, the patient benefits from the therapeutic effects. And as long as the therapeutic benefits

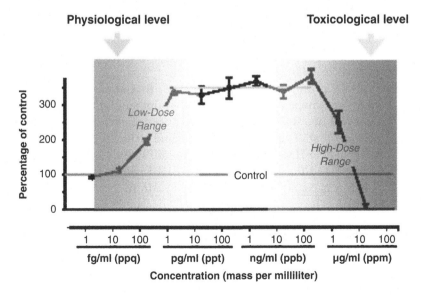

Figure 10.1　Dose–response curve.

outweigh the toxicity of the medication, the dose can be increased. At some dose, the benefits begin to wane and the toxicity increases, at which point any higher doses will not be useful for the patient (Figure 10.1). The critical characteristics of dose–response curves are that they are quite common in health care research, and that the correlation between dose and benefit will be zero. Thus, as long as researchers restrict their examination of the relationships between their measures to the correlation coefficient, they will never be able to detect a dose–response relationship (Meehl, 1978). So, there is enormous power in looking at your data.

Example 3. Clinical Inquiry About Taking Newborn Temperatures

Identifying the Problem

Newborns undergo profound physiologic changes at the moment of birth. Thermoregulation is an important first step for the newborn infant to adjust to extrauterine life. The World Health Organization (WHO, 1997) views thermoregulation as an essential component of caring for the newborn infant. Nurses caring for neonates are responsible for monitoring newborn temperatures and providing care that decreases heat loss and prevents overheating. Common practice involves taking rectal temperatures on full-term newborns, even though risks are associated with this practice, including perforation of the gastrointestinal tract (Fonkalsrud & Clatworthy, 1965).

The evidence behind this practice was questioned, and a literature review and query of similar institutions was conducted. Many institutions were using axillary temperature measurements, whereas others were still using the rectal method, suggesting inconsistencies in practice. The safest and most effective practice of obtaining a temperature in newborn infants continues to be controversial (Friedrichs et al., 2013). Thus, the question remains unanswered. Is the evidence for using rectal temperature in full-term infants strong enough to continue with this practice?

Methods to Address the Problem

The team designed an agreement study to determine the reliability of the electronic thermometer measuring temperature in the axilla compared with the rectum in full-term newborn infants. The specific research questions included the following: (a) Do axillary temperatures agree with rectal temperatures, allowing axillary temperatures to be considered the preferred alternative to rectal temperatures? (b) Is there a preference in one axilla over the other based on the levels of agreement? A study protocol was developed and within the first hour of arriving to the newborn nursery, right and left axillary temperatures were obtained first, followed by the rectal temperature.

Demographic characteristics were reported using descriptive statistics (means and standard deviations). To examine the relationship between rectal and axillary temperatures, regression analyses were conducted. To assess the agreement between rectal and axillary temperatures, a graphical representation of the temperature data was analyzed using a Bland–Altman approach (Altman & Bland, 1983; Bland & Altman, 2007). The Bland–Altman approach looks at how closely scores agree and then examines clinical/demographic factors to see if any of them might have influenced the amount of disagreement that was found. The amount of disagreement is found by examining a scatterplot, where the distance between the points (each point represents a matched pair of observations) is the distance between the point and the equivalue line (Figure 10.2).

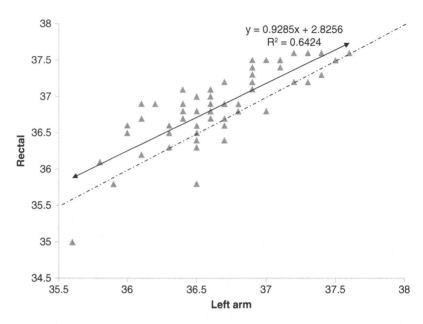

Figure 10.2   Bland–Altman analysis.

Pearls From the Toolbox
This study is an excellent illustration of the use of graphical representation of data to help explain relationships that may exist in the data. In this case, the Bland–Altman analysis (Altman & Bland, 1983) showed that both axilla could serve as sites for obtaining temperature data without loss of validity. In addition, this is also an excellent example of the use of a purposive sample. This study only works with newborns and so one is required to only choose participants from a select group, rather than from the general population. The comparison of rectal and axillary temperatures would not make sense in an adult sample.

Lessons Learned From This Project
Importantly, the clinicians challenged the status quo and searched for evidence supporting the clinical practice of rectal temperature taking in full-term newborns. The three basic tenets of evidence-based practice (research, clinical expertise, and patient preference) were used to investigate and draw conclusions for practice change. Results demonstrated that using the left axillary temperature measurements in full-term newborns was a safe alternative to rectal temperatures. This example reinforces the value of questioning current clinical practice by presenting evidence that may or may not support current practice.

The Statistical Toolbox

In most statistics courses, students only learn about the first tool (hypothesis testing) in the statistical toolbox. But for clinical inquiry research, it is important to use all three of the tools (Table 10.2). So, a quick and dirty guide to conducting statistical analysis is to use the tools in the following order. First, you should look at your data. If the data are nonlinear or have a funny distribution, this can make the statistics you calculate, even simple descriptive ones, completely useless. Again, you should think of the dose–response relationship.

Second, you should look at simple descriptive statistics. Remember how Florence Nightingale approached her data. She presented simple statistics that told her story. And finally, if there is clear evidence that you have an effect, but you want to present more compelling evidence to that effect, you should use hypothesis testing procedures to convince readers, or the audience, that your findings are real, as opposed to random findings.

One big advantage to this three-step process is that very often, our interventions or treatments just do not work. When this happens, it is usually easier to see this with a picture than it is to try to discover it from looking at summary statistics. There is much to be gained from learning what does not work, not the least of which is that it may, eventually, lead us to discover what does work.

Example 4: Using the Whole Toolbox

Cardiovascular disease (CVD) is the leading cause of death and disability in the United States with a disproportionate burden on racial/ethnic and underserved populations (Go et al., 2013). Moreover, CVD is the leading cause of death for older adults and the death rate attributable to CVD is greater for African Americans compared with Caucasians (Go et al., 2013). Sheltered homeless people constitute another vulnerable population that experiences significant health disparities (National Alliance to End Homelessness, 2013). This is particularly significant for clinicians working in such communities. The Heart Healthy Program (HHP) is an example of an APN-led initiative in such an underserved community setting. This example was the development and implementation of a HHP to improve the cardiovascular health of two underserved populations using the American Heart Association's Life Simple 7/My Life Check (MLC) tool (Murphy, Coke, Staffileno, Robinson & Tillotson, 2015).

Methods to Address the Problem
Two inner city community sites were targeted for this program. One was a senior center servicing African American older adults, and the other was a residential facility for women with histories of substance abuse and homelessness. The determination of a tool to measure cardiovascular health was the first step in identifying important data to collect. Once that was established, a protocol was developed for data collection and analysis.

The American Heart Association's Life Simple 7/MLC tool was identified as the measurement tool. The MLC tool provides a measure of overall cardiovascular health with a total score ranging from 0 to 10 based on four behavioral factors (maintaining a healthy weight, assessment of eating patterns, physical activity patterns, and smoking status) and three biomarker levels (blood pressure, blood cholesterol, and blood glucose). The MLC is a computer-based tool with an algorithm that calculates a weighted score using points based on multivariate associations with cardiovascular health (Murphy et al., 2015). Preprogram health data were collected to calculate the MLC scores.

All three statistical tools were used to describe the population and evaluate the outcomes of the HHP. Descriptive statistics (means and standard deviations) were used to describe the demographic characteristics (age, gender, and race). The mean MLC score was calculated both before and after the program was implemented to conduct hypothesis testing to determine if the program improved health. Then, the effect size of the changes was calculated based on the mean scores to evaluate whether cardiovascular health improved as a result of the program. Specific data on each health factor were displayed in a table along with a chart that graphically displayed the percentage change in the mean aggregate MLC scores for each population's overall change in cardiovascular health. All this can be found in Murphy et al.'s (2015) referenced publication.

Pearls From the Statistical Toolbox
This aforementioned example is a good example of the use of all three of our statistical tools. Hypothesis testing was used to determine if there was significant improvement among the participants from pre- to post-intervention, descriptive statistics were used to characterize the participants in this project, and charts were used to visually describe the improvement in cardiovascular health. Not all translational research projects use all three of our tools, but in the previous example they were used very effectively.

Lessons Learned From This Project
Program evaluation plan is an essential step in planning and implementing an evidence-based program to improve cardiovascular health. In this example, the first step was the determination of a tool to measure cardiovascular health. Using an established tool that was developed by the American Heart Association was useful in that the tool had been applied to multiple epidemiological data sets. Pre- and post-program data collected were used to calculate the MLC score. Descriptive statistics, specifically percentage change, were useful to determine the effectiveness of the program. The benefits of the HHP were seen in the older adults who exhibited a 37.1% improvement in their MLC score. A similar benefit was not observed in the women at the residential shelter who experienced a 10.2% decrease in their MLC score. This may be due to a constellation of social, environmental, and mental health factors that are not yet fully understood (Murphy et al., 2015).

The Statistician: The Story of How This Statistician Got to Become a Faculty Member in an Academic Nursing Unit

This section of the chapter ends with the story of how the statistician (L.F.) coauthoring this chapter became a full-time faculty member in nursing. He first started working at the Rush University College of Nursing, because he needed employment. The college needed a part-time statistician to run numbers and help with research, and he needed someone to pay half of his salary.

Through Luther Christman, who was the dean at the college at that point, he was expertly tutored on the intricacies of nursing research. Since nursing research is much more complicated than this, he states his view of three key principles that underlie nursing research. The first principle is that the goal of nursing research is getting the patient better, or making his or her life better. Nursing theory guides research with a holistic paradigm focused on optimizing wellness.

The second principle is that nursing interventions tend to be relatively simple and effective. Thus, they tend to be very cost effective. So, for example, it is simpler to help patients develop positive health behaviors to avoid disease than it is to treat most diseases once they are contracted. One big advantage of this principle is that it should make nursing research more useful to fund.

The third principle is that nursing research embraces both specialization of nursing knowledge and collaboration with researchers from a wide range of non-nursing fields. This is also consistent with Christman's (1965) view of nursing specialization as the path to expansion of knowledge in nursing. The ability of nurses to work with scholars from many different fields is one mechanism for advancing the breadth and depth of nursing knowledge.

This conceptualization of nursing research was what "hooked" this statistician (L.F.) on to the importance of conducting nursing research. This is the way the research was meant to be conducted. Intra-professional PhD–DNP (Doctor of Nursing Practice) research is very important as nursing goes forward in this century. Opportunities to make a difference through clinical inquiry are exciting. Data are plentiful; thus, using rigor in analysis is paramount, which often demands statistical services from a trained statistician. Tips on working with statisticians are described next.

WORKING WITH STATISTICIANS: WHAT NURSE SCHOLARS NEED TO KNOW

Working with statisticians, either as consultants or as collaborating researchers, can be a daunting experience. Statisticians seem to speak their own special language (e.g., *heteroscedasticity)* and very often do not seem to speak the language of nurse scholars very well. These issues can be quite frustrating when collaborating to conduct a research project. So, the purpose of this section is to present some guidelines to help a nurse scholar determine (a) if he or she needs the help of a statistician at all and (b) how to select the right statistician to work with. The good thing about putting a little work into this process at the start is that one can generally return to the same statistician for future projects. The time invested in the initial selection process can be time well spent.

Why write about this? There is actually quite a bit of literature on the role of statistical consultants in a number of social contexts (e.g., Bancroft, 1971; Boen & Zahn, 1982; Kimball, 1957; Kirk, 1991; Zabell, 2013); however, the interesting thing about the literature is that all of it was written by statisticians and directed to other statisticians. Although there is no problem with statisticians honing their communication skills, they do not have as difficult a task in selling themselves as consultants as the substantive scholar (e.g., doctorally prepared nurse) has in figuring out which statistician will be helpful. So with all due respect to my statistical colleagues and to their efforts to become a little more user friendly, it is dubious that becoming a user-friendly statistician is anywhere near as scary as being the user that the statistician is trying to befriend. And this, in a nutshell, is the purpose of this section—to introduce the innocent user to some of the perils and joys of working with a statistical expert.

When Is a Statistician Needed?

There are a couple of times when a statistician may not be needed. When primarily collecting narrative or qualitative data, a statistician either may not be needed at all or may only be needed for a very brief meeting or phone call. Generally, the statistics in narrative studies are fairly straightforward. The exceptions are mixed methods and narrative analyses where a scholar wants to examine inter-rater agreement. Many narrative analyses can be conducted without the benefit of a statistician.

The second type of study that may not require the aid of a statistician is one where the nurse scholar can conduct his or her own analyses. Amos Tversky is an example of a scholar who conducted his studies without a statistician. Tversky was a widely respected scholar whose papers were usually made up of two-by-two contingency tables that did not even present probability values with them (Twersky & Kahneman, 1981). He simply presented the frequencies and let the reader draw his or her own conclusions.

Tversky was a very eminent scholar. (For the rest of us, who are a bit less eminent, editors often want to see those probability statements. For us, it is often possible to conduct our own analysis.) There are often three ways to figure out how to conduct one's own analyses. The first is to find other published articles that are doing pretty much what you are doing, and seeing what statistical tests those authors use. Very often, nurse scholars already know how to run simple analyses. However, if it turns out that other articles are using complex or sophisticated models, this is a good indication that you might need to speak to a statistical expert.

The second method of learning about statistical modeling is to use the Internet. Although this should not be the sole source of statistical information, Wikipedia, for instance, is an excellent source of information on explaining simple statistical models in terms that may be understandable before delving deeper. Readers need to be aware that Wikipedia may not have correct information on complex or sophisticated models. But the Internet is a good place to start to learn about statistical modeling.

The third and final method of learning about statistical modeling is using a statistics textbook. Many statistical textbooks have been published over the years, but a recommended one for the non-statistician is written by Schmuller (2013) and is titled *Statistical Analysis With Excel for Dummies*. This little book has several virtues. For one, it is relatively inexpensive. For another, the author is an excellent writer and statistician. The book has simple examples of how to conduct simple statistical analyses using Excel. Because Excel is a commonly available computer program, it is a practical software application for many nurse scholars to use for data entry. The book also presents discussions of the many concepts that are central to statistical modeling (e.g., the normal distribution).

So, now that we discussed when we don't need a statistician, when do we actually need a statistician? Often, the first time one may speak to a statistician is when data are collected, but one cannot figure out how to analyze them in order to make some sense of the data. This was actually this author's (L.F.) journey to becoming a statistician (Box 10.2)

Another example when scholars often use a statistician is when writing or revising an article. Very often, editors or reviewers will recommend that you use a specific type of analysis, which may not be familiar, or specifically advise consultation with a statistician. In either case, it can be very helpful to speak with a statistician about these issues. Now, very often, statistical students can be helpful in collaborating on articles. Depending on the complexity of the study and data collected, it may be best to speak with a statistician who has a degree in statistics (either a master's or a doctorate).

Consulting with a statistician is needed when applying for a research grant, especially a federally funded grant. Many funding agencies want to see a statistician on these grants. In addition, it is usually best to get a statistician who has a

---

BOX 10.2   This Statistician's Story of His Journey to His PhD in Statistics
When I was working on a master's degree, I became interested in assaults that occurred in prisons. I was able to collect a substantial amount of data on assaults by extracting information from the incident reports that one prison produced to describe these assaults. The database included location, severity, time, and actors involved with each assault. Unfortunately, after collecting these data, I did not know how to analyze them.   I ended up visiting a senior statistician. He took a look at my data and said, "You know, if you want to keep analyzing data like this, you should probably get a doctorate in statistics." And I did exactly that. So, when you do not know what to do with your data, ask a statistician. It can help.

doctorate, a history of working on federal grants, and a history of publishing research in the substantive area with which the grant is concerned. In general, grant writing is the area where it is the most imperative to develop a relationship with a senior statistician.

What to Look for When Choosing a Statistician

There are two key elements to look for when seeking a statistician—competence and understandability. A competent statistician is needed to conduct the required analyses. Understandability is needed with the statistician so that he or she conducts an analysis that actually answers the question that you want answered. The tricky bit is finding these two qualities in the same individual. This is not always an easy task.

Let us consider whether there is a licensure of the certification process for ensuring competence. Well, at present there is not. The American Statistical Association (ASA) has, on occasion, put forth the idea of licensing statisticians, but it has never come to pass. Part of the problem is that statistics has become an increasingly complex field of study. The advent of the microcomputer and the Internet has caused an enormous proliferation of different statistical models that are used to assess everything from physical activity levels related to electronic monitors to the genetic diversity of the human microbiome.

So, if there are no licenses or certificates, how does one know how competent a statistician is? The first piece of information to look at is the statistician's curriculum vitae (CV) or résumé. In this document, there are three things that you can look at: education, publications, and grants. Of these, education is probably the most important. Statisticians coming out of top flight programs are probably going to be a little more skilled than those coming out of lower ranked programs. This is not a foolproof criterion, so you should look at the whole scholar before hitching your fortunes to someone.

The other excellent way to find a competent statistician is through referrals from colleagues. This method is a bit more dicey than looking at a résumé or CV. The problem with referrals is similar to finding a clinical expert. Are patients good judges of good clinicians? Not always. The problem is similar with statisticians. A colleague can think that a statistician is wonderful, but only because he or she does not understand the clinician's flaws. But referrals are quite useful nonetheless. They are good for assessing competence, but they are even better for assessing understandability.

To elaborate on understandability, it is ideal to always work with statisticians who communicate clearly. This is vitally important for answering the most important questions. Generally, you should consider statistical hypotheses as the blueprints for any analysis. But it is no trivial matter to ensure that the statistical hypotheses that are tested are the ones that will answer the most important questions.

Improved understandability is one reason for trying to maintain a stable relationship with the same statistician over time. In general, the statistician will learn more about your research over time, and will, as a result, be better able to address the questions of interest. Again, the areas of inquiry that use statistical modeling have proliferated to such an extent that just being able to keep current of these fields can be quite time consuming. So, the ideal statistician is one with whom one maintains a long-term collaboration.

The other issue with understandability is that many statisticians go into mathematical modeling, because they may be more comfortable with numbers than they are with prose. One suggestion is that it is often helpful to try to communicate with the statistician both verbally and in writing. Very often, they do better in one medium than the other.

Part of the problem is the way that statisticians are trained. One paradigm for training statisticians is using the "urns full of colored marbles" analogy. Learning statistics with examples involving pulling samples of marbles from an urn in order to infer the nature of the population of marbles that are found in that urn could be problematic when humans rather than marbles are being studied in health research. Sometimes, it may take a while to get over marble training and to adapt to the study of human beings.

When Do You Need to Call a Statistician?

In general, you should call in the statistician as early as possible. Statistical data analysis is much easier to conduct when you know what data you will need, and the format that makes it easy to analyze. The problem here is that you can start out working on a project thinking that you will not need a statistician, and then discover later on that you do need one. One of the big advantages of developing a long-term relationship with a statistician is that often you can just call him or her, explain what you are doing, and have the statistician decide if you would benefit from some early advice. And how available this type of advice is to come by is a function of how easy it is to speak with a statistician.

How Much Should a Statistician's Time Cost?

Statisticians work either as salaried employees of an organization or as independent consultants. Organizations often hire statisticians; in this case, their cost may not be apparent, at least until they are requested to be on a grant. The difficulty that salaried statisticians have is that often colleagues imagine that their time is free, and thus can make use of it any way they like. This is actually not the case: Statisticians are not free. And when organizations do not limit access to them, they can develop overwhelming workloads that make their professional lives unpleasant.

The misuse of the statistician's time is pretty common. This author (L.F.), while still a graduate student, took a job doing statistical analyses in a medical research lab.

The director of the lab found out that L.F. actually enjoyed performing statistical analyses, and he started sending him requests for statistical analyses, all of which were handwritten on sheets of yellow legal paper. The faster L.F. performed the analyses, the more yellow-sheeted requests he received, until, finally, he had an inbox on his desk with several inches of these requests piled up there, very few of which were ever to be conducted.

Statistical analysis and modeling is a resource that you do not want to abuse. This is the other reason why we like to recommend that nurse scholars at least consider conducting their own analyses where possible. It makes for a more efficient use of the statistician's time when you really do need it.

But for the sake of clarity, the ASA (2014) reports salaries for academic statisticians. For the 2013 to 2014 survey, the salary for an assistant professor was around $83,000 for a 9-month contract and about $110,000 for a 12-month contract. These salaries rise to $92,000 and $127,000 for an associate professor and $110,000 and $147,000 for a full professor. This translates to a base salary of about $55 per hour for an academic salaried statistician.

If seeking a statistical consultant, the fees vary widely. Almost all ethical statisticians should provide a cost estimate up front. And although fees vary widely, in general, you should expect to pay at least $100 per hour for a PhD statistician, with fees ranging upward from there. Highly sought after consultants can charge as much as $500 per hour for their time, with many charging more. In general, a master's-level statistician will charge at least $75 per hour and statistical consultants without advanced degrees start out at about $50 per hour. If money is an issue, most statistical consultants will use a sliding scale for researchers with limited resources, and many will perform pro bono work if the research represents a societal good. Most either help students pro bono or for very small amounts of money, and many work for charitable and nonprofit organizations for reduced fees.

How Much Expertise Is Needed From the Statistician?

As discussed earlier, there are three levels of a statistician: PhD statisticians, master's statisticians, and statisticians without an advanced degree in statistics. The relative costs of each are quite different, and so it probably behooves one to use just as much expertise as is needed and not pay for more expert assistance than needed.

PhD statisticians have years of training and can work either in academia or in industry. Ideally, they have a deep understanding of a few areas of statistics and an ability to work in a much broader variety of areas of statistics. One good example of an area where a PhD statistician can prove useful is in the analysis of social networks. Social network analysis (SNA) involves analysis of how interconnected social networks are, as well as how engaged in the network each person is. Generally, if the nurse scholar is interested in examining the impact of social networks on a person's health, a PhD statistician would be needed to figure out how to conduct these sorts of analyses. The other area where a PhD statistician is needed is in the arena of submitting grants, and sometimes in the submitting of papers.

Master's statisticians are not quite as well trained as PhD statisticians, but they are very skilled. The past 20 years have seen a proliferation of programs designed to provide students with master's-level training in statistics. These statisticians generally receive advanced training in terminal master's programs and then receive additional on-the-job training at the workplace. Often, they will be hired for a *stable of statisticians* sort of structure, where the stable of master's-level statisticians is overseen by one or two PhD statisticians. In such contexts, the master's-level statisticians can generally do one or two things very well (e.g., analyze randomized controlled trial [RCT] data), and have a reasonable knowledge of other areas of statistics. Master's-level statisticians can help write papers, although it may be a bit of a stretch to have them help write a grant, unless they have extensive experience doing so.

Statisticians without advanced degrees are, ideally, gifted analysts who can possess a somewhat unpredictable set of skills. Part of the unpredictability is that their training may not be curriculum based; as a result, they may not be intended to produce a specific type of statistical expertise. So the individual learns a lot of the material by the seat of his or her pants, so to speak. Ideally, these statisticians have a firm grasp of relatively simple, parametric models such as regression analysis or the analysis of variance, which can prove very useful for implementing evidence-based practice. Occasionally, a statistician without an advanced degree will have a publication history, and can be a material help in publishing papers. Thus, look at the type of analyses conducted in their published scientific papers for more insight into their analytical expertise. It is also important to remember that these levels of expertise are meant as guidelines, rather than as strict rules. An example of how misleading the degree a person possesses can misinform the reader is based on the 1964 Surgeon General's report (U.S. Public Health Service [PHS], 1964) on the health effects of smoking. The statistician on this report had only a master's degree, but the discussion of how one uses statistical analysis to draw causal inferences is absolutely brilliant and instrumental in changing the way that U.S. health care professionals look at smoking.

This 1964 report was lucidly written, because the master's-level statistician on the report was William G. Cochran, who, as it turns out, is one of the foremost experts on statistical modeling and causality. Cochran had a distinguished career, and the 1964 report was just at the start of it, before he had received his doctorate. And this is the moral of this story: The skills of the scholar are more important than the degree. It is true today, and it has always been true.

How Should a Statistician Be Accessed?

How do you actually get access to a statistician in an academic or other research setting? There are several models for getting a statistician to work with you; each model has its own strengths and weaknesses. The most effective method is to have a statistician on faculty or staff who is dedicated to working with members of the faculty. This is especially important in nursing, because nursing research tends to be a little difficult for many statisticians to understand.

The second method of providing statistical expertise is to use a stable of statisticians. Sometimes, this particular method of delivering statistical services is referred to as the *Center for Statistical Excellence*. One advantage of the Center for Statistical Excellence is that it avoids having to find a new statistician: If the one designated to your project cannot continue working on the project for a sundry of reasons (e.g. illness, other priorities), other statisticians are available to take his or her place. Another advantage is that it could be less expensive, because you can have a head statistician who has a PhD, and other master's-level statisticians who work in collaboration with the head to make sure their work is of high enough quality. But there can be problems as well.

One problem with the Center for Statistical Excellence is that the statistician who helps you is often a bit of a hired gun, who does the work for one project and then moves on after being hired by the next scholar. Sometimes, this arrangement can mean that the statistician who works with the scholar does not really have much understanding of the phenomenon that is being studied. One can view statistics as a technical skill, and the models that the statistician uses as being interchangeable from one research context to another, but there are clear limits to this mode of thinking. The nurse scholar does not get the opportunity to build a relationship with a statistician who understands the conceptual underpinnings of the program of research. So, from the next project onward, it is back to square one explaining the conceptual theoretical underpinnings of nursing research. It can be exhausting and not very efficient.

The third structure for providing statistical resources is to set up a list of recommended statisticians who have been used by the school or facility and are known and trusted. This approach is especially useful in organizations where there are insufficient resources to hire a full-time or part-time statistician, but the need for statistical services still exists. The biggest advantage of this method of obtaining statistical resources is that if you do not especially like the interactions you had with the statistician, you do not have to use him or her again. Furthermore, if the consulting work amounts to a substantial amount of money over a year, then the statistician may be motivated to try to keep the various nurse researchers happy in order to facilitate future work. The downside to the recommended statistician choice is that most statisticians who work as consultants charge more, on an hourly basis, than one would have to pay in salary. So, for instance, if the PhD statistician would earn $60 per hour for his or her labor, as a consultant, he or she will generally charge two or three times more for hourly compensation. If you are using the statistician an awful lot, this can get very expensive. But if this occurs, you may be able to offer the statistician a job, and transition him or her into dedicated statisticians.

The last method of obtaining statistical help is the "I'm afraid you're on your own, professor" approach. I do not know how many nursing programs use this approach, but it does not have much to recommend it, especially since the recommended statisticians approach discussed earlier is so much more useful. If you are working in this sort of an environment, I would recommend giving a copy of this chapter to your resource allocation decision maker. The amount of effort required to get a list of recommended statisticians (survey nurse researchers whom they have worked with successfully, obtain the CVs or résumés of the statisticians) seems so little compared to the substantial costs that can be associated with working with a difficult statistician that it seems logical to put this decision into the "no-brainer" category. Now that this opinion has been put into print, there is no doubt that it will be contradicted, but that is the nature of scholarship.

CONCLUSION WITH WORDS OF WISDOM FROM THE STATISTICIAN HIMSELF

This chapter closes with some final words on selecting a statistician from our statistician author himself (L.F.). The earlier discussion is concerned with the basic toolbox for statistics and choosing the best possible colleague to work with on nurse scholarship. I will throw one more quality that I look for in all colleagues, be they statisticians or short-order cooks. Friedrich Nietzsche famously said, "I would only believe in a god who could dance" (Nietzsche & Ludovici, 1911). I am less demanding of my colleagues than Nietzsche is of his gods, but I do like to work with colleagues who can laugh. This enterprise of finding new meaning is supposed to be fun. I realize that it has serious, real-world implications for the health of our patients, and that all of that is very important, but the simple act of discovering how the world, this giant puzzle we are able to inhabit, works is pure fun.

And so I close this chapter with Plato's parable of how we learn about the world as it is. When your soul was first created, the gods took you up on Mount Olympus and showed you the world as it really is. And then you drank from the river of forgetfulness (Halliwell, 2007). And to Plato, the discovery of new knowledge as we progress through our lives is actually just the jogging of your soul's memory to remember what the god showed you, way back when. So I close this particular chapter with the wish that you may enjoy the rediscovery of all of the truth that we already know and the hope that a statistician can help you with that rediscovery.

REFERENCES

Altman, D. G., & Bland, J. M. (1983). Measurement in medicine: The analysis of method comparison studies. *Statistician, 32*, 307–317.

American Heart Association Life Simple 7. Retrieved from http://www.heart.org/HEARTORG/Conditions/My-Life-Check—Lifes-Simple-7_UCM_471453_Article.jsp

American Statistical Association. (2014). Academic salary survey. *Amstat News*. Retrieved from http://magazine.amstat.org/blog/2014/01/01/academic-salary-survey-2

Bancroft, T. A. (1971). On establishing a university-wide statistical consulting and cooperative research service. *The American Statistician, 25*(5), 21–24.

Bland, J. M., & Altman, D. G. (2007). Agreement between methods of measurement with multiple observations per individual. *Journal of Biopharmaceutic Statistics, 17*(4), 571–582.

Boen, J. R., & Zahn, D. A. (1982). *The human side of statistical consulting*. Belmont, CA: Lifetime Learning Publications.

Centers for Disease Control and Prevention. (2013). *The state of aging and health in America 2013*. Atlanta, GA: Centers for Disease Control and Prevention, U.S. Department of Health and Human Services. Retrieved from http://www.cdc.gov/aging.

Christman, L. (1965). The influence of specialization on the nursing profession. *Nursing Science, 3*(6), 446–453.

Cohen, J. (1988). *Statistical power analysis for the behavioral sciences*. Hillsdale NJ: Lawrence Erlbaum Associates.

DeLean, A., Munson, P. J., & Rodbard, D. (1978). Simultaneous analysis of families of sigmoidal curves: Application to bioassay, radioligand assay, and physiological dose-response curves. *American Journal of Physiology-Gastrointenstinal and Liver Physiology, 235*(2), G97–G102.

Fisher, R. A. (1935/1971). *The design of experiments* (9th ed.). New York, NY: Macimillan Publishers.

Fonkalsrud, E. W., & Clatworthy, H. W. (1965). Accidental perforation of the colon and rectum in newborn infants. *New England Journal of Medicine, 272*, 1097–1100.

Friedrichs, J., Staffileno, B., Fogg, L., Jegier, B., Hunter, R., Portugal, D., & Peashey, J. (2013). Axillary temperatures in newborn infants. *Advances in Neonatal Care, 13*(5), 361–368.

Gilje, F., Lacey, L., & Moore, C. (2007). Gerontology and geriatric issues and trends in U.S. nursing programs: A national survey. *Journal of Professional Nursing, 23*(1), 21–29.

Go, A. S., Mozaffarian, D., Roger, V. L., Benjamin, E. J., Berry, J. D., Borden, W. B., & Bravata, D. M. (2013). American Heart Association Statistics Committee and Stroke Statistics Subcommittee. Heart disease and stroke statistics–2013 update: A report from the American Heart Association. *Circulation, 127*(1), e6–e245.

Halliwell, F. S. (2007). The life-and-death journey of the soul: Interpreting the myth of Er. In G. Ferrari (Ed.), *The Cambridge companion to Plato's Republic* (pp. 445–473). Cambridge, UK: Cambridge University Press.

Katz, S., Down, T. D., Cash, H. R., & Grotz, R. C. (1970). Progress in development of the index of ADL. *Gerontologist, 10*, 20–30.

Kimball, A. W. (1957). Errors of the third kind in statistical consulting. *Journal of the American Statistical Association, 52*(278), 133–142.

Kirk, R. E. (1991). Statistical consulting in a university: Dealing with people and other challenges. *The American Statistician, 45*(1), 28–34.

Krill, C., Staffileno, B. A., & Raven, C. (2012). Empowering staff nurses to use research to change practice for safe patient handling. *Nursing Outlook, 60*(3), 157–162. doi:10.1016/j.outlook.2011.06.005

Lee, S., Staffileno, B. A., & Fogg, L. (2013). Influence of staff education on the function of hospitalized elders. *Nursing Outlook, 61*(1), E2–E8.

Meehl, P. E. (1978). Theoretical risks and tabular asterisks: Sir Karl, Sir Ronald, and the slow progress of soft psychology. *Journal of Consulting and Clinical Psychology, 46*(4), 806.

Murphy, M. P., Coke, L., Staffileno, B. A., Robinson, J. D., & Tillotson, R. (2015). Improving cardiovascular health of underserved populations in the community with life simple 7. *Journal of the American Association of Nurse Practitioners, 27*(11), 614–623.

National Alliance to End Homelessness. (2013). *Mental and physical health.* Retrieved from http://www.endhomelessness.org/pages/mental_physical_health

Neyman, J., & Pearson, E. S. (1992). *On the problem of the most efficient tests of statistical hypotheses.* New York, NY: Springer.

Nietzsche, F. W., & Ludovici, A. M. (1911). *Thus spake Zarathustra: A book for all and none* (Vol. 11). Foulis. Germany: Ernst Schmeitzner Publisher.

Palmer, I. S. (1977). Florence Nightingale: Reformer, reactionary, researcher. *Nursing Research, 26*(2), 98–89.

Schmuller, J. (2013). *Statistical analysis with excel for dummies.* Hoboken, NJ: John Wiley & Sons.

Silverstein, B., & Howard, N. (2006). *Lifting patients/residents/clients in health care.* Washington State 2005 (Report to the Washington State Legislative House Commerce and Labor Committee). Washington State: Department of Labor and Industries.

Snedecor, G. W., & Cochrane, W. G. (1989). *Statistical methods* (8th ed.). Ames, IA: Iowa State University Press.

Stranges, E., & Friedman, B. (2009). *Trends in potentially preventable hospitalization rates declined for older adults, 2003–2007.* HCUP Statistical Brief #83. December 2009. Rockville, MD: Agency for Healthcare Research and Quality. Retrieved from http://www.hcup-us.ahrq.gov/reports/statbriefs/sb83.pdf

Swedish Medical Center. (2007). Safe patient handling risk assessment tool. Retrieved from http://www.washingtonsafepatienthandling.org/images/Swedish_Hospital_Risk_Assessment_Tool.pdf

Tukey, J. W. (1977). *EDA: Exploratory data analysis.* Reading, MA: Addison-Wesley.

Tversky, A., & Kahneman, D. (1981). The framing of decisions and the psychology of choice. *Science, 211*(4481), 453–458.

U.S. Public Health Service. (1964). *Smoking and health*. Report of the Advisory Committee to the Surgeon General. DHEW publication (PHS).

World Health Organization. (1997). *Thermal protection of the newborn: A practical guide*. Geneva, Switzerland: Author.

Zabell, S. (2013). Paul Meier on legal consulting. *The American Statistician*, 67(1), 18–21.

CHAPTER ELEVEN

LOGIC MODELS

SHIRLEE M. DRAYTON-BROOKS, PAULA GRAY, AND MARIA ELAYNE DESIMONE

OBJECTIVES

After reading this chapter, readers will be able to:

1. Define and describe logic models
2. Discuss how logic models can be used as an important tool to enhance health program planning, implementation, evaluation, and dissemination activities
3. Explain the steps in building a logic model
4. Create a logic model

Logic models are important tools that nurse scholars can use to design, implement, and evaluate new programs and projects. A *logic model* is a common term for a one-page graphic depiction that serves as a road map of the proposed program or project. The overall objective of this chapter is to provide nurse scholars with a thorough understanding of what logic models are and how to create them. Examples of logic models are shown in this chapter to demonstrate to the reader that there is no one format and that scholars must tailor their logic models carefully to what they want to communicate. Successful programs of nursing scholarship will benefit from using logic models as tools in translating knowledge from nursing science and practice into feasible, fundable programs and projects that aim at improving health and health care systems. Logic models are an important tool to enhance program planning, implementation, and dissemination activities.

LOGIC MODEL DEFINED

The Centers for Disease Control and Prevention (CDC, 2010) defines a logic model as a visual "snapshot" of a program (or project) that communicates the intended relationship between program goals, activities, outputs, and intended outcomes (Figure 11.1). Logic models communicate underlying concepts and assumptions, the situation, condition, or problem. Useful for project or program planning and evaluation purposes, logic models graphically describe the theory, or logic, and

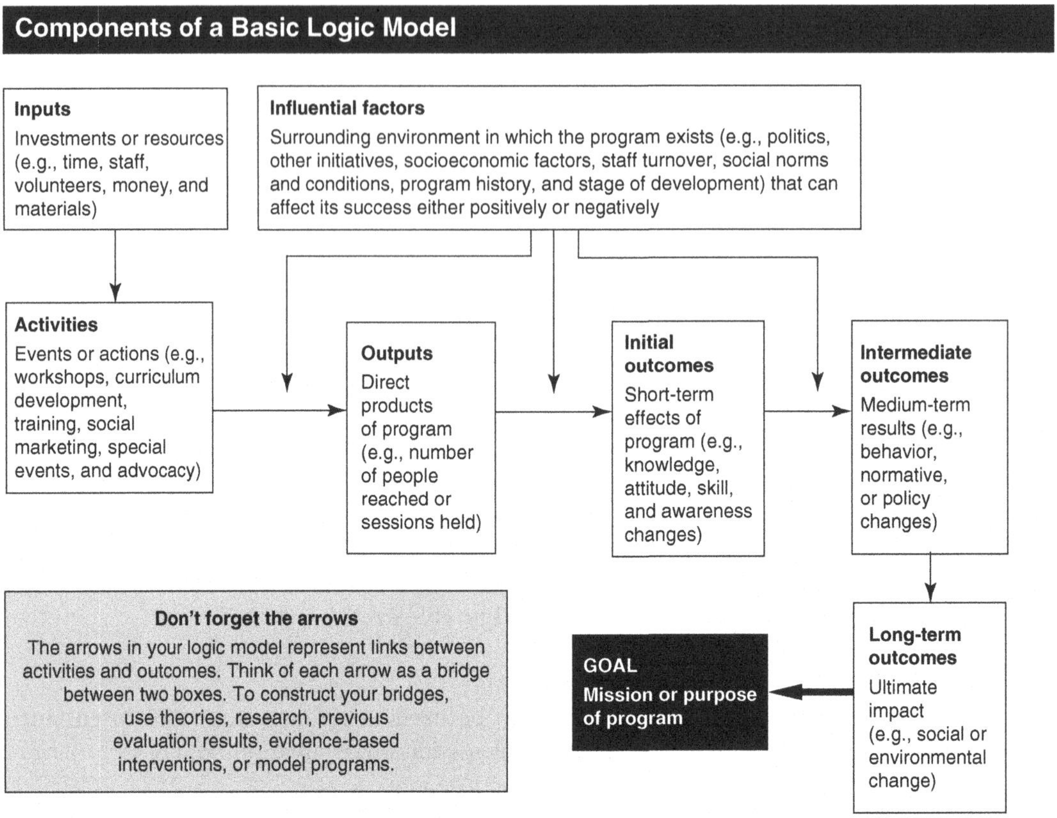

Components of a Basic Logic Model

Inputs
Investments or resources (e.g., time, staff, volunteers, money, and materials)

Influential factors
Surrounding environment in which the program exists (e.g., politics, other initiatives, socioeconomic factors, staff turnover, social norms and conditions, program history, and stage of development) that can affect its success either positively or negatively

Activities
Events or actions (e.g., workshops, curriculum development, training, social marketing, special events, and advocacy)

Outputs
Direct products of program (e.g., number of people reached or sessions held)

Initial outcomes
Short-term effects of program (e.g., knowledge, attitude, skill, and awareness changes)

Intermediate outcomes
Medium-term results (e.g., behavior, normative, or policy changes)

Don't forget the arrows
The arrows in your logic model represent links between activities and outcomes. Think of each arrow as a bridge between two boxes. To construct your bridges, use theories, research, previous evaluation results, evidence-based interventions, or model programs.

GOAL
Mission or purpose of program

Long-term outcomes
Ultimate impact (e.g., social or environmental change)

Figure 11.1 Components of a basic logic model.
From the Centers for Disease Control and Prevention (2010). Reprinted with permission.

activities depicting how a program is intended to work. It provides a picture of the program or a desired change. Logic models provide a systematic approach to understand program development, program change, and program evaluation. Logic models comprise "logical linkages" that describe how desired results are being achieved. Further, logic models provide a plausible, consistent picture of planning processes, efforts, necessary resources, and the steps used to enable a project or program to achieve desired outcomes. Often used as a tool for programs that are designed to solve difficult problems, logic models serve as a vehicle to illustrate efficiency and effectiveness of programmatic activities and performance measures (U.S. Bureau of Health Professions, 2011).

Logic is basically reasoning based on sound judgment. A model is a depiction of patterns, a representation of actions, or images that reflect how concepts or components fit together. A logic model defines patterns and relations in a simple or complex graphic of planning, implementation, coordination, and evaluation. Resources needed such as equipment, activities of personnel, and necessary faculties to accomplish a task are often depicted. Logic models can provide a logical framework to examine results; particularly if the resources are available, structures are in place, and the best research evidence is applied, then the desired outcomes should be achieved. According to the CDC (2010), a basic logic model presents inputs connected to activities, outputs, initial outcomes, intermediate outcomes, and long-term outcomes. These elements are linked to influential factors from the environment and to the mission and purpose for a program (Figure 11.1).

THE IMPORTANCE OF LOGIC MODELS

Logic models are widely used in health care to guide practice improvement initiatives and to evaluate outcomes. The demand for quality and accountability in the delivery of health care to the public has been highlighted in significant Institute of Medicine (IOM) reports (IOM, 1999, 2001, 2005, 2010, 2011). To improve health care quality, very intentional, well-planned logical approaches to problem solving, decision making, and practice improvement are necessary. Consumers demand that health care reflects the six IOM aims; the expectation is that health care is safe, effective, patient centered, timely, efficient, and equitable (IOM, 2001). Furthermore, consumers only want to fund programs that are meaningful, cost effective, efficient, and of the highest quality. The public demands accountability for quality and results. The expectation is that programs for health care quality improvement and outcomes are based on the best evidence. It is also expected that accountability is assured by logical planning processes and evaluation with valid and reliable performance measures. Nurse scholars across practice settings (e.g., administration, education, and clinical practice) collaborating together must have knowledge and skills necessary to design, implement, and evaluate system change. Logic models provide a tool to support effective health care system enhancement.

Population health care needs in the United States and globally have changed drastically, due to growing demographic diversity and an increasing number of older adults living longer while experiencing multiple chronic conditions. Technological advances have led to increasing health care complexity, whereas health disparities and significant social determinants continue to persist even in the context of evidence-based practice (CDC, 2013). Since the landmark 1999 IOM report on medical errors, great emphasis has been placed on practice improvement in care delivery. According to that IOM (1999) report *To Err Is Human: Building a Safer Health Care System*, between 44,000 and 98,000 Americans die each year due to medical errors. The national cost of preventable adverse events was estimated to be approximately $37.6 billion each year; about $17 billion of those costs are associated with preventable errors, and about half of the expenditures for preventable medical errors are for direct health care costs. Since 2001, there has been an increased emphasis on safety and quality in health care with particular attention to medication and surgical site errors.

The National Association of Healthcare Quality (2012, p. 1) called for "leaders to implement protective structures to assure accountability for integrity in quality and safety evaluation and comprehensive, transparent, accurate data collection, and reporting to internal and external oversight bodies." In 2013, the World Health Organization (WHO) identified patient safety and quality as a global public health concern, noting that in developed countries 10 patients may have been harmed; whereas in the hospital, 14 out of every 100 patients admitted to a hospital acquired an infection (WHO, 2014). The WHO also noted that 20% to 40% of all health spending is wasted due to poor-quality care (2014). Logic models are being widely used in health care to inform evidence-based practice and quality improvement research (Carroll & McKenna, 2001). Governmental agencies and private agencies use logic models to guide research, performance measurement, and strategic planning as they can be useful conceptual maps to describe theory, causal chains, and intended relationships among interventions and results. The ability to use logic models to clearly communicate the design, implementation, and intended evaluation outcomes of evidence-based practice and research in a plausible manner is an important skill for practice improvement experts and researchers.

REASONS FOR USING LOGIC MODELS

Although there are many reasons to support using logic models, three compelling reasons are given so nurses are better equipped to create logic models in their scholarly work. These reasons are to (a) lobby for curricular changes to include the skill of developing logic models in nursing education, especially for Doctor of Nursing Practice (DNP) students who are expected to lead change for health care improvements; (b) provide workshops for nursing practice leaders so they have these requisite skills in writing competitive program proposals; and (c) request an expert review of their logic model that provides a critical picture that must be focused, thorough, and concise in communicating what is being proposed.

Logic Models Serve as Focused, Concise, and Thorough Road Maps

Imagine planning to take a trip. A travel plan would need to be developed. Travel resources such as a suitcase with appropriate clothing and toiletries would be obtained. A road map might be purchased, and the destination would be studied to maximize the experience. Using this road map analogy, a logic model serves as a graphic depiction of how to get to the desired destination. As a picture with all the component parts, it can be shown during dissemination activities to guide and communicate change.

Nurses contemplating changing practice must use an organized, systematic approach that can be communicated to others in a concise, focused, and thorough manner. Creating a logic model provides such a tool. Nurse scholars must be able to think through the process, organize approaches, and put "pen to paper" to concisely create a diagram that clearly describes the *what*, *why*, and *how* about proposed programs or projects in ways to create a visual that supports successful proposals. External funders of health programs often require submission of a logic model in program proposal grant applications.

METHODS OF CREATING LOGIC MODELS

Nursing Practice Problems

There are several steps that should be considered when building a logic model. Each must be carefully considered to develop an evidence-based, plausible, and useful logic model. The first step is to perform a thorough assessment of the problem and examine the need for change or improvement. One should identify the cause of the problem, perhaps in collaboration with the interprofessional team. A root cause analysis using a fishbone diagram (Zastrow, 2015), a human factor analysis, or an organizational analysis may be used to assess the problem in context. Consider also interviews and focus groups with stakeholders, both internal and external, to the organization and, perhaps, from the public to understand these important perspectives. To further understand the problem, questionnaires and surveys to gather data may be used as appropriate. Once you have assessed the problem, appraise the research evidence related to the problem or the desired practice change. Examine what others are doing as well as the best evidence-based practice related to the problem, condition, or situation. This effort is completed through a thorough evaluation and synthesis of the available research to effectively guide change.

Develop a PICOT Question

To initiate a health care practice change, a "PICOT" question should be developed that reflects the population (P) of concern, intervention (I) or issue of concern, comparison (C) of the intervention or the problem issue, outcome (O), and the time frame (T) (Melnyk & Fineout-Overholt, 2015). The level of the available evidence about the problem should be evaluated. Levels of evidence can range from the highest level (e.g., meta-analysis of randomized controlled trials [RCTs]) to evidence from a panel of experts. The validity of the research studies examined must be appraised from content to construct, including the examination of significance and the sample size and power (Craig & Smyth, 2012). One should determine whether a program or project is replicable.

As you work on creating your logic model, be explicit about the assumptions of your model as well as about the existing or anticipated structure, processes, and outcomes. Do not rely on simply one model; rather, test out different combinations of relationships, shapes, and directions of logic.

When you determine the purpose, goals, objectives and sub-objectives, time frames, and the change, be aware that the project, practice improvement project, or program should be consistent with the institutional values and mission. Determine who will comprise the stakeholder group and include them in the processes. Often, sustained change may require interprofessional collaboration and multiple networks of communication and support. Linkages to specific activities, needed resources, outcome indicators, and/or performance measures, both summative and formative evaluations, must be clearly articulated. Performance measures should be designed to be useful to monitor a project or program and to manage results. Link each input or action to specific outputs, outcomes, or efficiency measures such as cost in dollars, improved health outcomes, or more efficient use of resources. Delineate productivity in time and product quality.

Determining Simple Versus Complex, Nonlinear Logic Models

Determine whether the logic model should be simple, complex, linear, or nonlinear. Clearly demonstrate multiple linkages or just simple cause–effect relationships. If the problem is difficult to solve with no clear solutions, one can expect that the model will be very complex. Remember, innovation is needed with wicked problems since problems will surface that may not be foreseen (Rittel & Webber, 1973). If the logic model needs to be complex with multiple components that demonstrate nonlinear linkages, or cyclical to reflect dynamic connections, it may be best to communicate nonlinearity.

A logic model can be built from left to right, bottom to top, stepwise, linear, or cyclical. The use of shapes, squares, columns, cylinders, spheres, or funnels must be decided. Logic models may be in a flow chart format, vertical, horizontal, or in a table format with clear linkages. Use arrows, directional or multidirectional, to delineate the flow of energy and expected change. Show structures, core processes, and outputs or outcomes to include the use of arrows; otherwise, a logic table and not a dynamic logic model may be illustrated. Several software programs are available to help design logic models. The use of software such as DoVIEW, Microsoft VISIO, and Inspiration can make formatting and creating logic models easier.

Outcome Measures

Provide clear and appropriate outcome measures collected during a defined period. Stakeholders can be used to judge the extent to which each component or branch of the logic model is valid and if the best performance indicators are being examined. After a logic model is designed, it is crucial to have stakeholders or external examiners evaluate the depiction for face validity of the outcomes as well as to verify whether the model is meaningful, the results are achieved, the resources are sufficient, and, finally, intended populations or products are reflected in the results.

PRESENTATION OF THEORY-DRIVEN LOGIC MODELS

Planning for practice improvements should be theory driven. Whether explicit or implicit, the nurse scholar's world view influences the theories they choose. The chosen theory should guide the development of the logic model. In this section, many examples of theory-driven logic models are presented, guided by systems theory, change theory, and Donabedian's (1966) classic health care quality theory. Additionally, logic models guided by complexity science and the field of health program planning and evaluation are presented.

Logic models often have limitations. A logic model can be superficial instead of providing depth and rationale. There is a tendency to depict simple relationships that may be far more complex than illustrated. Logic models present only a snapshot of reality that may not be true or free from contextual influences. The designer of a logic model may believe that the depiction is sound, but the relationships may not be evidence based. The designer may believe patterns reflect sound reasoning and clear connections; however, stakeholders may not agree. Logic models may imply cause and effect that cannot be validated. Finally, logic models may present a stagnant linear depiction of activities, instead of complex, dynamic, and changing concepts and elements.

Logic Models and Systems Theory

Logic models are often guided by Ludwig von Bertalanffy's General Systems Theory (Drack, Apfalter, & Pouvreau, 2007). Systems may be simple with inputs, throughputs, outputs, and feedback; alternatively, systems may be complex, fluid, and adaptive. A logic model may describe inputs; core processes at the individual, group, and organization level; and outputs (Figure 11.2). Systems theory can serve as a guide to support illustration of logical linkages. According to systems theory, the whole is

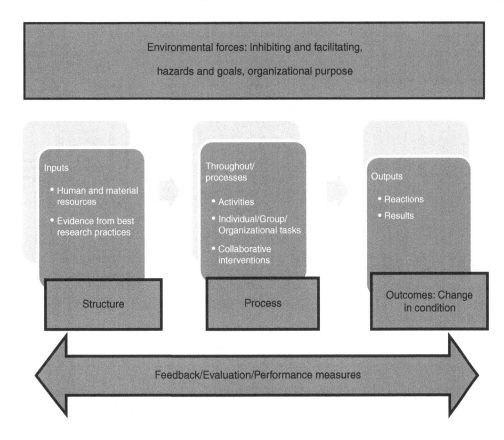

Figure 11.2 Example of a systems-based logic model.

greater than the sum of its parts (Drack et al., 2007). A logic model, therefore, may infer a dynamic system of interrelated parts. Models may be depicted as linear or as complex and nonlinear. Inputs are resources, materials, and energy through work that go into a system. Core processes refer to the work, activities, and tasks that must be performed by individuals, groups, or even an organization. Outputs are results and outcomes of a system that may be in the form of materials and work. Outputs may be illustrated in a logic model to show how a system fulfills its purpose and targeted goals. Outputs may provide feedback that illustrates the alignment of results with the environmental goals, public need, and expected performance measures. A logic model may provide a graphic depiction of individual, group, or organizational-level responsibilities, tasks, and even outcomes. Linkages between macro- and micro-systems may also be illustrated in a logic model.

Logic models describe input, activities, outputs, short-term, intermediate, and long-term outcomes as the CDC model illustrates in Figure 11.1. According to McLaughlin and Jordan (1999), resources include human and financial resources; activities include actions that are necessary to produce program outputs, the products, goods, and services provided to the program customers; and outcomes are characterized as changes or benefits resulting from activities and outputs. Logic models often present a linear approach linked to external influences and related programs (McLaughlin & Jordan, 1999). The model in Figure 11.2 provides a simple

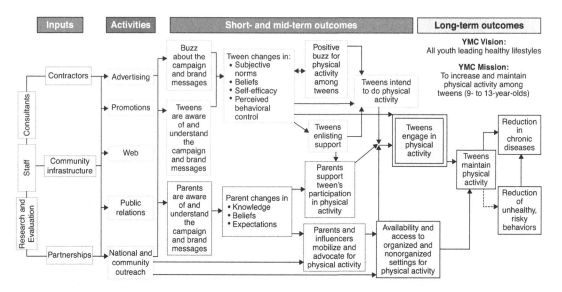

Figure 11.3   Centers for Disease Control: The VERB™ campaign logic model: A tool for planning and evaluation.

YMC, Youth Media Campaign.

From Huhman, Heitzler, and Wong (2004). Reprinted with permission.

logic model. It is clearly linked to a linear systems approach in which short-term outcomes are associated with program outputs and are the antecedents to intermittent outcomes, as well as in which long-term outcomes follow the benefits accrued through intermediate outcomes. McLaughlin and Jordan (1999) describe five stages to building a logic model. In Stage 1, the logic model designer collects relevant data from multiple sources. In Stage 2, the problem, the context, and linkages to the needs of consumers are clearly defined. Stage 3 involves defining the elements, or categories, in the model and its logical flow. In Stage 4, the model is conceptualized and graphically depicted to portray details, which also includes measures of performance. Stage 5 verifies the logic model, including measures of success with stakeholders. The VERB campaign logic model in Figure 11.3 illustrates the components of a program to enhance physical activity.

Logic Models and Change Theory

A logic model may be designed to provide a quick picture of planned change. In Figure 11.4, a sample plan of a change model is presented. Kurt Lewin, a renowned German social scientist, developed a three-prong theory to explain, guide, and evaluate change (Shirey, 2013). Through his research in group dynamics, he studied factors that influence change. Lewin identified three stages needed to effectively plan change (Shirey, 2013). In the first stage, the unfreezing stage, the need for change is thoroughly assessed. The need for change is clear and the inputs from people and key stakeholder groups, resources, and activities needed for change are determined. The forces that inhibit and facilitate change are determined. Lewin believed that facilitating forces must be in place so that there is enough force to overcome inhibiting forces. In the second stage, the movement stage, change is implemented and processes are evaluated and refined. In the third stage, refreezing, successful

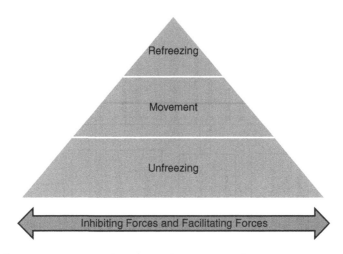

Figure 11.4 Illustration of Lewin's theory of planned change.
Adapted from Shirey (2013).

change is subjected to ongoing evaluation, sustained (refreezed) or changed again (unfreezed) based on the assessment of need and the ongoing evaluation of the outcomes.

Logic models have been referred to as theory of change, or program change, plans. Health care system changes may include short-term and/or intermediate outcomes; a change in attitudes, awareness, skills, or knowledge behavior; a change in people; or even a change in practice. The impact may have long-term outcomes that change public health and social conditions of populations. Figure 11.5 provides a logic model that illustrates a project using The Joint Commission's recommended situation, background, assessment, and recommendation (SBAR) technique to improve nurse-to-nurse communication in falls prevention. The situation, inputs, and outputs in the form of activities and participation, as well as short-term, medium, and long-term outcomes, are depicted.

Logic Models to Enhance and Evaluate Quality: The Donabedian Model Approach

There is increased emphasis on continuous quality improvement in health care as patients experience adverse events due to medical errors. Logic models provide a tool to support logical program planning and evaluation to assure health care quality, safety, and efficiency. Donabedian provided a logic model to evaluate quality medical care. The Donabedian model was first introduced in 1966 in a publication titled *Evaluating the Quality of Medical Care*. The model was designed as a conceptual framework to assure quality of health services program planning, evaluation, and research. The model comprises three concepts that can be used to infer that quality is achieved. According to Donabedian (1966), the measurement of quality in care is not exact and outcomes must be examined while also considering structures and processes. Donabedian understood that health care is complex and cannot be examined in fragmented parts. There are problems, hazards, and contributing factors that must be considered.

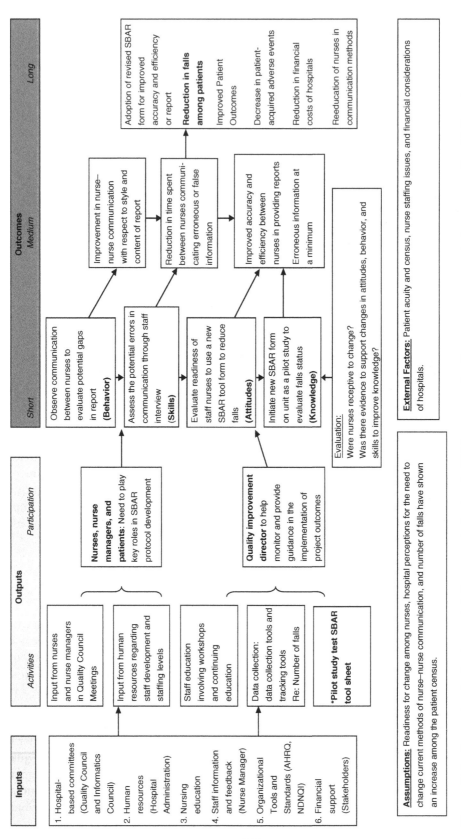

Figure 11.5 Example of a logic model: The use of electronic SBAR communication among nurses to improve patient falls outcomes.

AHRQ, Agency for Healthcare Research and Quality; NDNQI, National Database of Nursing Quality Indicators; SBAR, situation, background, assessment, and recommendation.

Source: Pineda (2015). Reprinted with permission of author.

In the Donabedian model (1966), *structure* refers to resources and administrative support necessary to develop and achieve results. Process includes the method or activities used to execute structure. Outcomes are results, impact, or changes that may be attributed to processes and to structures of health care. Structures provide the foundation, investment, and resources that go into the program development and are essential to carry out a quality program. Health care delivery must build on evidence and best research findings. How do we know we have achieved the desired results? It is through impact analysis performed by evaluation of performance measures and research that provides evidence that we have achieved desired results. Although only a rational graphic depiction, from a practice improvement perspective, logic models present a valid argument to achieve a conclusion that can support quality in health care.

Quality is often measured by outcomes in health care. Quality is a function of the structures (S), the processes (P), and the outcomes (O); all areas are interrelated and must be examined together.

$$Q = f (P, S, 0)$$

Figure 11.6 illustrates a logic model that was used to guide a diabetes telehealth self-management care program. This model was used to show how the activities of the practice change, telehealth visits, would improve diabetic patients' self-management

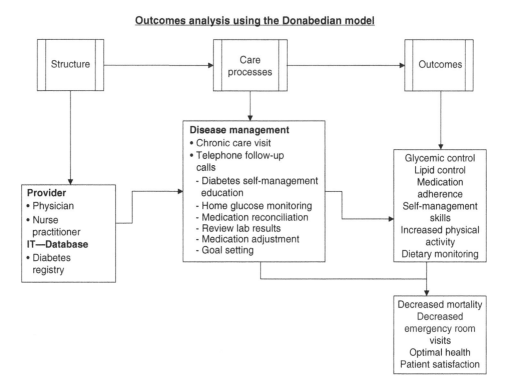

Figure 11.6 Example of a Gray's (2013) logic model of a diabetes telehealth self-management care program.

of their disease and optimize their health outcomes. To achieve this outcome, the following steps were taken:

- *Structure*: Patients with this problem (diabetes) are identified via the diabetic registry (produced by information technology) in primary care practices.
- *Care processes*: The use of telehealth (virtual visits) is enacted to educate and support these diabetic patients.
- *Outcomes:* The primary measured clinical outcome was the glycemic levels of these patients. Other evaluated outcomes included the patient's anecdotal statements regarding improvements in their self-management skills and patient satisfaction with weekly diabetes care-management telephone calls.

Another example of a Donabedian guided logic model is shown in Figure 11.7. This logic model was created to explain an integrated learning outcome assessment model for a DNP academic program. The linkage between the institution mission, values, goals, educational standards, external forces, and the needs of populations served by program graduates is depicted. The structure identifies the important

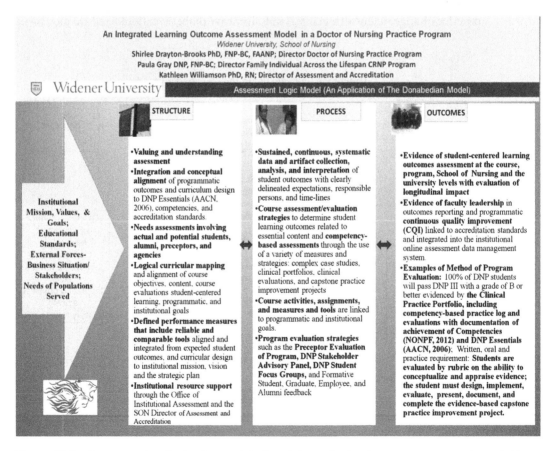

Figure 11.7 An example of a logic model of an integrated outcome assessment model in a Doctor of Nursing Practice program guided by Donabedian.

Source: Drayton-Brooks, Gray, and Williamson (2014). Reprinted with permission of authors.

structure needed for a comprehensive student-centered learning outcomes approach. This includes a culture that values assessment and logical curricular mapping, valid and reliable measurement tools, and instructional resources. The process explicates the comprehensiveness of data collection. The outcomes identify the evidence that student-centered learning outcomes, program outcomes, and course outcomes have been achieved. The emphasis on continuous quality improvement and linkages to expected program outcomes, competencies, and standards is highlighted.

Problem-Solving and Logic Models: Simple, Complex, and Wicked Problems

Logic models are useful when trying to understand and solve complex, untamed, and wicked problems. One approach to problem solving is to apply root cause analysis (Zastrow, 2015) to a problem and develop a specific type of logic model called a fishbone diagram (Catchpole, 2013), which is illustrated in Figure 11.8. The head of the diagram (see the far right side of the diagram) depicts the effect or the problem, whereas the branches represent the causes of the problem and why the problem exists. As causes are assessed, the "why" question is asked to build the subdivisions, interconnections, and links to branches. To understand the problem, a root cause, the effect or problem, is established at the head of the diagram that will look similar to a fish. Each causal factor represents the branches or bones of the fish. In Figure 11.8, the fishbone diagram illustrates multiple causes of health disparities. The first major branch, or bone, is socioeconomic. It is positioned close to the head of the fish. To check the logical flow of the diagram, examine the cause of each linkage and question why this is a cause. You must examine the logic of the

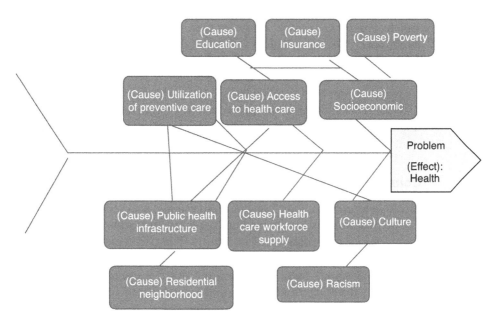

Figure 11.8 Example of a logic model depicting a fishbone root cause analysis of health disparities.
Adapted from Ishikawa (1968).

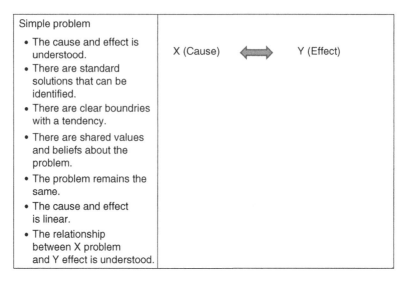

Figure 11.9   Illustration of a simple problem.

diagram, because each bone should be linked to a reason or research evidence. The root cause may be attributed to people—knowledge, skills, attitudes, or social processes and resources.

Simple Problems

When developing a logic model, an assessment of contributing factors and hazards is among the first steps. The problem must be clearly examined. A problem may be simple, complex, or tame. However, a problem may be "wicked" and demand different approaches to problem solving and decision making. A simple problem is fairly well understood, and the way to achieve the desired result is usually understood as well (Figure 11.9). A simple problem may be supported by many research studies that support an easy solution. The problem solving and decision making for a simple problem is understood. For example, a problem with a car, such as a flat tire, might be a simple problem. The cause may be related to a nail causing tire malfunction. If the tire is repaired, the simple problem is fixed.

Complex Problems

A complex problem, found in complex systems, also comprises many components. Complex problems are unpredictable, have no standard solution, and are often multidimensional (illustrated in Figure 11.10). Complex systems are often open, and the problem tends to be multicausal. Building logic models to solve complex problems demands that researchers and practice improvement scholars engage in complexity thinking. Leaders must understand that there is no clear problem-solving approach. Therefore, simple problem approaches are not appropriate. Exchange of people, energy, resources, and other components that comprise a complex system must be expected when working in complex systems that are nonlinear with complex problems (Chaffee & McNeill, 2007).

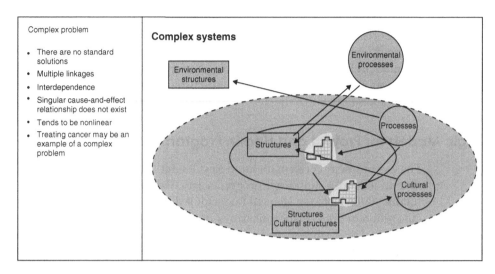

Figure 11.10 Logic model example depicting complex problems of complex systems.

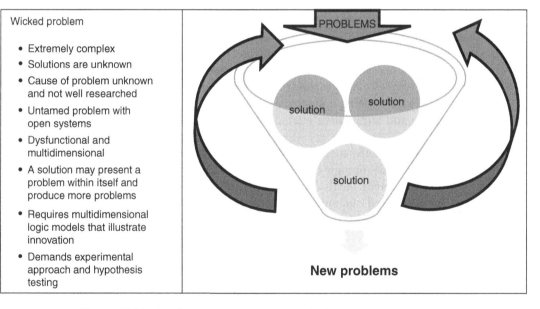

Figure 11.11 Logic model example depicting wicked problems.
Source: Conklin (2006).

Wicked Problems

A problem can change and grow. Sometimes, the problem is not understood until a solution has been developed (Conklin, 2006). Wicked problems are extremely complex (Figure 11.11). Problem-solving approaches may further exacerbate the problem. The problem is not often understood, but when there is an identified solution, another unexpected problem may surface from the solution (Conklin, 2006).

An example of a wicked problem is the national deficit, expenditures, and the economic crisis in the United States. The problem-solving approach to a wicked problem requires innovation. Problem solving may be derived from what worked best in a similar problem. There should be objective indicators to evaluate outcomes. Wicked problems require well-thought-out structures, many resources, and people working in collaboration, since the best problem-solving approaches are not understood.

Logic Models for Project and Health Program Proposals

The Government Performance and Results Act (GPRA), enacted in 1993, mandates that all federally supported programs articulate what they are doing with federal funding (Office of Management Budget [OMB], 1993). Each federal program has specific program performance measures requiring that grantees must prepare progress and annual performance reports. Many program grant applications to the federal government (e.g., Health Resources and Services Administration [HRSA], CDC) require submission of a logic model. The situation or problem, which the program or project addresses, must be clearly explicated to form the foundation on which to build the logic model. Activities or processes must be clearly stated and the program effectiveness, based on clearly articulated performance measures, must be reported.

Federally funded projects are held accountable to document and report their results. The goals, objectives, and outcomes must be clearly described. Linkages to the organization's mission and legislative purpose of the funding agency must be clearly described and substantiated. The expectation is that salient consumer needs are addressed and are evaluated by performance measures that explain the project's progress. A logic model serves as a tool to communicate a logical plan to describe what is being done in a project and how it is functioning through guided formative and summative evaluations (Chapter 1 describes evaluation in more detail).

Often under the methodology section of a funding proposal, a strategic program logic model or logic tables (Figure 11.12) illustrate program goals, objectives, and sub-objectives. Goals clarify specific program targets to guide progress toward achieving desired outcomes. Inputs, such as people and ideas, are highlighted. In addition to interprofessional collaboration, inputs may include finances, human

Sub-objective	Person(s) Responsible	Inputs, Processes/ Activities/Approaches	Time Table Year I				Year II				Year III				Evaluation Methods/Outputs Outcome Indicators
			Q1	Q2	Q3	Q4	Q1	Q2	Q3	Q4	Q1	Q2	Q3	Q4	
Recruit a student services coordinator (12 month 1 FTE)	Program director	Advertise on university website and HigherEdJobs.com by Dec 31, 2014 Targeted military and/or minority December 31, 2014	X												The DNP/IPE student services coordinator and the administrative assistant is hired by December 31, 2014 Summative Recruitment/retention/ enrollment/preceptor site/ career job coordinator position and administrative assistant are recruited and filled

Objective 1. To further develop, enhance, implement, and evaluate an innovative FNP program with emphasis on underserved rural communities.

Figure 11.12 Example of a logic table showing an objective, sub-objective, activities, timeline, and outputs.

FNP, family nurse practitioner.

beings, and resource capital. Processes are the necessary tasks and activities that will be done to achieve the intended results. Assumptions reflect beliefs about the program and benefits, functions, and staff performance. External factors such as values, beliefs, socioeconomics, and politics are often depicted in a logic model. A timeline is included to show the time frame in which program activities will occur.

The project evaluation provides feedback to examine the effectiveness of activities and to map the degree to which the project is achieving stated goals and objectives. To establish project effectiveness, project objectives should be clearly measurable, focused, applicable to the overall goal, and linked to performance measures. According to the IOM (2005), performance measures often lack comprehensiveness in focus; lack a composite measure of recommended services and population; and lack systems-based inputs. There are also narrow time limits and narrow focus of accountability (IOM, 2005). Designers of logic models should guard against these potential deficiencies. Performance measurement should articulate the following:

- What is being done
- Who the participant is
- Why the processes are important
- When activities will be performed
- Outputs with specific outcomes that are expected

Specifically, performance measures or indicators can be used to gauge the extent to which the outcomes meet the program's purpose, goals, and specific project objectives and their sub-objectives. Overall, logic models should be plausible with verifiable processes to measure effectiveness and manage results.

Logic Models for Program Evaluation

Logic models can be used to describe and measure specific outcomes of the program and the evaluation process. The CDC has a framework for program evaluation, well illustrated in projects such as the state birth defects surveillance program (Boulet, Mai, O'leary, & Silverman, 2007). According to the CDC (1999), program evaluation is a systematic way to improve and account for public health actions. Evaluation should involve procedures that are useful, feasible, ethical, and accurate. A strong evaluation plan ensures that the value of a program's efforts can be determined and judgments about its value can be made based on evidence. According to the CDC (1999), a sound program evaluation plan should be able to answer the following questions:

- What will be evaluated? (e.g., what is "the program" and in what context does it exist?)
- What aspects of the program will be considered when judging program performance?
- What standards (i.e., type or level of performance) must be reached for the program to be considered successful?
- What evidence will be used to indicate how the program has performed?
- What conclusions regarding program performance are justified by comparing the available evidence with the selected standards?
- How will the lessons learned be used to improve public health effectiveness?

Healthier Worksite Initiative Logic Model

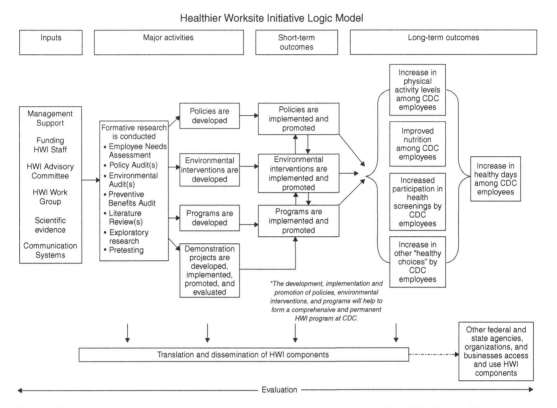

Figure 11.13 An example of a program evaluation logic model: The CDC's Healthier Worksite Initiative.

CDC, Centers for Disease Control and Prevention; HWI, Healthier Worksite Initiative.

An excellent example of a program evaluation logic model was created by the CDC's (2010) Healthier Worksite Initiative, shown in Figure 11.13. It provides answers to all the questions listed earlier. The program is described, the evaluation design is clear, and the results that will be examined are listed. There is a process evaluation that will examine whether the intended changes are achieved. The listed long-term outcomes reflect the impact evaluation to demonstrate benefits of the Healthier Worksite Initiative to CDC employees and other federal and state agencies linkages, illustrating that the resources spent are worth the cost. The logic model's depiction makes it apparent that there will be an analysis, interpretation, and a report of results.

Training Resources for Logic Models

Listed here are a variety of resources that enable one to learn more about logic models and how to create them.

- *Centers for Disease Control and Prevention Evaluation Working Group: Resources*
  http://www.cdc.gov/eval/resources/index.htm
- *Centers for Disease Control Healthier Worksite Initiative*
  www.cdc.gov/nccdphp/dnpao/hwi/programdesign/logic_model.htm

- *Centers for Disease Control Physical Activity Evaluation Handbook*
  http://www.cdc.gov/nccdphp/dnpa/physical/handbook/pdf/handbook.pdf
- *Centers for Disease Control Stacks*
  http://stacks.cdc.gov/view/cdc/11569
- *Environmental Protection Agency (2013): Online logic model course*
  www.epa.gov/evaluate/lm-training
- *Innovation Network (2006): Logic Model Workbook*
  www.wkkf.org/resource-directory/resource/2006/02/wk-kellogg-founda
  tion-logic-model-development-guide
- *TAD & Network (2012)*. Constructing logic models and performance measures. www.tadnet.org/pages/589
- *University of Wisconsin (2003): Extension, Program Development, Evaluation*
  www.uwex.edu/ces/pdande/evaluation/evallogicmodel.html
- *University of Wisconsin-Extension, Cooperative Extension (2008)*. Developing a logic model: Teaching and training guide.
  www.uwx.edu/ces/pdande.html
- *W. K. Kellogg Foundation (2007) Logic Model Guide*
  www.wkkf.org/resource-directory/resource/2006/02/wk-kellogg-founda
  tion-logic-model-development-guide

SUMMARY

A logic model is an iterative tool that is useful to help guide the development of programs designed to improve health care quality and health outcomes. Logic models can be used for quality improvement, program development, and ongoing program and project evaluations. PhD and DNP nurse scholars in practice and research require skill in building logic models that promote evidence-based systems change, innovations in health care, and performance evaluation to be sure that goals, strategies, and results are aligned. There are several steps that should be considered when building a logic model. Each must be carefully considered to develop an evidence-based, plausible, and useful logic model.

REFERENCES

Boulet, S., Mai, C., O'leary, L. A., & Silverman, B. (2007). *Logic models for planning and evaluation; A resource guide for the CDC State Birth Defects Surveillance Program cooperative agreement*. Retrieved from http://stacks.cdc.gov/view/cdc/11569

Carroll, J., & McKenna, J. (2001). Theory to practice: Using the logic model to organize and report research results in a collaborative project. *Journal of Family and Consumer Science*, 93(4), 63–65.

Catchpole, K. (2013). Spreading human factors expertise in healthcare: Untangling the knots of people and systems. *BMJ Quality and Safety*, 22(10), 793–797.

Centers for Disease Control and Prevention. (1999). *Framework for program evaluation in public health* (MMWR, 48[No. RR-11]). Retrieved from http://www.cdc.gov/eval/framework/index.htm

Centers for Disease Control and Prevention. (2010). *Healthier worksite initiative*. Retrieved from http://www.cdc.gov/nccdphp/dnpao/hwi/programdesign/logic_model.htm

Centers for Disease Control and Prevention. (2013). *Healthy People 2020 progress reviews*. Retrieved from http://www.cdc.gov/nchs/healthy_people/hp2020/hp2020_progress_reviews.htm

Chaffee, M. W., & McNeill, M. M. (2007). A model of nursing as a complex adaptive system. *Nursing Outlook, 55*, 232–241.

Conklin, J. (2006). *Dialogue mapping: Building shared understanding of wicked problems*. Somerset, NJ: Wiley.

Craig, J. V., & Smyth, R. L. (2012). *The evidence-based practice manual for nurses* (3rd ed.). Philadelphia, PA: Elsevier, Ltd.

Donabedian, A. (1966). Evaluating the quality of medical care. *Milbank Memorial Fund Quarterly, 44*(3), 166–203.

Drack, M., Apfalter, W., & Pouvreau, D. (2007). On the making of a system theory of life: Paul A Weiss and Ludwig von Bertalanffy's conceptual connection. *Quarterly Review of Biology, 82*(4), 349–373.

Drayton-Brooks, S., Gray, P., & Williamson, K. (2014). Learning outcome assessment model applying the Donabedian model. *Poster presented at the National Organization of Nurse Practitioner Faculties 40th Meeting in Pittsburgh, Pennsylvania*.

Environmental Protection Agency. (2013). *Online logic model course*. Retrieved from http://www.epa.gov/evaluate/lm-training

Gray, P. A., Drayton-Brooks, S., & Williamson, K. M. (2013). Diabetes follow-up support for patients with uncontrolled diabetes. *Nurse Practitioner, 38*(4), 49–53.

Huhman, M., Heitzler, C., & Wong, F. (2004). *The VERB™ campaign logic model: A tool for planning and evaluation*. Retrieved from http://stacks.cdc.gov/view/cdc/4067

Institute of Medicine. (1999). *To err is human: Building a safer health system*. Retrieved from http://www.iom.edu/Reports/1999/To-Err-is-Human-Building-A-Safer-Health-System.aspx

Institute of Medicine. (2001). *Crossing the quality chasm: A new health system for the 21st century*. Washington, DC: The National Academies Press.

Institute of Medicine. (2005). *Pathways to quality health care: Performance measurement accelerating improvement*. Retrieved from http://www.iom.edu/Reports/2005/Performance-Measurement-Accelerating-Improvement.aspx

Institute of Medicine. (2010). *Future directions for the national healthcare quality and disparities reports*. Retrieved from http://iom.nationalacademies.org/Reports/2010/Future-Directions-for-the-National-Healthcare-Quality-and-Disparities-Reports.aspx

Institute of Medicine. (2011). *Health IT and patient safety: Building safer systems for better care*. Retrieved from http://iom.nationalacademies.org/Reports/2011/Health-IT-and-Patient-Safety-Building-Safer-Systems-for-Better-Care.aspx

Innovation Network. (2006). *Logic model workbook*. Retrieved from http://www.innonet.org/client_docs/File/logic_model_workbook.pdf

Ishikawa, K. (1968). *Guide to quality control*. Tokyo, Japan: JUSE.

McLaughlin, J. A., & Jordan, G. B. (1999). Logic models: A tool for telling your program's performance story. *Evaluation and Program Planning, 22*(1), 1–14.

Melnyk, B. M., & Fineout-Overholt, E. (2015). *Evidence-based practice in nursing and healthcare* (3rd ed.). Philadelphia, PA: Wolters Kluwer.

National Association of Healthcare Quality. (2012). *National call to action to improve adverse events report: PSOs part of the solution*. Retrieved from http://www.centerforpatientsafety.org/category/preventable-errors

Office of Management Budget. (1993). *The Government Performance and Results Act (GPRA)*. Retrieved from https://www.whitehouse.gov/omb/mgmt-gpra/index-gpra

Pineda, R. (2015). *The use of electronic SBAR communication between nurses to improve patient falls outcomes*. An unpublished Doctor of Nursing Practice capstone project, Widener University.

Rittel, H. W. J., & Webber, M. M. (1973). Dilemmas in a general theory of planning. *Policy Sciences, 4*, 155–169.

Shirey, M. R. (2013). Lewin's theory of planned change as a strategic resource. *Journal of Nursing Administration, 43*(2), 69–72.

TAD & Network. (2012). *Constructing logic models and performance measures.* Retrieved from http://www.tadnet.org/pages/589

U.S. Bureau of Health Professions. (2011). *Bureau of Health Professions: Performance measure update.* Retrieved from http://bhpr.hrsa.gov/grants/areahealtheducationcenters/ta/Trainings/materials/ta201bhprperformmeasures.pdf

University of Wisconsin. (2003). *Extension, program development, evaluation.* Retrieved from http://www.uwex.edu/ces/pdande/evaluation/evallogicmodel.html

University of Wisconsin-Extension, Cooperative Extension. (2008). *Developing a logic model: Teaching and training guide.* Retrieved from http://www.uwex.edu/ces/pdande/evaluation/pdf/lmguidecomplete.pdf

W. K. Kellogg Foundation. (2007). *Logic model guide.* Retrieved from http://www.wkkf.org/resource-directory/resource/2006/02/wk-kellogg-foundation-logic-model-development-guide

World Health Organization. (2014). *10 facts on patient safety.* Retrieved from http://www.who.int/features/factfiles/patient_safety/en

Zastrow, R. L. (2015). Root analysis in infusion nursing: Applying quality improvement for adverse events. *Journal of Infusion Nursing, 38*(3), 225–231.

INDEX

Printed in the United States
By Bookmasters